TRACHEOSTOMY
A MULTIPROFESSIONAL HANDBOOK

Claudia Russell
Tracheostomy Practitioner
Addenbrooke's Hospital
Cambridge

Basil Matta
Consultant Anaesthetist
Addenbrooke's Hospital
Cambridge

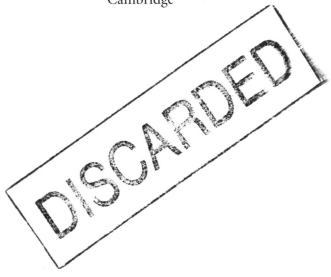
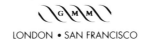

LONDON • SAN FRANCISCO

www.greenwich-medical.co.uk

© 2004
Greenwich Medical Media Limited
137 Euston Road
London
NW1 2AA

870 Market Street, Ste 720
San Francisco, CA 94102

ISBN 1 84110 1524

First Published 2004

A catalogue record for this book is available from the British Library

Typeset by Mizpah Publishing Services, Chennai, India

Printed in Malta by the Gutenberg Press

CONTENTS

LIST OF ABBREVIATIONS

ACT	Aid for Children with Tracheostomies
AH	Absolute Humidity
ASA	American Society of Anesthesiologists
ASB	Assisted Spontaneous Breathing
ATC	Automatic Tube Compensation
BiPAP	Biphasic Positive Airway Pressure
BLS	Basic Life Support
CCN	Children's Community Nursing
CHART	Continuous Hyperfractionated Accelerated Radiotherapy
COPD	Chronic Obstructive Pulmonary Disease
CPAP	Continuous Positive Airway Pressure
CSF	Cerebral Spinal Fluid
DISS	Diameter Safety System
DLA	Disability Living Allowance
EBRT	External Beam Radiotherapy
FEES	Fiberoptic Endoscopic Evaluation of Swallowing
FRC	Functional Residual Capacity
HAI	Hospital Acquired Infection
HCAI	Health Care Acquired Infection
HCP	Health Care Professional
HCWs	Health Care Workers
HHME	Hygroscopic Heat and Moisture Exchanger
HHMEF	Hygroscopic Heat and Moisture Exchanging Filter
HME	Head and Moisture Exchanger
HMEF	Heat and Moisture Exchanging Filter
HVLP	High-Volume Low-Pressure Cuffs
ILMA	Intubating Laryngeal Mask Airway
ISB	Isothermic Saturation Boundary
LMA	Laryngeal Mask Airway
MDR-TB	Multi-Drug-Resistant *Mycobacterium tuberculosis*
MLT	Minimal Leak Technique
MOV	Minimal Occlusive Volume

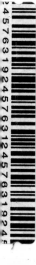

MRSA	Methicillin-Resistant *Staph. aureus*
MSSA	Methicillin-Sensitive *Staph. aureus*
MTB	*Mycobacterium tuberculosis*
NBM	Nil by Mouth
NPPV	Non-invasive Positive Pressure Ventilation
PDT	Percutaneous Dilatational Tracheostomy
PEEP	Positive End Expiratory Pressure
PEG	Percutaneous Entero-Gastrostomy
PICU	Paediatric Intensive Care Unit
PPE	Personal Protective Equipment
Ppl	Intrapleural Pressure
PSV	Pressure Support Ventilation
RH	Relative Humidity
RSV	Respiratory Syncytial Virus
SEN	Statement of Education Needs
SIMV	Synchronised Intermittent Mandatory Ventilation
SLT	Speech and Language Therapist
vCJD	variant Creutzfeldt–Jakob Disease

LIST OF CONTRIBUTORS

Lucy Andrews
Children's Community Nurse
South Cambridgeshire Primary
  Care Trust

Kate Bamkin
Carer
Suffolk

Claudine Billau
Superintendent Physiotherapist
Sandwell and West Birmingham
  NHS Trust

Rachel Brooks
Clinical Nurse Specialist Infection
  Control
Addenbrooke's Hospital
Cambridge

Lorraine de Grey
Specialist Registrar in Anaesthetics
Addenbrooke's Hospital
Cambridge

Vicky Gravenstede
Dietician
Addenbrooke's Hospital
Cambridge

Pippa Hales
Specialist Speech and Language
  Therapist
Addenbrooke's Hospital
Cambridge

Hilary Harkin
ENT Nurse Practitioner
Guy's and St Thomas' NHS
  Trust
London

Lisa Hooper
Clinical Specialist in Physiotherapy
  for Neurosciences
Addenbrooke's Hospital
Cambridge

Teresa Johnson
Paediatric Practice Development
  Nurse
Addenbrooke's Hospital
Cambridge

Basil Matta
Consultant Anaesthetist
Addenbrooke's Hospital
Cambridge

Jasmine Patel
Specialist Registrar
Intensive Care Unit
Manchester Royal Infirmary
Manchester

Carol Phillips
Parent
Suffolk

Tim Price
ENT Registrar
East Anglia Deanery

Tova Prior
Clinical Research Fellow
Meyerstein Institute of Oncology
Middlesex Hospital
London

Claudia Russell
Tracheostomy Practitioner
Addenbrooke's Hospital
Cambridge

Simon Russell
Consultant Clinical Oncologist
Addenbrooke's Hospital
Cambridge

Claire Scase
Tracheostomy Support Nurse
Addenbrooke's Hospital
Cambridge

Rakesh Tandon
Consultant Anaesthetist
Addenbrooke's Hospital
Cambridge

Cheryl Trundle
Senior Infection Control Nurse
  Specialist
Addenbrooke's Hospital
Cambridge

Francis Vaz
Specialist Registrar in Otolaryngology
South East Thames Deanery

PREFACE

A multidisciplinary team approach has improved the care of patients with tracheostomies. These dedicated teams, comprised of doctors, nurses, speech therapists, physiotherapists and dietetic staff, have to work closely and in a co-ordinated collaborative manner to ensure all the needs of these patients are met so that outcomes are optimised. In this handbook, we have outlined upper airway and respiratory basic anatomy and physiology, how it is altered by the introduction of a tracheostomy. Where possible, we have based our management plans on high quality evidence and outcome research. However, in many instances, such data is lacking and the treatment plans we have provided are inevitably tinged with local bias.

Claudia Russell
Basil Matta
January 2004

ACKNOWLEDGEMENT

We would like to thank all the contributors who have devoted their time to produce their chapters on time. We would also like to thank Greenwich Medical Media for their patience, belief in the project and for agreeing to take on this project. We must not forget several manufacturers who have willingly answered endless queries and requests about tracheostomy products. In particular, our special thanks goes to Sims Portex Ltd, Kapitex Healthcare Ltd, Tyco Healthcare and Rüsch Ltd for providing the illustrations, photographs, technical data and their excellent support from their sales and marketing staff.

ANATOMY AND PHYSIOLOGY OF THE RESPIRATORY TRACT

Lorraine de Grey

Respiration is the utilisation of oxygen by the body in the production of energy. Much of the metabolism occurs by aerobic means, i.e. it requires the presence of oxygen.

The respiratory tract has evolved into a complex series of tubes whose primary function is to allow the exchange of gases across all aerobic cells.

Maintaining an adequate supply of oxygen to cells requires four basic steps:

1. Oxygen is taken up from the air by the blood.
2. Oxygen is carried by blood.
3. Tissues receive adequate perfusion with blood.
4. Oxygen passes from the blood to cells.

Carbon dioxide is a product of metabolism in the cells and transfer of carbon dioxide from blood to the air together with step one above are the main functions of the respiratory tract.

A good knowledge of the basic anatomy is an essential prerequisite to understanding the complex physiology of the respiratory tract. In this chapter, I shall start with the central control of respiration and proceed to give an intertwined description of function and anatomy.

RHYTHMIC CONTROL OF BREATHING

Central control of respiration has evolved such that there is an automatic and subconscious control of inspiration and expiration.

This may however be overridden by voluntary actions or the reflex actions of swallowing and speech.

Table 1: Factors influencing the medullary respiratory centre	
Central factors	**Peripheral factors**
Cortex	Peripheral chemoreceptors
Hypothalamus	Pharyngeal mechanoceptors
Pons	Vagal afferents
Central chemoreceptors	Non-respiratory reflexes

Broadly speaking the respiratory cycle may be divided into:

1. *Inspiratory phase*, during which pharyngeal dilator muscles start to contract, shortly followed by increasing activity of the inspiratory muscles.
2. *Expiratory phase I*, during which there is a decreased activity of the inspiratory muscles.
3. *Expiratory phase II*, during which inspiratory muscles show no activity and the expiratory muscles may be recruited if forcible expiration is necessary.

The neurones central to the repetitive and involuntary movements of respiration are concentrated in the *medulla oblongata*. This is under the influence of a variety of factors, summarised in Table 1.

The motor neurones are divided into two groups.

1. The *dorsal respiratory group*, the main function of which is in relation to the timing of the respiration. It lies in close relation to the tractus solitarius and is made up mainly of the inspiratory neurones, crossing over to the anterior horn cells of the other side.
2. The *ventral respiratory group*, also known as the expiratory group is controlled by the nucleus retroambigualis. The dilator functions of the larynx, pharynx and tongue are controlled by the nucleus ambiguous and the inspiratory muscles are controlled mainly by the nucleus para-ambigualis.

The pons undoubtedly contributes to the fine-tuning and modification of the respiratory rhythm but is no longer considered to be the dominant pneumotaxic centre.

CENTRAL CHEMOCEPTORS

These respond to changes in the pH of cerebral spinal fluid (CSF), which in turn is dependent upon pCO_2. Compensatory changes are seen in respiratory and metabolic alkalosis or acidosis.

If pCO_2 is kept abnormally high the CSF pH gradually returns to normal due to changes in CSF bicarbonate levels. Whether this is an active or passive distribution remains uncertain, but the gradual resetting results in a prolonged period of hyperventilation.

PERIPHERAL CHEMOCEPTORS

The carotid bodies

These are placed close to the bifurcation of the common carotid artery whence they have a very rich blood supply. Carotid bodies respond to

1. Falls in partial pressure of oxygen (but not content).
2. Decrease of hydrogen ion concentration.
3. Oscillations of partial pressures of carbon dioxide (in response to the rate of rise as well as to its concentration).
4. Hypotension (<60 mmHg).
5. Hyperthermia.
6. Drug: Sympathomimetics (acetylcholine, nicotine) and cytochrome chain inhibitors (cyanide, carbon monoxide).

Baroceptor reflexes – These are found in the carotid sinus and the aortic arch. They are sensitive to changes in the circulation; a decrease in pressure causes hyperventilation, while a rise causes respiratory depression.

Pulmonary stretch reflexes – These are involved in the classic inflation and deflation reflexes (Hering–Breuer reflexes). There are three main types of receptors.

- *Stretch receptors* are mainly in the airways.
- *Slowly adapting receptors* are in the tracheobronchial smooth muscle.
- *Rapidly adapting receptors* are in the superficial mucosal layer. Afferents are conducted by the vagus or occasionally the sympathetic nervous system.
- Their role in man is minimal.

J receptors – These are C-fibre endings in close relationship to the capillaries of the bronchial and the pulmonary microcirculation. They are activated by tissue damage and produce bradycardia, hypotension, apnoea, bronchoconstriction and increased mucus secretion.

Upper respiratory tract reflexes

The upper respiratory tract has developed a number of reflexes to protect itself from 'foreign material'.

In the *nose* – Water can trigger apnoea; irritants cause sneezing; cold receptors trigger bronchoconstriction.

In the *pharynx* – Mechanoceptors cause activation of pharyngeal dilator muscles, whilst irritants can cause bronchodilatation.

In the *larynx* – Mechanical stimulation via the superior laryngeal nerve causes cough, laryngeal closure and bronchospasm.

In addition the cough reflex has evolved. This involves the inspiration of a volume of air into the lungs followed by contraction of the lungs against a closed glottis. This results in forced expiration through narrowed airways allowing a forceful jet of air to expel irritant materials out into the pharynx. The pressure generated may be as high as 300 mmHg.

THE ROLE OF THE SPINAL CORD IN CONTROL OF RESPIRATION

Messages from the upper control centres are transmitted to the lower motor neurones via three groups of fibres in the spinal tracts.

1. In the **ventrolateral** cord – nerve fibres originating from the dorsal and ventral respiratory groups of the medulla.
2. In the **dorsolateral** and **ventrolateral** quadrants of the cord – transmitting nerve fibres relating to the voluntary control of breathing especially speech.
3. A disparate group of fibres innervating the diaphragm, controlling its rhythmic contraction.

All of these fibres converge onto the anterior horn cells in the spinal cord from which emerge the lower motor neurones.

There are two *efferent* fibres

- The alpha fibres passing directly to the neuromuscular junction of the spinal cord.
- The gamma fibre that ends directly on the intrafusal part of the muscle spindle.

Contraction of the intrafusal fibres causes stimulation of the annulospiral endings. These will send off an impulse via the dorsal root that will then cause an excitatory effect on the alpha fibres, thus closing a reflex loop.

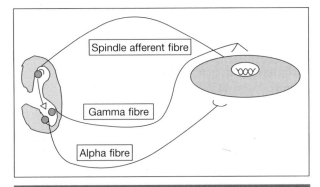

Spindle afferent fibre

Gamma fibre

Alpha fibre

Fig. 1: Diagrammatic representation of lower motor neurone fibres reflexes.

The muscles of respiration

The chest wall is a moderately flexible anatomical entity that contains all the structures surrounding the lungs and pleura. The chest wall behaves as an elastic container when relaxed. In the absence of any pressure difference across the chest wall, it comes to its unstressed volume, which is roughly 75% of total lung capacity.

If the chest wall muscles were to be relaxed (as in quiet expiration), when the pleural pressure is below atmospheric, the chest wall is pulled inwards. When the pleural pressure rises above atmospheric pressure (Pw is positive), the chest wall bows out. In certain disease states the chest wall may stiffen, causing a restrictive ventilatory defect.

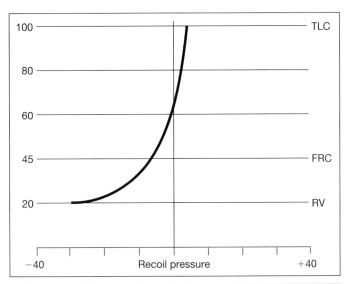

Fig. 2: Compliance curve of relaxed chest wall.
FRC = Functional residue capacity, RV = Residual volume,
TLC = Total lung capacity.

The only active phase of the respiratory cycle is the phase of inspiration under resting conditions.

The *inspiratory muscles* include:

1. The *diaphragm*: The normal expiratory excursion is about 1.5 cm and occurs as the insertion and origin of the diaphragm pull against each other.
2. The *intercostals*: External intercostals are primarily inspiratory; Internal intercostals are primarily expiratory.
3. The *scalenes*: These are active in inspiration by lifting up the rib cage to counteract the diaphragmatic pull.

4. *Sternocleidomastoid*: They are potent accessory muscles during forced inspiration.

These muscles work to overcome two main sources of resistance:

- The work against elastic recoil.
- The work against resistance to gas flow.

The optimal rate and depth of respiration is in proportion to the resistance offered by either during the respiratory cycle. The work of breathing is measured in Joules.

The *expiratory muscles* include:

1. Rectus abdominis
2. External obliques
3. Internal obliques
4. Transversalis

The elastic recoil of the expanded chest cavity drives the phase of expiration. Expiratory muscles are normally silent in quiet breathing and usually chip in when the minute volume is in excess of 40 l/min.

The pressure difference across the chest wall will have no relationship to its size if the respiratory muscles are being used either to move the chest or to keep it at a particular volume.

The pleura

The lungs are paired organs lying within the thoracic cavity. The left lung has two lobes, and the right has three. The left lung is smaller than the right because of space occupied by the heart.

The lungs are encased with the chest wall. Within this, it lies in *the pleura* – a thin membrane which lines the walls of the thoracic cavity – *the parietal pleura* and the lung surfaces – *visceral pleura*.

These two sides are continuous, meeting at the lung hilum; they are directly opposed to one another, and the entire potential space within the pleura contains only a few millilitres of serous pleural fluid.

Anatomically, the parietal pleura starts at the dome of the pleura overlying the apex of the lung reaching as high as the lower edge of the neck of the first rib, then moving medially to form the costal pleura.

This can be traced down to the inner margin of the first rib. It then proceeds down just behind the sternoclavicular joint to the median plane behind the sternum where the left and right sides are in contact with each other down to the fourth costal cartilage.

It sweeps laterally on the right side down to the posterior surface of the xiphisternum while on the left side; it sweeps up to 25 mm away from the midline to the sixth costal cartilage.

On each side it sweeps laterally so as to cross the tenth rib in the mid-axillary line and is just below the twelfth rib at the costo-vertebral junction. The visceral pleura adhere tightly to the surface of the lung being reflected off the structures in the hilum.

The surrounding forces exert an *Intrapleural pressure* (Ppl) within the pleural space. During quiet breathing, the pleural pressure is negative; that is to say, *below* atmospheric pressure.

The pressure gradient in the erect person drops exponentially down the lung decreasing 1 cm H_2O for every 3 cm drop. This has a profound effect on many features of pulmonary function including airways closure, ventilation/perfusion ratios and gaseous exchange.

The lungs are totally separated from the abdomen by a sheet of skeletal muscle – the *diaphragm*, which is dome shaped before lung expansion but flattens during breathing in.

During active expiration, the abdominal muscles are contracted to force up the diaphragm and the resulting pleural pressure can become positive. Positive pleural pressure may temporarily collapse the bronchi and cause limitation of airflow.

Anatomy of the upper airway

This describes the portion of the airway that lies above the vocal cords and includes:

1. The nasal passages (septum, turbinate, and adenoids)
2. The oral cavity (teeth and tongue)
3. The pharynx (tonsils, uvula, and epiglottis)
4. The glottis

Breathing normally occurs through the nose or mouth and the direction it takes is under voluntary control utilising the soft palate, tongue and lips.

Normally the mouth is closed and the tongue is applied to the hard palate to allow nasal breathing. This is the physiological way to breathe, as the nose is specially adapted for this function. The nose provides:

1. Hairs to filter off particulate matter.
2. Humidification and warming of the air over the increased surface area provided by the turbinates.

The mouth is brought into play when the respiratory minute volume is greater than 35 l/min. Forced mouth breathing is affected by a functional anatomical change that arches the soft palate upwards and backwards against the band of the superior constrictor of the pharynx, effectively closing off the nasopharynx.

The *pharynx* has two components: The *oropharynx*, i.e. the throat area and the *nasopharynx* is an extension of the throat upwards towards the nasal passages. The opening into the airways from the oropharynx is called the *glottis*, which is closed off during swallowing by a small flap called the *epiglottis*.

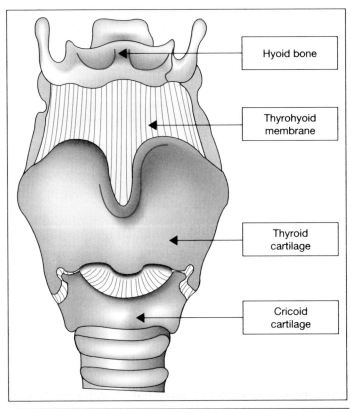

Hyoid bone

Thyrohyoid membrane

Thyroid cartilage

Cricoid cartilage

Fig. 3: Laryngeal anatomy.

After the glottis, the air enters the *larynx*, a structure of cartilage and ligaments that forms the Adam's apple. The entire structure is supported by muscles that suspend the larynx from a small bone in the neck called the hyoid.

Within the larynx are folds of cartilage that form the vocal cords. Air flowing over these cords causes them to vibrate and so produce sound. Their tension determines the tone or pitch of the sound; small muscles that pass from the cords to the cartilage of the larynx capsule can alter this.

Innervation of the upper airway

The upper airway is innervated by three main cranial nerves:

Trigeminal nerve (Cranial nerve V): Branches of the trigeminal nerve innervate the nose and the anterior two thirds of the tongue.

Glossopharyngeal (Cranial nerve IX): Branches of the glossopharyngeal nerve innervate the posterior third of the tongue, roof of pharynx and tonsils.

Vagus (Cranial nerve X): The two major divisions of the vagus nerve in airway innervation are the superior laryngeal and the recurrent laryngeal nerves.

Sensory innervation
1. *Trigeminal nerve* – the sensory innervation of the nasal mucosa arises from two divisions:

   – The anterior ethmoidal nerve supplies the anterior septum and lateral wall;
   – The nasopalatine nerves from the sphenopalatine ganglion innervate the posterior areas.

2. *Glossopharyngeal nerve* – supplies the posterior third of the tongue, soft palate, epiglottis, fauces and the pharyngo-oesophageal junction.
3. *Superior laryngeal nerve* – the internal branch of the vagus nerve innervates mucosa from the epiglottis to and including the vocal cords.
4. *Recurrent laryngeal nerve* – a branch of the vagus nerve innervates mucosa below the vocal chords to the trachea.

Motor innervation
1. The *external branch of the superior laryngeal nerve* is responsible for innervation of the cricothyroid muscle.
2. The *recurrent laryngeal nerve* provides a motor supply to all the muscles of the larynx (posterior and lateral cricoarythenoid muscles) except the cricothyroid muscle.

   – The lateral cricoarythenoid adducts the cords
   – The posterior cricoarythenoid abducts the cords

Unilateral damage to the recurrent laryngeal nerve causes hoarseness. Bilateral damage causes respiratory distress and stridor whilst chronic damage can cause aphonia.

Anatomy of the lower airway

This describes the portion of the airway below the vocal cords. In an adult, the vocal cords are the narrowest portion of the airway.

The lower airway can be divided into:

The larynx is found at the level of the fourth to the sixth of the cervical vertebrae. Protection of the airway remains its most important function. However it has developed further as the organ of speech. The larynx is made up of nine cartilages:

1. Unpaired (thyroid, cricoid, and epiglottis). The cricoid cartilage is the only complete cartilaginous ring the respiratory system. It lies below the thyroid cartilage.
2. Paired cartilages (arytenoids, corniculate, and cuneiform).

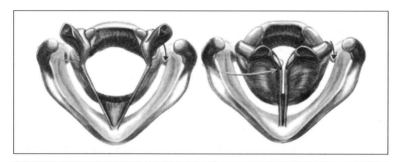

Fig. 4: Diagrammatic representation of the closure of the vocal cords.

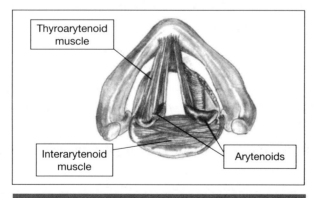

Fig. 5: Superior aspect of the larynx.

The larynx also has two groups of muscles:

1. Muscles that open and close the glottis (lateral cricoarytenoid, post cricoarytenoid, and transverse arytenoid).

2. Muscles that control the tension of the vocal ligaments (cricothyroid, vocalis, and thyroarytenoid).

The cricothyroid membrane is another important structure found in the lower respiratory tract. This membrane connects the thyroid cartilage and the cricoid ring. It is a thin membrane without major vessels and may be used for obtaining emergency airway access in emergency cricothyroid puncture.

THE TRACHEOBRONCHIAL TREE

Classically, the tracheobronchial tree has been described as extending from the trachea (generation 0), doubling with each generation to the alveolar sacs (generation 23).

The trachea is essentially a fibromuscular tube that is supported by 20 U-shaped cartilages and enters the chest cavity at the superior mediastinum. It bifurcates at the carina at the level of T4.

The mucosa lining the trachea is columnar ciliated epithelium. Co-ordinated beating of cilia causes an upward stream of mucus and foreign bodies.

The trachea divides into two main bronchi, which are asymmetrical, the right being one-third wider and a little shorter than the left. The right bronchus slopes more steeply (25 degrees off the vertical) than the left (45 degrees off the vertical), so that foreign bodies of whatever shape, are statistically more likely to enter the right bronchus. The same rule naturally applies to the endotracheal tube that is inserted down too far into the trachea.

Each main bronchus divides into three *lobar bronchi*, which in turn divide into *lobar bronchi* that give off segmental bronchi. Each of these supplies a segment of the lung.

Cartilage supports the main, lobar and segmental bronchi. It is U-shaped in the main bronchi and helical lower down, with helical bands of muscle completing the geodesic plates.

Bronchi down to the fourth generation are regular enough to be named separately:

	UPPER LOBE – RIGHT	UPPER LOBE – LEFT
1	Apical bronchus	Apical bronchus
2	Posterior bronchus	Posterior bronchus
3	Anterior bronchus	Anterior bronchus

	MIDDLE LOBE – RIGHT	**LINGULA – LEFT**
4	Lateral bronchus	Superior bronchus
5	Medial bronchus	Inferior bronchus
	LOWER LOBE – RIGHT	**LOWER LOBE – LEFT**
6	Apical bronchus	Apical bronchus
7	Medial basal	–
8	Anterior basal bronchus	Anterior basal bronchus
9	Lateral basal bronchus	Lateral basal bronchus
10	Posterior basal bronchus	Posterior basal bronchus

Small bronchi span generations 5–11. The true bronchi are typified by the close proximity of the pulmonary artery and pulmonary lymphatics in a sheath. They rely on the cartilage in their walls for patency combined with a positive transmural pressure gradient at this level and a negative intrathoracic pressure.

Between generations 12–16 *bronchioles* form; they are characterised by a lack of cartilage maintaining their patency by the elastic recoil of the lung parenchyma in which they are embedded. In the terminal bronchioles due to the rapid and multiple branching of the bronchioles, the surface is at least 100 times more than at the level of the large bronchi. Nutrition down to this level is from the bronchial circulation.

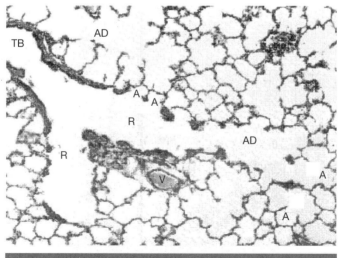

Fig. 6: Cross-section of respiratory bronchioles.

Generations 17–19 make up the *respiratory bronchioles*. It is beyond this point that gaseous exchange occurs.

- The lining epithelium starts off as cuboidal and ends up as flat alveolar.
- There is a well-demarcated muscle layer that bands over the opening of the alveolar ducts and mural alveoli.
- The calibre of the advancing generations remains unchanged at about 0.4 mm to provide a total cross-sectional area of several hundred cm^2.

Generations 20–22 make up the *alveolar ducts*. They arise from the terminal respiratory bronchioles. They have no walls than the mouths of the mural alveoli; about half the alveoli arise from the ducts.

Generation 23 are the *alveolar sacs*. They are blind ending sacs, about 17 alveoli arising from each alveolar sac. Around half of the alveoli arise from the alveolar sacs.

THE ALVEOLI

The primary function of the respiratory system is gaseous exchange. This occurs at the level of the alveoli.

1. There are 200–600 million in total, with a mean diameter of 0.2 mm.
2. Their size is proportional to the lung volume except at maximal inflation when vertical gradient in size disappears. This vertical gradient is dependent on gravity. The reduction in size of alveoli and the corresponding reduction in calibre of the smaller airways in the dependent parts of the lung have important implications in gas exchange.

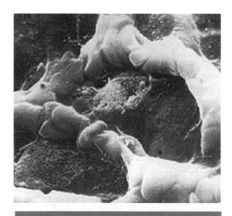

Fig. 7: Electron microscopic picture of alveoli.

3. Alveoli are polyhedral in shape, this shape being determined by elastic fibres in the alveolar septum. The septa are perforated by the pores of Kohn, which allow collateral ventilation.
4. The alveolar septum has a network of fibre forming a mesh from the peripheral fibres to the bronchioles, supporting capillaries that thread in and out of the meshwork.
5. The cells rest on a basement membrane. This is made of collagen IV (which provides great strength), as well as heparin sulphate, laminin, and entactin (these promote cell attachment and protein permeability).

There are a number of special cells in the alveoli:

1. *Capillary endothelial cell:* These are continuous with the general circulation. They have a featureless cytoplasm apart from plasmalemmal vesicles (caveolae) and may be involved in pinocytosis. They serve to further increase the surface area and have enzymes on their surface. Fairly loose junctions connect the cells.
2. *Alveolar epithelial cells – Type I:* These cells form continuous sheets and meet at tight junctions. These junctions help to prevent the escape of large molecules. This maintains the oncotic pressure gradient that protects against pulmonary oedema, while allowing the passage of macrophages and polymorphs in response to chemotactic stimuli.
3. *Alveolar epithelial cells – Type II:* These are the stem cells from which the type I cells arise. They have large nuclei and microvilli, are round in shape and are situated at the junction of the septa.
4. *Alveolar brush cells – Type III:* They are uncommon and their function is uncertain.
5. *Alveolar macrophages:* These may lie freely on the surface of the alveolar epithelial cells where they scavenge dust particles. They combat infection by phagocytosis, use of oxygen-free radicals and enzymes. Neutropils may also appear especially in the lungs of smokers.
6. *Clara cells:* This is a type of non-ciliated bronchiolar epithelium that secrete at least three proteins including antiproteases and a surfactant apoprotein.
7. *APUD cells:* These are known to produce a range of hormones elsewhere but their role in the respiratory system is uncertain.
8. *Mast cells:* There are numerous mast cells that lie in the alveolar septa and also freely in the luminal airways – they play a role in bronchoconstriction.

Surfactant

There is a potential danger that on breathing out, the walls of alveoli may touch and adhere to each other. Contact between moist surfaces produces powerful adhesion because of surface tension. Respiratory movements are unable to overcome these forces and it is **Surfactant**, a product of specialised cells lining the alveoli that prevents alveoli from deflating totally following expiration.

The main function of surfactant is to reduce the surface tension throughout the lung. It also indirectly prevents lung oedema and also influences the rate of alveolar collapse thereby contributing to its general compliance.

Surfactant is a complex substance produced by the Type II alveolar cells. It lines the alveoli and smallest bronchioles.

Surfactant consists of:

- ~90% phospholipids (mainly dipalmitoyl phosphatidyl choline and phosphatidyl glycerol).
- ~10% protein.

The fatty acids are saturated and straight. These tend to pack better in expiration therefore making the actual surface tension vary in different parts of the respiratory cycle. Cholesterol, phosphatidyl inositol, phosphatidyl serine and phosphatidyl ethanolamine are also present.

The protein component increases the speed with which the surface film is reconstituted. Most of the proteins are 26–38 kDa although a group of hydrophobic 11 kDa proteins also play a role.

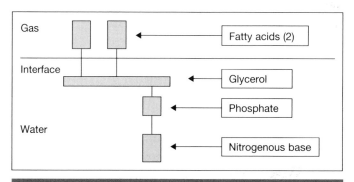

Fig. 8: Schematic diagram of surfactant.

The pressure inside a bubble is subject to the law of Laplace's law viz;

$P = 4T/r$ (for a sphere with two liquid-gas interfaces, like a soap bubble)

$P = 2T/r$ (for a sphere with one liquid-gas interface, like an alveolus)

(P = pressure, T = surface tension and r = radius).

That is, at a constant surface tension, small alveoli will generate bigger pressures within them than will large alveoli.

One would therefore expect the smaller alveoli to empty into larger alveoli as lung volume decreases. However, surfactant differentially reduces surface tension (more so at lower volumes) and this leads to alveolar stability avoiding alveolar collapse.

Surfactant is formed relatively late in foetal life; thus premature infants born without adequate amounts experience respiratory distress and may die.

Elastic forces in the lung

The lungs exhibit a phenomenon of compliance that is the ability to change volume with pressure as demonstrated by all elastic organs.

This can be explained by hysteresis – a phenomenon whereby the inflation pressure falls exponentially from its initial value to a lower value attained after inflation. Rather more than expected pressure is required in inflation while less recoil pressure is available during deflation.

The lungs exhibit two forms of compliance:

- Dynamic compliance
- Static compliance

$$\text{Dynamic compliance} = \frac{\text{Change in volume gradient}}{\text{Change in initial transmural pressure}}$$

$$\text{Static compliance} = \frac{\text{Change in volume gradient}}{\text{Change in ultimate transmural pressure}}$$

There are a variety of factors affecting the lung compliance:

1. *Changes in surfactant activity* – the surface tension is greater at larger lung volumes and during inspiration. It is the single most important factor determining hysteresis. It is also important in maintaining alveolar patency thus reducing alveolar recruitment during normal respiration.
2. *Recent ventilatory history* – compliance is maintained by continuous rhythmic cycling and the effect is dependant on tidal volume as well as the total lung volume.
3. *Restriction of chest expansion* – artificial reduction with strapping reduces lung volume; the compliance remains reduced until a single deep breath reinflates the lung – the 'physiological sigh'.
4. *Bronchial smooth muscle tone* – has a role in dynamic compliance but not in static compliance.
5. *Age* – this has no effect on compliance, confirming that the lung 'elasticity' is largely determined by surface forces.
6. *Stress relaxation* – this explains the principle that on pulling an elastic body to a fixed increase in length, this will result in an initial maximal tension that declines exponentially to a constant value.

7. *Emphysema* – causes increased static lung compliance, but the dynamic compliance is reduced.
8. Other lung diseases such as pulmonary fibrosis, consolidation, and fibrous pleurisy, adult respiratory distress syndrome – decrease both static and dynamic compliance.

AIRFLOW IN THE RESPIRATORY TRACTS

Air will flow from a region of high pressure to one of low pressure – the velocity of flow is in direct relation to the pressure difference.

Air therefore flows in during inspiration because the alveolar pressure is less than the pressure at the mouth; conversely the air flows out during expiration because alveolar pressure exceeds the pressure at the mouth.

Different parts of the airways anatomy have a variety of mechanisms to counteract and maintain patency throughout the respiratory cycle. This allows easy, continuous and repetitive gaseous exchange to occur efficiently with minimal energy expenditure.

The pharynx in inspiration is subject to a negative pressure of a few kilopascals that would normally tend to pull the tongue backwards and cause the pharynx to collapse.

This is countered in an active manner using musculature – mainly the genioglossus to effectively prevent changes in pharyngeal anatomy in all the phases of respiration.

The nasopharynx is also kept patent by the tensor palati, palatopharyngeus and palatoglossus.

Passage of air in the relatively larger airways creates eddies and is described as:

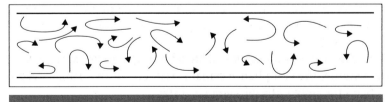

Fig. 9: Turbulent flow.

Driving pressure is proportional to the square of the flow rate and is described in this formula:

$$\Delta P = KV^2$$

where P is the driving pressure, K is a constant and V is the air flow.

This means that to double the airflow one needs to quadruple the driving pressure.

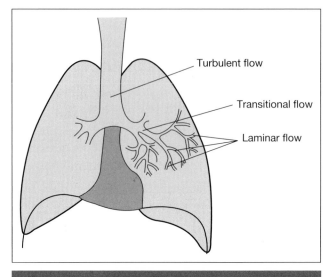

Fig. 10: Locations of flow patterns.

Turbulent flow is found mainly in the largest airways, like the trachea.

When flow is low velocity and through narrow tubes, it tends to be more orderly and streamlined and flows in a straight line. This type of flow is called *laminar flow*.

Unlike turbulent flow, laminar flow is directly proportional to the driving pressure, such that to double the flow rate, one needs only double the driving pressure.

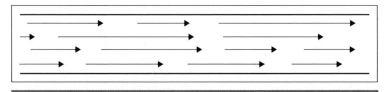

Fig. 11: Laminar flow.

Poiseuille's Law can describe laminar flow:

$$\Delta P = v(8\rho l/\pi r^4)$$

During quiet breathing, laminar flow exists from the medium-sized bronchi down to the level of the bronchioles. During exercise, when the airflow is more rapid, laminar flow may be confined to the smallest airways.

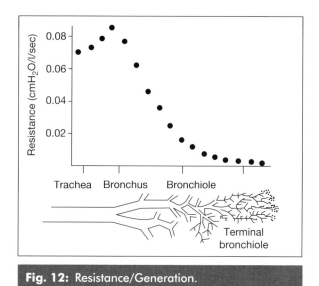

Fig. 12: Resistance/Generation.

Transitional flow, which has some of the characteristics of both laminar and turbulent flow, is found between the two along the rest of the bronchial tree.

LUNG VOLUMES

At rest, an adult breathes in about 500 ml of air (7–8 ml/kg body weight) with each breath. This is referred to as the **tidal volume.**

Hence 5–6 l of air are breathed in and out each minute. This is enough to meet the needs of the cells of the body at rest, which require around 250 ml per minute. During exercise, oxygen requirements may reach as much as 4 l per minute. To keep up with demand, the volume of air inspired per minute may reach as high as 80 l per minute.

However even at rest, we can consciously increase the volume breathed in, or further deflate the lung. Thus there are *inspiratory* and *expiratory reserve volumes.*

In addition, the lung contains a volume of gas even after maximal expiration has occurred, as deflation of the alveoli is incomplete and some gas fills the dead space, i.e. there is *a residual volume* of gas within the lungs – around 1.5 l in adults.

Consequently, the gases within the lung into which inspired air will pass when we breathe in will be the volume represented by the expiratory reserve plus the residual volume; this is the *functional residual capacity* (FRC) – around 2.5 l in an adult. This is equal approximately to half the maximum capacity of the lungs called the *total lung capacity.*

If we inflate the lungs maximally and then breathe out maximally, the volume of gas expired from the lungs represents the maximum volume of gas that can possibly be expelled from the lung in a single breath; this is called *the vital capacity* – around 4 l in an adult.

If we add the vital capacity to the residual volume, then this gives the total lung capacity – around 5–6 l in an adult.

Lung volumes and capacities are measured using a machine called a spirometer. Such measurements may be of particular importance in patients undergoing partial or complete lung resections, and in patients with chronic obstructive or restrictive ventilatory defects.

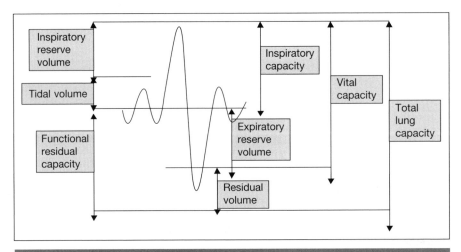

Fig. 13: Lung volumes and capacities.

Factors affecting the functional residual capacity:

1. Body size – linearly relates to height although obesity reduces FRC.
2. FRC is greater in females than males by 10%.
3. Diaphragmatic muscle tone – residual end-expiratory tone is a major factor while in the supine position keeping the FRC around 400 ml above the volume in the anaesthetised position. The diaphragm also protects the lungs from the abdominal contents and limits the FRC change from 500 to 1000 ml between the supine and the upright positions.
4. FRC is increased in asthma and emphysema.

Pleural pressure

Pleural pressure can be estimated in human subjects using an oesophageal balloon.

The size of the lung is determined by the difference between the alveolar pressure and the pleural pressure, or the transpulmonary pressure – the larger the difference, the bigger the lung.

As a result of gravity, in an upright individual, the pleural pressure at the base of the lung base is greater (less negative) than at its apex.

When the individual lies on his back, the pleural pressure becomes greatest along his back. Since alveolar pressure is uniform throughout the lung, the top of the lung generally experiences a greater transpulmonary pressure and is therefore more expanded and less compliant than the bottom of the lung.

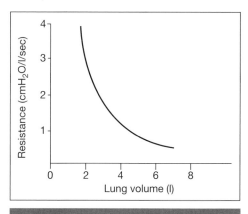

Fig. 14: Resistance/Volume.

DEAD SPACE

This is the fraction of the tidal volume that serves no function in gaseous exchange. This is determined by the equation:

$$V_A = f(V_T - V_D)$$

V_A = alveolar ventilation V_T = tidal volume

f = respiratory frequency V_D = dead space

Dead space consists of:

1. *Apparatus dead space* – only occurs when an external breathing apparatus is used. This is further complicated by the fact that the inhaled gas composition

may be variable: end-expiratory gas, mixed expired gas or even expired dead space gas. This makes the actual gas interchange at the functioning alveolar surface difficult to assess. This may be of importance when using various breathing circuits during anaesthesia.

2. *Anatomical dead space* – made up of the conducting air passages. It is not constant and is subject to a number of variables including:

   – Age – usually sees an increase in the anatomical dead space.
   – End-inspiratory lung volume – the volume in the air passages varies in relation to the lung volume.
   – Size – volume of air in passageways (ml) ~2.2 × wt in kg.
   – Posture – sitting > supine
     Neck extended > normal position > neck flexed.
   – Tracheostomy – bypasses all extra thoracic dead space (65–70 ml).
   – Hypoventilation (tidal volumes of <250 ml) – reduced dead space by laminar flow of the gases allows easier passage into the alveoli.

3. *Alveolar dead space* – this is the inspired gas that passes through the anatomical dead space to the alveolar surface but does not take part in gaseous exchange, due to a lack of perfusion. It is of little significance normally, but may increase appreciably in some situations:

   – Pulmonary embolism/pulmonary artery obstruction during surgery – the alveolar dead space rises in relation to the degree of occlusion of the pulmonary circulation.
   – Ventilation of non-vascular air space in chronic lung diseases.
   – Pulmonary hypoventilation – whether due to low output circulatory failure or during anaesthesia results in less perfusion for the non-dependant parts with a subsequent increase in the alveolar dead space?

Posture in itself does not affect the dead space to any significant degree except when under anaesthesia. In the patient lying on one side, the upper lung will be preferentially ventilated resulting in an increase in the dead space.

4. *Physiological dead space* – this is the sum of the alveolar and the anatomical dead spaces and is shown by the Bohr equation:

$$V_D/V_T = (PaCO_2 - PECO_2)/PaCO_2$$

Factors influencing the physiological dead space include:

   – Age – V_D/V_T increases with age.
   – Sex and body size – V_D/V_T ratios slightly greater in males and V_D raises 17 ml for every 10 cm of height.
   – Posture – drop from 34% to 30% from the erect to the supine positions.

- Smoking – can increase the ratio by ~30%.
- Pulmonary disease – as above.
- Anaesthesia – V_D/V_T is 30–35% below the carina; prolonged use of PEEP increases dead space.

Pulmonary circulation and ventilation

The total pulmonary circulation at rest is measured as 0.5–1.0 l (10–20%) of the total blood volume, but will equal the systemic circulation and can rise to as much as 25 l/min without a significant rise in pressure.

The ability to control pressure by tone is significantly less in the pulmonary circulation than in the systemic circulation, as a result of which gravity dictates the distribution of blood flow with a mismatch of circulation in the more dependant areas of the lung.

Factors affecting pulmonary blood volume include:

1. Systole – when inflow exceeds outflow.
2. Valsalva manoeuvre (decreases pulmonary blood flow).
3. Posture – change from supine to erect decreases blood flow by 27%.
4. Vasoconstrictor drugs or catecholamines push blood from the systemic into the pulmonary circulation.

While the systemic circulation shows a drop of pressures from 90 mmHg to 2 mmHg as it courses through from the arteries, until it gets to the right atrium, the drop in pulmonary pressure is much smaller and falls from 17 mmHg in the pulmonary arteries to 6 mmHg in the left atrium.

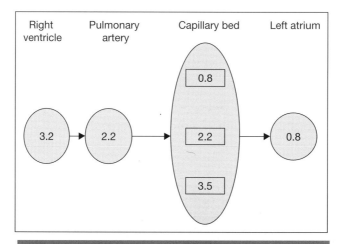

Fig. 15: Pulmonary circulation pressures (kPa).

FACTORS AFFECTING PULMONARY VASCULAR PRESSURES

Several factors have an influence on the pressure in the pulmonary circulation. They include:

1. Cardiac output – there is normally an increase in volume without a rise in pressures by recruitment of vessels and by passive dilatation. There is a limit to this and in cases where left to right shunting occurs as in ventral and atrial septal defects as well as in patent ductus arteriosus, pulmonary hypertension occurs.
2. Changes in intra-thoracic pressure – intra vascular pressures rise reflecting rises in intra-thoracic pressures. This is seen in the Valsalva manoeuvre (forced expiration against a closed glottis). There are also rhythmic changes with the normal respiratory cycle. The upright position is also associated with a decreased intrathoracic pressure).
3. Chronic hypoxia.
4. Pulmonary thromboembolism.
5. Mitral stenosis and incompetence.
6. Pulmonary vascular resistance.
7. Autonomic control.
8. Changes in oxygen and carbon dioxide tension.

Gas exchange across the alveolus

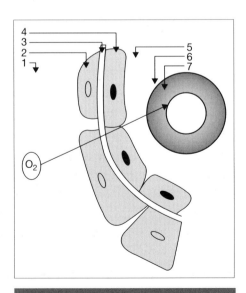

Fig. 16: Passage of O_2 molecule across its diffusing membrane.

1 = Alveolus.

The average diameter of an alveolus is 200 μm. Mixing is probably complete within 10 min. The process is slower for heavier gases but as oxygen, nitrogen and carbon dioxide are roughly similar, it is unlikely to affect the process significantly.

2 = Alveolar epithelium – There are 4 separate lipid bilayers measuring a total of 0.5 μm.

3 = Basement membrane.

4 = Capillary endothelium.

5 = Pulmonary capillary. These are usually about 7 μm, so there is not much fluid plasma as the RBC squeezes through.

6 = RBC membrane – the erythrocyte diameter is 14 times the thickness of the alveolar/capillary membrane.

7 = Cytoplasm.

The *uptake of oxygen by haemoglobin* is the rate-determining step in the uptake of oxygen from alveolar gas by the erythrocyte.

Mathematically the rate of oxygen diffusion can be defined as:

$$O_2 \text{ diffusing capacity} = \frac{\text{Oxygen uptake}}{\text{Alveolar } O_2 - \text{mean pulm. cap. } PO_2}$$

Ventilation and perfusion

In the ideal situation, the ventilation and perfusion of all parts of the lung would be equally and perfectly matched. There are however variations in both parameters in different parts of the lung.

The pulmonary circulation is a low-pressure system. As a result it is subject to a variety of pressures, namely the alveolar pressure, flow rate and the vascular resistance, that determine the relative amount to which each part of the lung is perfused. The interplay of pressures is mainly dependant on gravity.

In *Zone 1*, the alveolar pressure is greater than the arterial pressure therefore keeping the vessel closed, preventing flow.

In *Zone 2*, the arterial pressure rises thanks to the effect of gravity and therefore, it exceeds the alveolar pressure and flow occurs in relation to this pressure difference. The distal venous pressure in normal subjects has no role to play in determining the flow in this zone.

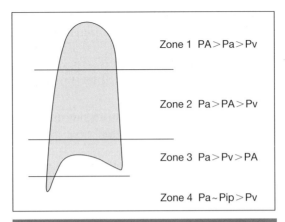

Fig. 17: Ventilation and perfusion.

In *Zone 3*, the venous pressure is greater than the alveolar pressure and the flow rate is determined solely as a result of the difference between the arterial and venous side of the circulation.

In *Zone 4*, (seen only at reduced lung volumes) the interstitial pressure increases to reduce blood flow by the occlusion of the larger blood vessels.

A number of factors can affect the perfusion of the lung:

1. Central factors – cardiac failure.
2. Position – in the supine position, the difference between the top and bottom of the lung is only 30 cm so that the uppermost part of the lung equates to Zone 2 and the bottom of the lung to Zone 3.
3. Effect of inflation of the lung: The larger blood vessels are opened up due to traction of the surrounding lung tissue but the smaller vessels are collapsed as the lung expands in ventilation. In the collapsed lung, the driving force is the PO_2; the alveolar PO_2 is controlled by the pulmonary arterial PO_2 and as a result in the short term will not lead to a decreased blood flow although in the longer term the blood flow will inevitably decrease.

Distribution of ventilation

In the normal subject the main influence on ventilation is position and the manner of ventilation.

- The right lung is slightly better ventilated than the left in both the erect and supine positions.
- The lower lung is better ventilated than the upper lung in the lateral position except in the ventilated patient with an open chest who will have a better ventilation of the upper lung.

- The rate of ventilation is also important. With ventilatory rates of <1.5 l/s, the ratio of ventilation of the lower to the upper parts of the lung is 1.5:1.
- The rate of alveolar filling is expressed as a *time constant* that is the time required to inflate the lungs if the initial rate of gas flow were maintained through inflation. The time constant varies for different alveoli, dependant on their compliance and resistance.
- If the time constants were equal for all alveoli then there would be no distribution of gases as its distribution would be independent of rate duration or frequency of respiration.
- However if the time constants were different then gaseous distribution occurs, dependant on the rate, duration and frequency resulting from a decreased dynamic compliance with increased frequency of respiration.

Ventilation/perfusion ratios

If ventilation occurs to areas of lung that are not perfused, then it can have no role to play in gas exchange.

Taking the lung as a whole, the rate of ventilation is ~4 l/min and the pulmonary blood flow is ~5 l/min making a V/Q ratio of 0.8. If all parts of the lung were equally ventilated and perfused this would be the case all over the lung.

There is a differential perfusion and ventilation from the unventilated to the unperfused alveoli in the lung.

The below diagram gives an indication of the V/Q ratios from the completely unperfused (dead space) on the left to the unventilated (shunt) at the far right, going through various degrees of relative perfusion to ventilation (with the ideal as shown on the graph marked at 1.

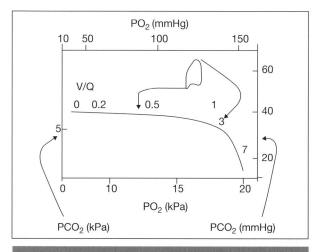

Fig. 18: V/Q ratios in different areas of the lung.

In practical terms in the young the V/Q ratio varies from 0.5–2.0, increasing in its range to 0.3–5.0 in the elderly.

Summary of learning objectives

1. The carriage of oxygen and carbon dioxide to and from tissues, and the exchange of these gases with air, is vital for life.
2. At rest, a person breathes in and out 5 l of air per minute. During exercise this may increase to up to 100 l per minute. This done by increasing both frequency and depth of ventilation.
3. Low airway resistance and a high elasticity allow for a very efficient system.
4. Spirometry can be used to measure lung volumes and capacities.
5. Gas exchange occurs across lung alveoli; the rest of the airway comprises a 'dead space'.
6. Breathing is mainly involuntary but can be changed consciously, and is controlled by the rhythmical discharge of nerve impulses from the respiratory centres.
7. Blood gas composition is monitored continuously by chemoreceptors that respond to changes in either oxygen or carbon dioxide/pH content.
8. The upper airway has evolved to produce humidification and warming of inspired air. It also has the important property of phonation.
9. The lower airway can be divided into 23 generations.
10. Surfactant is a phospholipid that acts to lower the surface tension, and prevents alveoli from deflating totally following expiration.
11. Dead space is the volume of inspired air that does not take part in gas exchange. It can be divided into physiological and anatomical dead space.
12. The significance of ventilation/perfusion matching is that areas of the lung may pathologically exhibit diminished ventilation or perfusion, leading to abnormal oxygenation of blood.

REFERENCES

1. Lumb AB, Nunn JF. *Nunn's Applied Respiratory Physiology 4th Edition*. London: Butterworth-Heinemann, 1993.
2. McMinn RMH. *Last's Anatomy Regional and Applied*, 9th edn. London: Churchill Livingstone, 1994.
3. Clancy J, McVicar AJ. *Physiology and Anatomy: A Homeostatic Approach*. London: Arnold, 2002.
4. John Hopkins School of Medicine. *Interactive Respiratory Physiology*. www.airflow.htm.
5. Mallory GB. *The Influence of the Physiology of the Upper Airway on the Lower Airway*. www.CIPA.htm.
6. Johnson DR. *Introductory Anatomy: Respiratory System*. www.IntroductoryAnatomyRespiratorySystem.htm.

WHAT IS A TRACHEOSTOMY?

Tim Price

NOMENCLATURE

The term tracheotomy refers to the formation of a surgical opening in the trachea. It refers strictly to a temporary procedure. Tracheostomy on the other hand refers to the creation of a permanent stoma between the trachea and the cervical skin.[1,2] The two terms are however in common use and are interchangeable depending on which side of the Atlantic you find yourself on. In this text the term tracheostomy will be used.

HISTORY

Tracheostomies have been performed since ancient times and the first known reference can be found in Rig Veda, the sacred Hindu scripture which dates back to 2000 BC. In 1620 Habicot published the first book on tracheostomies.[2]

In the 1800s tracheostomy gained in popularity, as it became a recognised way of treating patients with Diphtheria. At the time there were two ways of performing a tracheostomy. The first was the 'high' method in which the trachea was entered through the larynx, usually dividing the cricoid cartilage. The second way was the 'low' tracheostomy in which the trachea was entered directly. This was felt to be very difficult and there was a taboo about dividing the thyroid gland in order to gain access to the trachea. Tracheostomies therefore tended to be performed by the 'high' method. There were significant problems associated with this method especially laryngeal stenosis and a high mortality rate.

Chevelier Jackson in 1923 published his work on tracheostomies and was the first person to recognise that dividing the cricoid cartilage during a 'high' tracheostomy leads to stenosis. The modern practice of placing the tracheostomy below the first tracheal ring significantly reduced these complications and it was largely due to Jackson's teachings that the mortality rate dropped from 25% to 1–2% and the incidence of stenosis, particularly in children, decreased.[2]

INDICATIONS FOR TRACHEOSTOMY

Diphtheria is now largely a historical disease but the indications for tracheostomy continue to evolve. The indications fall into five broad categories, with some overlap between them:

1. Mechanical obstruction of the upper airways.
2. Protection of tracheobronchial tree in patients at risk of aspiration.
3. Respiratory failure.
4. Retention of bronchial secretions.
5. Elective tracheostomy, e.g. during major head and neck surgery a tracheostomy can provide/improve surgical access and facilitate ventilation.

Examples of each category can be found (see Chapter 3, Surgical Tracheostomy).

PHYSIOLOGY

There are significant benefits for the patient having a tracheostomy but altering the physiology of respiration also has its own drawbacks.

The advantages of a tracheostomy tube are that they reduce the upper airway dead space by up to 150 ml (50%). This means that there is a significantly reduced effort in breathing compared to the naso- or oropharyngeal route. There is consequently significantly reduced airway resistance and increased alveolar ventilation [alveolar ventilation = tidal volume − dead space volume].[1,3,4]

The tracheostomy tubes are more comfortable than endotracheal tubes and therefore, better tolerated by patients, who consequently require less sedation. Patients also have the potential to eat and talk with the tube in situ.

The disadvantage of bypassing the upper airways is that the warming, humidification and filtering of air do not take place before the inspired air reaches the trachea and lungs. This results in the drying out of the tracheal and bronchial epithelium. The epithelium responds by increased production of mucus. There is also increased production of mucus in response to a foreign body (the tube) within the trachea.[3] The increased amount, together with the increased viscosity of the mucus may result in mucus plugs or crusts as the mucus desiccates. This can lead to blockage of the airways and/or the tracheostomy tube.

The normal mucociliary clearance mechanism is also disrupted. Firstly, by the mechanical presence of the tube obstructing the upward movement of mucus and secondly, by the metaplastic change of the ciliated epithelium to squamous epithelium, in response to the dry inspired air.

The presence of the tube also causes a degree of disruption to the normal swallowing mechanism by splinting the larynx and preventing normal upward movement of the larynx on swallowing. The cuff may also compress the oesophagus, which is immediately behind the trachea.[5] Thus the effectiveness of the patients swallow may be significantly reduced (see Chapter 11, Swallowing).

Aspiration and pooling of secretions above a cuffed tube may also be a problem. The normal cough reflex and the positive intralaryngeal pressure on expiration, is lost.[3,6] The loss of the ability to close the vocal cords and produce a positive intralaryngeal pressure also results in a less effective cough and the result is some retention of secretions within the bronchial tree.[7–9]

The patient cannot talk when intubated but this problem can be overcome with special fenestrated tracheostomy tubes or speaking valves (see Chapter 12, Communication). Strategies for dealing with the specific problems relating to the tracheostomy tubes, outlined above, can be found (see Chapters 6 and 7, Tracheostomy Tubes and Tracheostomy Management in the Intensive Care Unit).

ALTERNATIVE METHODS OF SECURING A SAFE AIRWAY

Non-invasive positive pressure ventilation (NPPV)

This is where a tight fitting face mask is applied over the nose and mouth and the patient's respiration is assisted by a ventilator. This method is only possible in patients who have normal upper airways. In appropriately selected patients with acute respiratory failure (e.g. COPD), this method is effective for short periods of time (± 24 h). This method avoids the potential risks, including possible mortality, from a surgical airway. However, dealing with bronchial secretions while the face mask is applied is problematic and difficulties with swallowing are encountered with this method.[2,10] It is quite often uncomfortable for the patient and may not be tolerated for long periods.

Laryngeal mask airway (LMA)

The LMA consists of a tube connected to a miniature inflatable mask. This is inserted into the patient's pharynx and the mask is inflated. The epiglottis is pushed forwards and the oropharyngeal airway is opened up and a low-pressure seal is formed around the larynx. This method is not suitable for emergency airway management as the patient is at risk of aspiration of stomach contents.

Endotracheal intubation

Securing an airway by passing an endotracheal (ET) tube via the oro- or nasotracheal route is the most commonly used method and is the treatment of choice in the vast majority of patients with airway/breathing problems, even those with a degree of upper airway obstruction.

The intubated patient is unable to speak, or swallow properly and the tube is very uncomfortable in an awake patient. They therefore require a degree of sedation in order to keep them comfortable. The ET tubes cause trauma to the upper airways and larynx and in up to 80% of patients there is visible tissue injury immediately after extubation.[2] This is largely due to pressure, causing ulceration of the delicate laryngeal mucosa. These ulcerated areas can become infected and this may lead to perichondritis and ultimately to stenosis. In the majority of cases the injury is minor and does not lead to any long-term problems for the patient. However, in prolonged intubation (>2–3 weeks), there may be serious complications, with long-term laryngeal injuries. See Chapters 3 and 5, Surgical Tracheostomy and Difficult Airway for further information on complications and management strategies.

Transtracheal needle ventilation

This method is used to rapidly obtain a surgical airway after failed mask ventilation and endotracheal intubation. A 12- to 14-gauge (16- to 18-gauge in children), plastic sheathed intravenous cannula is pushed into the tracheal lumen via the cricothyroid ligament. In the midline, the cricothyroid ligament is a very safe route to the airway as there are usually no structures between the skin and the ligament. This area is therefore referred to as a bloodless field.

The cannula is then connected to an oxygen supply at 15 l/min, with either a Y-connector or a side hole cut in the tubing attached to the cannula. Intermittent insufflation can then be achieved by placing the thumb over the open end of the Y-connector or the hole in the tubing. Commercially available kits are now available in most A&E Departments or operating theatres. This method of ventilation can be used for up to 45 min, buying sufficient time to convert to a more definitive surgical airway.[11] This technique is hazardous for patients with total upper airway obstruction as the lack of air exit may result in a pneumothorax.

Cricothyroidotomy (minitracheostomy, laryngotomy)

In this procedure a scalpel blade is used to incise the cricothyroid ligament and the blade is then turned through 90 degrees to hold the wound open while a small ET or minitracheostomy tube is inserted into the trachea. This is extremely effective in the emergency situation and the patient can be ventilated for up to 24–48 h with this tube in situ. If ventilation is needed for longer then the cricothyroidotomy should be converted to a formal tracheostomy as there is an increased risk of subglottic laryngeal stenosis and voice problems.[2–3] The procedure is contraindicated in children under 12 years because of the risk of damage to the cricoid cartilage in younger children.[11]

Tracheostomy

This is the definitive surgical airway. The methods of performing a tracheostomy, the indications and complications are covered (see Chapters 3 and 5, Surgical Tracheostomy and Difficult Airway).

BENEFITS OF A TRACHEOSTOMY

Patients with tracheostomies tend to have fewer days of mechanical ventilation because of the improvements in the respiratory physiology, as alluded to earlier. This is especially true in trauma patients.[12] They have a lower risk of laryngotracheal injury than patients with ET tubes, largely because of anatomical factors. They have improved secretion clearance as suction is easy and less strength is required for expectoration. This may be linked to the lower incidence of pneumonia and respiratory infections seen, especially in trauma victims.[12]

The airway is more secure than with an ET tube, particularly if the patient is transported to other parts of the hospital (e.g. X-ray or theatres) or not sedated and therefore able to move about in bed. Less sedation is required as the tube is more comfortable than an ET tube. The patients may also be able to swallow, so may be started on oral feeding sooner and mouth care is easier compared with an ET tube.

The most significant benefit from a patient's point of view is that they can communicate more easily, either by articulating or mouthing words or by using a speaking valve and/or fenestrated tube.

REFERENCES

1. Bradley PJ. Management of the obstructed airway and tracheostomy. In: Hibbert J (ed.). *Laryngology and Head & Neck Surgery*. In: Kerr AG, Booth JB (eds). *Scott-Brown's Otolaryngology*, 6th edn. Oxford: Butterworth-Heinemann, 1997; 5(7): 1–20.

2. Eavey RD. The history of tracheotomy. In: Myers EN, Johnson JT, Murry T (eds). *Tracheotomy Airway Management, Communication, and Swallowing.* San Diego: Singular Publishing Group, 1998; Chapter 1: 1–8.

3. Howard DJ. Emergency and elective airway procedures: Tracheostomy, cricothyroidotomy and their variants. In: McGregor IA, Howard DJ (eds). *Rob & Smith's Operative Surgery Head and Neck*, Part 1, 4th edn. Oxford: Butterworth-Heinemann, 1992; 1: 27–44.

4. Pritchard AP, Mallet J. *Tracheostomy Care. The Royal Marsden Manual of Clinical & Nursing Procedures*, 3rd edn. London: Blackwell Scientific Publications, 1994.

5. Flanagan K, Miller R, Laws-Chapman C. Bedside Evaluation of Swallowing, Eating and Drinking. In: Laws-Chapman C, Rushmer F, Miller R, Flanagan K, Prigmore S, Chabane C. Guidelines for the Care of Patients with Tracheostomy Tubes. St George's Healthcare NHS Trust, London, August 2000; 41.

6. Tippets D, Siebens A. Speaking and swallowing on a ventilator. *Dysphagia* 1991; 6: 94–99.

7. Dikeman KJ, Kazandjian MS. *Communication & Swallowing Management of Tracheostomized and Ventilator-Dependant Adults.* San Diego: Singular Publishing Group, 1996.

8. Nash M. Swallowing problems in the tracheostomized patient. *Otolaryng Clin N Am* 1988; 21(4): 701–709.

9. Gross RG, Dettlebach MA, Zajac DJ, Eibling DE. *Measure of Subglottic Air Pressure During Swallowing in a Patient with Tracheostomy.* Paper presented at the convention of the American Academy of Otolaryngology-Head and Neck Surgery. Sep 1992, San Diego.

10. Hoffman LA. Timing of tracheostomy: What is the best approach? *Resp Care* 1994; 39: 378–385.

11. Johnson JT. Alternatives to tracheotomy. In: Myers EN, Johnson JT, Murry T (eds). *Tracheotomy Airway Management, Communication, and Swallowing.* San Diego: Singular Publishing Group, 1998; Chapter 1: 1–8.

12. Alexander RH, Proctor HJ. *ATLS, Advanced Trauma Life Support Course for Physicians*, (Student Manual) 5th edn. American College of Surgeons, Chicago, 1993; 54–55, 69–73.

SURGICAL TRACHEOSTOMY

Tim Price

INDICATIONS

1. Mechanical upper airway obstruction.
2. Protection of tracheobronchial tree in patients at risk of aspiration.
3. Respiratory failure.
4. Retention of bronchial secretions.
5. Elective tracheostomy for major head and neck surgery.

These five categories are not strictly separate indications as there is substantial overlap between them. Therefore a patient may fall into more than one category and require a tracheostomy for a whole host of reasons.

MECHANICAL UPPER AIRWAY OBSTRUCTION

This group contains the largest number of examples and is best broken down further by employing the 'surgical sieve':

Cause	Examples
Congenital	Subglottic or upper tracheal stenosis, laryngeal web, laryngeal and vallecular cysts, tracheo-oesophageal anomalies or haemangioma of the larynx.
Infective	Acute epiglottitis, laryngotracheobronchitis, diphtheria or Ludwig's angina.
Malignancy	Advanced tumours of larynx, tongue, pharynx or upper trachea presenting with stridor.
Trauma	Gunshot and knife wounds to the neck, inhalation of steam or smoke, swallowing of corrosive fluid.
Vocal cord paralysis	Post-op complication of thyroidectomy, cardiac or oesophageal surgery, bulbar palsy.
Foreign body	Swallowed or inhaled object lodged in upper airway causing stridor.

This probably started off as the most common group of conditions requiring a tracheostomy but with advances in medical treatment options (e.g. antibiotics), and in intubation with an endotracheal tube, these conditions are now encountered less often by the ENT surgeon.

PROTECTION OF THE TRACHEOBRONCHIAL TREE FROM ASPIRATION

In chronic conditions where laryngeal or pharyngeal incompetence may allow aspiration and inhalation of saliva or gastric contents, a tracheostomy should be performed. A cuffed tube will prevent inhalation of fluids and the tube allows easy access to the trachea and the bronchi for suction. Examples include:

- Neurological diseases [polyneuritis (e.g. Guillain–Barre syndrome), motor neurone disease, bulbar poliomyelitis, multiple sclerosis, myasthenia gravis, tetanus, brain-stem stroke and bulbar palsy].
- Coma (in any situation where the Glasgow Coma Scale score is less than 8, the patient is at risk of aspiration as the protective reflexes are lost. That includes head injury, overdose, poisoning, stroke, and brain tumour).
- Trauma (severe facial fractures, may result in the aspiration of blood from the upper airways).

RESPIRATORY FAILURE

As already mentioned in Chapter 2, What is a Tracheostomy; the tracheostomy reduces dead space by 50% and results in less effort in breathing and increased alveolar ventilation. It also results in easy access to the respiratory tree for suctioning and removal of bronchial secretions. The following groups of patients are included:

- Pulmonary diseases (exacerbation of chronic bronchitis and emphysema, severe asthma, severe pneumonia).
- Neurological diseases (multiple sclerosis, motor neurone disease).
- Severe chest injury (flail chest).

RETENTION OF BRONCHIAL SECRETIONS

This may occur in a variety of conditions including chronic pulmonary disease, acute respiratory infection, decreased level of consciousness, and trauma to the thoracic cage or musculature with in-effective cough and retention of secretions.

ELECTIVE TRACHEOSTOMY

In major head and neck procedures where there are often major co-morbidity factors a tracheostomy is usually performed electively, in anticipation of post-operative problems with the airway or swallowing mechanism, which will place them at risk of aspiration.

This group also includes those patients on intensive care who have been intubated via the naso- or orotracheal route for a prolonged period. The precise length of time that a patient can be safely intubated in this manner is still the subject of some debate, but there is a direct relationship between the duration of intubation, and the incidence and severity of laryngeal complications (discussed in the previous chapters). The risk of complications greatly increases after intubation for more than 48 h.[1]

Early tracheostomy will speed up the weaning from mechanical ventilation. As a general rule though, endotracheal intubation is the treatment of choice and can be continued for 7–10 days with minimal risk. If it appears that assisted ventilation will be required for longer than 14 days, an elective tracheostomy should be performed.[1–3] Those patients who may possibly be extubated before this time may be assessed on a daily basis until such time as it becomes apparent which option is correct. No patient should be intubated for longer than three weeks however, as the incidence of laryngeal stenosis becomes unacceptably high. Figures of 12% and higher have been quoted.[3] The average intensivist will usually request a tracheostomy at 7–10 days in an attempt to speed up weaning because of the high demand for beds on intensive care wards.

PRE-OPERATIVE CARE AND ASSESSMENT

The operation of emergency tracheostomy has been dealt with in Chapter 5, Difficult Airway and Paediatric Tracheostomy is covered in Chapter 17, so we will confine ourselves to a description of the elective procedure, as in the ITU patient.

The first thing to do, if the patient is conscious, is to speak to the patient about what has been proposed. The procedure should be explained and the benefits and risks laid out for them. It is important to explain that they will not be able to speak initially but will be able to write on a pad, which will be provided for them. Once they no longer require mechanical ventilation then the tube can be changed to a fenestrated one or a speaking valve can be used. If it is truly an elective procedure, as part of a larger operation, then an introduction to someone with a tracheostomy should be considered so that they can speak to them about it and see for themselves what it entails. Once they have been fully informed then they can sign the appropriate consent form. Remember that in the UK, no adult can consent another adult for surgery. So, if the patient is unconscious one should discuss the procedure with the next of kin but do not get them to sign a consent form for the procedure as it is not legally valid. A separate consent form is available for the surgeon and intensivist to sign in this case (Form 4).

The patients clotting should be checked and any anti-coagulants stopped for the time of the procedure. The platelet count should ideally be 100×10^9/l but a count of, at least 50×10^9/l, is acceptable.[4,5] This may not be possible though for all cases.

The patient's neck should also be examined. This will enable one to anticipate difficulties when performing the surgery. For example, in relation to an enlarged thyroid gland or with limited neck extension, making it difficult to gain access to the trachea.

PERI-OPERATIVE CARE

The following description is intended to inform all grades of surgeon and will seem quite basic at times as we have assumed no prior knowledge of the procedure. Experienced surgeons may find some of the tips useful.

A good assistant is vital when performing the tracheostomy as good retraction of structures enables the operation to proceed more smoothly with potentially less intra-operative complications.

The patient should be positioned on the operating table with the neck extended. This is accomplished by placing a shoulder pad under the patient's shoulders. This results in extension of the neck and exposes more of the trachea as it is brought up out of the chest. The head should be supported in a head ring and the patient should be lying squarely on the table. If not the surgeon is likely to stray to one or other side of the trachea with potentially disastrous consequences. Care must also be taken not to over extend the neck, especially in the elderly as this may lead to subluxation or even fracture of a rigid cervical spine (Fig. 1).

The trachea and laryngeal cartilages should be palpated in order to establish where to make the incision. This should be a horizontal incision half way between the sternal notch and the cricoid cartilage, which can be felt just inferior to the cricothyroid ligament. This spot can be marked with a marking pen and the skin and beeper structures should be infiltrated with 0.5% Marcaine containing 1 : 200,000 adrenaline. This provides post-op pain relief and a dryer surgical field for the surgeon. The infiltration should be performed before the surgeon scrubs, as the adrenaline will then have adequate time to work (Fig. 2).

Check with the scrub nurse that an appropriate sized tube for the patient is available and that the cuff is patent on test inflation. A non-fenestrated tube should always be used in the initial period to allow positive pressure ventilation.

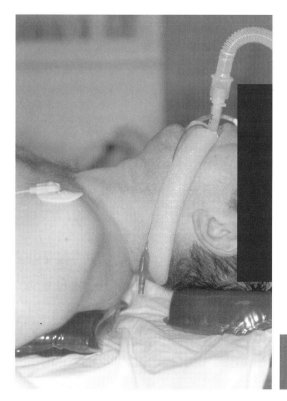

Fig. 1: Patient correctly positioned with shoulder pad and head ring.

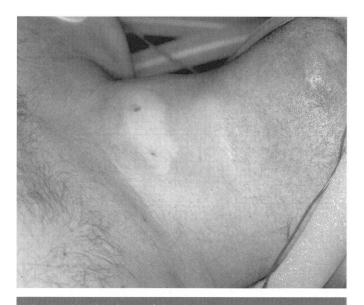

Fig. 2: The blanching of the skin is clearly seen.

There have been instances of air leaks despite the use of non-fenestrated inner tubes (personal observation). A second tube should be available as well as a selection of smaller, and larger tubes in case a problem arises. A catheter mount is also needed to enable the anaesthetic tube to be attached to the tracheostomy tube. Other essential items include a Travis self-retainer, a cricoid hook, a tracheal dilator and sutures (Figs 3, 4).

The neck must be prepared with an appropriate non-alcoholic, anti-septic, surgical skin preparation and the neck is then draped. The endotracheal tube should be taken over the top of the patient's head so that it is not in the surgical field and the anaesthetist can access it easily.

The patient should be draped using three small and one large sticky drape. A head drape should not be used, as it needs to be unwrapped in order to gain access to the ET tube and this cannot be done in a hurry, as it is cumbersome. Place one small sticky drape on either side of the neck, up to the angle of the jaw making sure that the anaesthetic tube is not stuck to the drape. The third drape is applied horizontally just under the chin. In this way the ET tube is not caught up in the drapes and the anaesthetist can get to it very easily (Figs 5, 6).

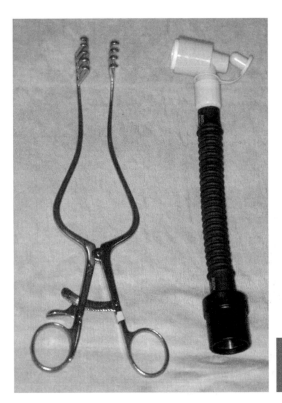

Fig. 3: Travis self-retaining forceps and anaesthetic catheter mount.

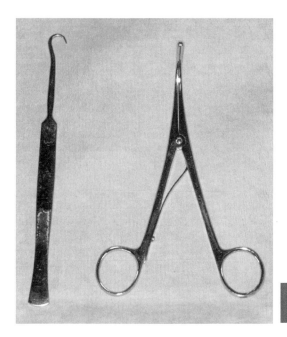

Fig. 4: Cricoid hook and tracheal dilators.

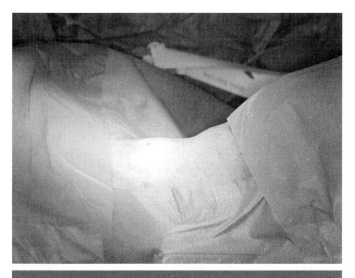

Fig. 5: Illustrates the positioning of the drapes.

The incision should be at least 6 cm long in the adult and should extend to the anterior border of the sternocleidomastoid muscles on either side. More experienced surgeons may choose to make a smaller incision but the wider the exposure, the easier the operation is to perform (Fig. 7).

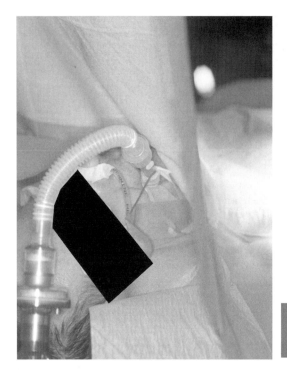

Fig. 6: Illustrates that the anaesthetist has easy access to the ET tube from above.

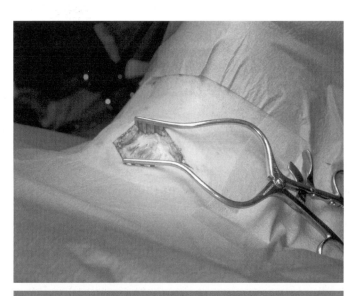

Fig. 7: The horizontal skin incision held open by a self-retaining forcep.

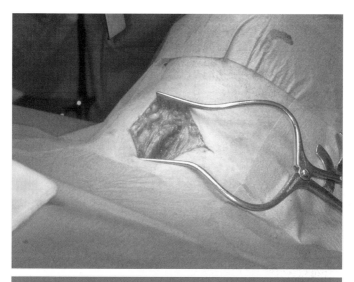

Fig. 8: The strap muscles are clearly seen with the bloodless plane visible in the midline.

The incision is made through the subcutaneous tissue and platysma, down to the deep cervical fascia. The anterior jugular veins will be encountered superficial to the deep cervical fascia on either side of the midline. If they are quite lateral, they do not need to be divided but can be retracted to the sides of the wound. Remember to use the full width of the skin incision as deeper layers are dissected, and note that the trachea is deeper than one imagines.

A self-retaining retractor can now be inserted and the dissection continued until the strap muscles are encountered. These should be separated in the midline. The assistant can do this using a pair of Langenbeck retractors. The dissection is continued with blunt ended dissecting scissors. If one stays in the midline, it is a relatively bloodless field and one continues deeper until the thyroid isthmus is identified (Figs 8, 9).

If the trachea is low in the neck and one is having difficulty accessing the upper trachea, then there are two strategies to bring the trachea further up into the neck. Firstly a Cricoid hook can be used. The hook is inserted into the trachea just under the cricoid cartilage and the trachea is gently pulled upwards into the incision. This usually works well but the hook is very sharp and the authors have experience of the hook cutting through a soft cricoid cartilage. An alternative strategy is to insert a deep Travis retractor and place the upper arm against the lower edge of the thyroid cartilage and the lower, against the upper edge of the sternum. When the retractor is

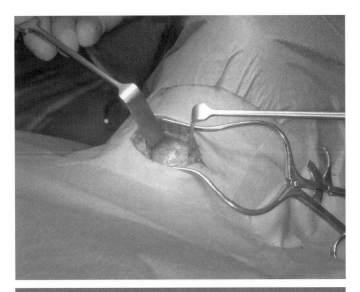

Fig. 9: With the strap muscles retracted, the thyroid isthmus is clearly seen.

opened the trachea is drawn upwards by the pull on the more robust thyroid cartilage.

The thyroid isthmus should be divided between two haemostats and the cut ends transfixed with 2/0 Vicryl suture. This is usually illustrated in textbooks with the haemostats applied from below. However, this is not usually possible as the presence of the sternum and clavicles prevents them being placed from below, especially in the short fat neck. There is also the problem of the inferior thyroid veins exiting from the lower border of the isthmus. Damage to these veins can cause bleeding which may be difficult to control.

In practice, a plane is dissected between the cricoid cartilage and the thyroid isthmus from above. Keeping to the surface of the cricoid cartilage and the trachea prevents bleeding from the isthmus. One should also not dissect lateral to the anterior surface of the trachea in order to avoid injury to the recurrent laryngeal nerves and other important lateral structures. The haemostats are then placed across the isthmus from above and the isthmus divided. This may need to be repeated depending on the thickness of the isthmus (Figs 10, 11).

The practice of pushing the thyroid isthmus inferiorly or superiorly in order to gain access to the trachea should not be used for a number of reasons. Firstly, this is not as easy as it sounds as the thyroid isthmus is firmly attached

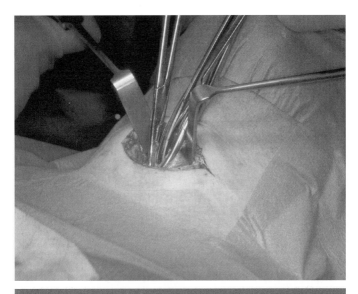

Fig. 10: The thyroid isthmus is divided between two haemostats.

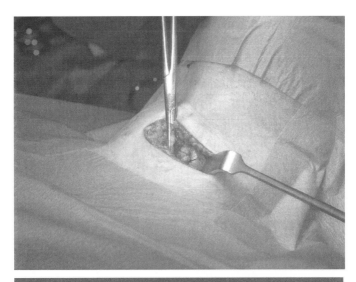

Fig. 11: The left side of the isthmus has been transfixed, with the second haemostat still in place.

to the anterior aspect of the 2nd and 3rd tracheal cartilages as the pre-tracheal fascia, which envelopes the thyroid gland, blends with the trachea at this point. So, some degree of dissection is always necessary in order to mobilise it, with the risk of bleeding. The isthmus may also cause problems with an early tube change as it may flop into the opening in the trachea and it may not be possible to get a new tube in.

Once the isthmus is divided the trachea will be exposed and the rings should be counted. Meticulous haemostasis is essential at this stage as it is difficult to visualise the depths of the wound once the tube is in situ. The surgeon should therefore pay attention to any bleeding at this stage by judicious use of bipolar diathermy. Beware of injury to the recurrent laryngeal nerves when using diathermy lateral to the trachea (Fig. 12).

The tracheostomy should be sited over the 2nd and 3rd or 3rd and 4th tracheal cartilages. The tracheostomy must not involve the first tracheal ring because of the high incidence of post-op, subglottic stenosis if it is divided. The trachea should be incised longitudinally in the midline through these cartilages or if the cartilages are heavily calcified, a window, big enough to take an appropriate sized tube, should be cut in the anterior aspect of the tracheal cartilages. Care must be taken not to dissect laterally as the recurrent laryngeal nerves may be damaged. A pair of heavy scissors may be necessary to cut through heavily calcified cartilages.

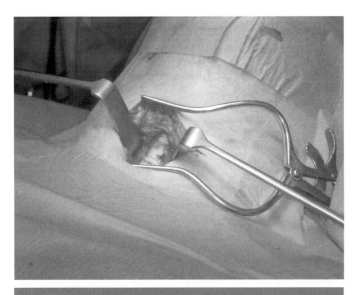

Fig. 12: The tracheal rings are clearly seen with the cricoid cartilage superiorly.

In the past a flap was raised in the tracheal wall. This was referred to as a Bjork flap and was based either inferiorly or superiorly. The edge of the flap was stitched to the skin edge, effectively exteriorising the trachea. This technique was developed during the Diphtheria epidemic to allow the safe management of large numbers of children, with tracheostomies, on an unsupervised ward. If the tube was accidentally dislodged in the early post-op period, it was not possible to intubate them via the endotracheal route, so a semi-permanent stoma, through which the children could breath, unassisted, needed to be formed.[6] In modern practice, patients are nursed on ITU or HDU with close supervision and can be rapidly intubated using an ET tube, if a tracheostomy tube proved impossible to re-insert.

There are also distinct problems with the Bjork flap. Firstly, if the sutures in the flap cut out on the first tube change, the flap may prevent the successful re-insertion of a tube. The stoma, which involves exteriorisation of the trachea, may also need to be closed surgically once the patient has been weaned-off of ventilatory support as it may not close spontaneously. Bjork flaps are also said to have a higher degree of tracheal stenosis than other methods.

Some authors advocate the use of a Bjork flap for reasons of safe reintroduction of a displaced tube and feel that the procedure is particularly useful for surgeons who only do tracheostomies occasionally.[2] We would dispute this as today formal surgical tracheostomies are only performed on the most difficult patients who are not suitable for the percutaneous method. These patients tend to have short fat necks and therefore it is very difficult to oppose the edge of the short tracheal flap to the skin edge, which may be several orders of magnitude longer. So for the inexperienced surgeon this is definitely not the best method of performing a tracheostomy. There is rarely any justification for a Bjork flap tracheostomy in today's practice[6] and it should be abandoned.

Stay or traction sutures, placed in the trachea, on either side of the incision are needed in children. The sutures are placed before the trachea is incised as it becomes very mobile afterwards which may make it difficult to place them accurately. These sutures enable traction to be applied to the trachea and at the same time the skin edges are retracted. This establishes an airway and facilitates the first tube change or assists with replacement of a tube that has come out in the early post-op period (see Chapter 18, Nursing Care of the Child with a Tracheostomy).

Some authors advocate the placement of stay sutures in adults.[2,7] This is not universally carried out and is not common practice in the UK. There are potential disadvantages in adults. The sutures may be difficult to place in the trachea if the cartilages are calcified. The sutures may also cut out when traction is applied as the tissues are not as yielding in the adult patient. The practice of placing the suture through the tracheal wall may also cause further ischaemia of the mucosa and subsequent scarring and stenosis. Certainly the use of silk sutures should not be advocated[7] because of the intense immune reaction that they provoke and the problems of bacteria being able to travel down from the wound surface along this multifilament material (capillarity). This could result in further wound infection with subsequent perichondritis and stenosis at the stoma site. Only strong monofilament suture material should be used, if at all.

When one is ready to make the incision in the trachea, the anaesthetist should be alerted so that he/she can be ready to withdraw the tube. Check that all the equipment is available and working before making your incision. Make especially sure that the right size tube has been selected. If the trachea is relatively deep to the skin edge, an adjustable flange tube is recommended as there is less likelihood of the tube being displaced in the early post-operative period.

Make every effort not to puncture the cuff of the tube. The easiest way to do this is to ask the anaesthetist to push the tube further down the trachea towards the carina before making the hole. Once the trachea is incised the tube is withdrawn under direct vision until the tip is just above the incision. It should not be removed as it can be rapidly advanced to secure the airway in the event of a problem. The cut edges of the trachea may bleed fairly briskly. Do not stop to deal with this but insert the tube and inflate the cuff to protect the airway. If a vertical incision has been made, tracheal dilators will be needed to enable the tube to be inserted into the tracheal lumen (Fig. 13).

The assistant should now hold the tube in situ until it is secured. Use a flexible suction catheter down the tube to suction any blood or mucus out of the trachea and connect the catheter mount to the tracheostomy tube and the anaesthetic tubing. Inflate the cuff of the tube with enough air to create a seal. The anaesthetist should confirm that there is good CO_2 return and that the patient is oxygenating well and that the air-pressures are adequate. Check the cuff on the tracheostomy tube is staying inflated as it can be punctured by a sharp edge of calcified cartilage. If it has, then change the tube.

Diathermy may now be used to control any bleeding, making sure that the gases/fumes produced are suctioned away with the sucker to prevent the chances of an airway fire.[8] This subject is covered later in the chapter, under the heading of Complications.

The wound should not be packed as there is always some leakage of respiratory secretions into the wound and a low grade wound infection. If a pack is inserted then there is a good culture medium to encourage a full-blown wound infection with subsequent wound breakdown and possible, long-term, tracheal stenosis. The author has experience of just such an event.

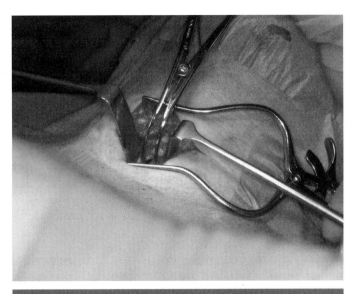

Fig. 13: The tracheal dilator is used to open the trachea after incising vertically through the tracheal rings.

The tracheostomy wound should be closed with monofilament, interrupted sutures to the skin. This is a loose closure and no more than two or three sutures are needed on either side of the tube. Tight closure may result in surgical emphysema especially if positive pressure ventilation is used. The sutures can be removed after seven days.

The tube itself should be secured with both tracheostomy ties and sutures. This will prevent the tube from falling out if someone is offended by blood on the ties and decides to change them in the immediate post-operative period!

The tube is sutured in place using a thick silk stitch. The stitch is placed through the loop provided for the ties and not through the plastic of the flange itself. The author has seen this practice lead to the flange tearing in the early post-operative period and it was no longer possible to secure the ties to the flange. The tube therefore had to be changed before a tract had formed, with all the potential hazards that go with early tube changes (see Complications). The sutures are tied with just enough slack to allow the Lyofoam dressing to be inserted between the skin and the tracheostomy tube (see Chapter 10, Wound Care). Only now can the assistant let go of the tube!

The tracheostomy tapes are tied around the neck only once the sand bag has been removed from behind the patient's shoulders and the neck has been flexed. If this is not done in this order then the tapes will be very loose once the neck is

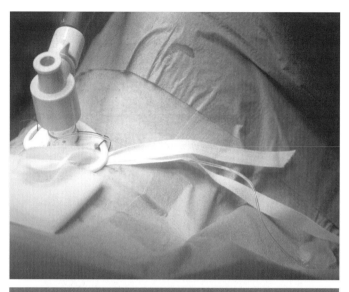

Fig. 14: The loop in the tracheostomy tape is passed through the flange. The silk suture holding the tube in place is also illustrated.

flexed and if the tube is not sutured in place, it will simply fall out. The easiest way to securely fasten the tapes to the flange of the tube is to make a loop with a long and short limb and pass this loop through the flange and then pull the ends of the tape through the loop and pull them tight (see Figures 14 and 15). This will lock the tape in place. Now pass the long ends of the tape under the patient's neck and tie securely to the opposite short ends. The tapes should be tied in such a way that only the tip of one finger can be placed between them and the skin of the neck and they should be tied with proper knots and not bows!

The tube should only be changed once a tract has formed between the trachea and the skin. This only occurs after 48–72 h, so the tube should not be replaced until at least three days have passed. There is no real reason to want to change a tube that is working well, any earlier. Therefore, one should wait to perform the first tube change on day 5 when a good tract would have formed and no problems should be encountered in replacing the tube.

If the tube needs to be changed because of a defective cuff then various methods of changing the tube over a 'guidewire' have been described.[9,10] These include passing a solid bougie into the trachea via the lumen of the tube and then removing the defective tube and introducing a new tube, over the bougie. This is probably the safest method to employ (see Chapter 13, Tracheostomy Tube Changes)

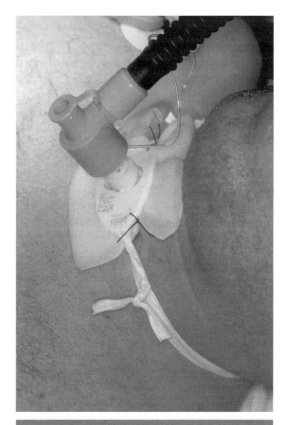

Fig. 15: The ends of the tracheostomy tape have been pulled through the loop and tied firmly around the patient's neck.

COMPLICATIONS OF SURGICAL TRACHEOSTOMIES

There are many complications associated with performing a tracheostomy. Most of them can be avoided with a meticulous surgical approach and dedicated post-operative care, administered by a multidisciplinary team. The complications can be intra-operative (including the first 24 h), early post-operative (1–14 days) or late (>14 days). Table 1 gives a comprehensive list of all the complications associated with tracheostomy.[1–3,11]

The incidence of overall complications depends on individual departments and ranges from 5 to 40%.[1,3] The most commonly occurring complications are haemorrhage, tube obstruction and tube displacement. The incidence varies depending on the papers quoted.[1,3] Death occurs in 0.5–1.6% and is most often the result of tube displacement. Emergency tracheostomy carries

Table 1: Complications of tracheostomy	
Stage	**Complication**
Intra-operative	Haemorrhage
	Airway fire
	Injury to trachea and larynx
	Injury to paratracheal structures
	Air embolism
	Apnoea
	Cardiac arrest
Early post-operative	Subcutaneous emphysema
	Pneumothorax/pneumomediastinum
	Tube displacement
	Tube blockage (crusts)
	Wound infection
	Tracheal necrosis
	Secondary haemorrhage
	Swallowing problems
Late post-operative	Haemorrhage
	Granuloma formation
	Tracheo-oesophageal fistula
	Difficult decannulation
	Tracheocutaneous fistula
	Laryngotracheal stenosis
	Tracheostomy scar

a two to five fold increase in the incidence of complications over an elective procedure.[1]

Intra-operative complications

Primary haemorrhage

Coagulation disorders must be corrected as far as possible pre-operatively. If the procedure is being performed under local anaesthesia then the surgeon should not proceed until the vasoconstriction is complete.[7] Significant bleeding can occur from the anterior jugular veins and from the thyroid isthmus. The surgeon needs to be meticulous when tying off these vessels and over sewing the divided ends of the thyroid isthmus. By not dissecting lateral to the trachea, damage to the internal jugular vein and the carotid artery are avoided.

Airway fires

This important and potentially catastrophic complication is not mentioned in any standard texts! Fires usually arise when diathermy is used in the presence of an open airway. That is to say, when there is a source of heat, an oxygen supply and an inflammable substance available. It is well known that the gases arising from diathermied fat will burn when made hot enough or if mixed with sufficient oxygen.[8] It is therefore essential that a dry field be obtained prior to opening the trachea. If there is heavy bleeding from the tracheal wall after inserting the tracheostomy tube, the anaesthetist should be informed so that ventilation can momentarily be suspended before using diathermy. The fumes created should be suctioned away while diathermy is in use. Bipolar diathermy is said to be safer because of less arcing, but this possibility still exists so care must be taken whatever method is used. If an airway fire should occur, empty a bowl of saline into the wound, stop ventilating the patient and use a carbon dioxide fire-extinguisher if the fire continues.[8]

Injury to the trachea and larynx
Careful haemostasis and good exposure will help to minimise the risks of damage to these structures. The most important sites of damage to recognise are the posterior tracheal wall and the cricoid and 1st cartilage ring. If the damage is recognised at the time of surgery careful apposition of the edges of the cartilage is necessary to minimise the risk of post-operative stenosis of the trachea and larynx. Injury to the posterior tracheal wall must be avoided, as a tracheo-oesophageal fistula is the ultimate result if this injury goes unrecognised. Both structures should be repaired separately.

Injury to paratracheal structures
Do not dissect lateral to the trachea. This will avoid damage to the recurrent laryngeal nerves, carotid artery, jugular vein and vagus nerve. Also avoid placing the tracheostomy too low or hyper-extending the neck, as the left brachiocephalic vein and right brachiocephalic trunk (incorrectly referred to as the innominate artery) could be damaged. This is especially so in children. The pleural domes can also be damaged in patients with emphysematous hyper-expansion of the lungs and in children. This would result in a post-operative pneumomediastinum or pneumothorax.

Air embolism
This rare complication will also be avoided by keeping to the midline and avoiding damage to the internal jugular vein.

Apnoea
This may occur in patients with very high $PaCO_2$ levels because of prolonged expiratory airway obstruction. For example, in a severe COAD patient with an acute pneumonia, or in partial upper-airway obstruction. When a tracheostomy tube is inserted, there is a sudden drop in the $PaCO_2$ level, which

results in apnoea. The reason for this is the respiratory drive, which is maintained by the high $PaCO_2$, is cut off and the patient stops breathing. The anaesthetist needs to be aware of this possibility and may need to use 5% CO_2 in oxygen to prevent this problem occurring.

Cardiac dysrhythmias and cardiac arrest

Patients may arrest intra-operatively because of other co-morbidity factors or the sudden swings in acid base balance, which occur with respiratory obstruction and its subsequent rapid correction. The sudden swing from respiratory acidosis to alkalosis also results in a rise in the potassium levels and this together with the raised levels of adrenaline may result in a cardiac arrest.[1]

Displacement or blockage of the tube, a tension pneumothorax or pneumomediastinum can also result in a cardio-respiratory arrest.[7]

Early post-operative complications

Subcutaneous emphysema

This can be very dramatic, especially if the patient is receiving positive pressure ventilation. It is most commonly caused by too tight a closure of the tracheostomy wound or an incorrectly sized tube allowing air to escape. It is important to allow the inevitable leak of some air, from the trachea, to escape to the surface of the skin. Therefore leave the wound loosely closed with only three or four sutures and make sure the tube is the correct size for the patient. If the situation does arise then address the above two points and cover the patient with antibiotics as cellulitis may ensue. The air will be re-absorbed spontaneously.

Pneumomediastinum and pneumothorax

This occurs with dissection low in the neck and damage to the pleural domes. This condition should always be suspected and a post-operative chest X-ray performed. This condition usually requires chest tube drainage if present.

Tube displacement

The most important factor to consider, when trying to avoid this potentially lethal complication, is the tube size. Make sure that you choose the appropriate size, allowing for some post-operative swelling of the soft tissues of the neck and that the tube is firmly sutured in place and the ties tied with the neck flexed. The easiest way to check for displacement of the tube if the patient is short of breath is to pass a flexible bronchoscope or nasendoscope down the lumen of the tube. This will usually enable you to manipulate the tube back into the lumen of the trachea.

Tube blockage/crusts

The increase in viscosity and the amount of mucus produced in response to a tracheostomy tube (see Chapter 2, What is a Tracheostomy?) may result in blockage of the bronchi or the tube. This is especially so if there is inadequate suction and humidification of the inspired air over the first few days as the mucus will dry out and form very hard crusts which can irreversibly block a tube (see Chapters 8 and 9, Humidification and Suctioning). If the patient is experiencing shortness-of-breath, or the nursing staff are having difficulty passing a suction catheter then this complication should be suspected. The first thing to do is to remove the inner cannula of the tracheostomy tube to check for crusts. Once this is out, a flexible endoscope can be passed down the lumen of the tube and an inspection made of the position of the tube and the presence of any crusts at the tip of the tube or within the trachea or major bronchi. If there are crusts present then firstly nebulised saline or 5 ml of saline trickled into the trachea via the tube, can be used in an attempt to soften the crusts and allow successful suction clearance. If this fails the tube may need to be removed and replaced or the crusts may need to be removed with long nasal packing forceps.

Wound infection

The tracheostomy wound always develops a low-grade infection with skin and respiratory tract organisms. This is usually a self-limiting infection and no treatment is needed. However, if there is any pressure necrosis of the skin from ill-fitting tubes and dressings then a more serious infection may occur. Sterile dressings should be changed when soiled to prevent prolonged contact of wet, contaminated dressings, with the skin.

The wound should never be packed for a prolonged period to control bleeding because this may provide a culture medium for infection, with wound breakdown and septicaemia.

Infection of the tracheal mucosa (trachiitis) may result if the trachea is allowed to dry out and this may lead to perichondritis and subsequent tracheal stenosis. Adequate humidification and correctly fitting tubes are essential to prevent this complication.

A paratracheal mediastinal abscess has been reported post-operatively but fortunately this is rare.[7]

Tracheal necrosis

This is usually the result of pressure necrosis caused by an inappropriately sized tube pressing on the posterior wall of the trachea or an inappropriately high pressure within the cuff of the tube. It is therefore important to check the position of the tube and to monitor cuff pressure to prevent it. The pressure necrosis predisposes to infection (perichondritis) and there may be erosion through the trachea into the oesophagus (tracheo-oesophageal fistula) or a vessel (tracheo-arterial fistula). The necrosis often leads to long-term tracheal stenosis.

Secondary haemorrhage

Minor bleeding from the skin edge may result when the vasoconstriction wears off. This is easy to control with a pressure dressing. More serious bleeding can occur from erosion of a vessel by the tube (tracheo-arterial fistula) or from an area of granulation tissue within the stoma or trachea. The granulation tissue is usually the result of local infection and or a tube, which is not fitting properly rubbing on an area of the trachea. Therefore, make sure that the patient is getting adequate humidification, the tube is fitting properly and that there is prompt treatment of any infection.

Erosion of a tube into a large vessel is invariably fatal and occurs in 0.4% of tracheostomies.[1] The vessel involved is most commonly the right brachiocephalic trunk and the reasons for this have been alluded to already. Suffice to say that the tracheostomy must not be placed too low in the trachea and that the tube is the appropriate size for the patient.

Swallowing problems

These have been covered (see Chapter 2, What is a Tracheostomy?). The problem may be overcome in patients who are not at risk of aspiration by deflating the cuff during meals or by down sizing the tube. The problem usually resolves spontaneously (see Chapter 11, Swallowing for further details).

Late post-operative complications

Haemorrhage

This has been covered in the previous section but can occur at any time.

Granuloma formation

Granulomas form in response to an ill-fitting tube or a chronic low-grade infection. They occur most commonly at the stoma but can also form in the lumen of the trachea. They usually cause minor bleeding on suctioning or changing the tube and occasionally they may cause difficulty in passing a suction catheter. Granulomas are treated by firstly removing a tube that is rubbing on the wall of the trachea, and replacing it with a better fitting tube. This removes the stimulus for their formation. They can then be cauterised with a silver nitrate cautery stick and topical antiseptic ointment applied. Failing this they can be treated with a CO_2 laser via a bronchoscope.[7]

Tracheo-oesophageal fistula

As mentioned above, this complication may result from primary trauma to the posterior wall of the trachea and the oesophagus at the time of surgery. It may also arise from pressure necrosis where the cuff pressure is too high or the tube is pressing on the tracheal wall. This is compounded by the presence of a large bore feeding tube in the oesophagus.[1] This is because the anterior wall of the oesophagus and the posterior wall of the trachea are pinched between these two unyielding surfaces. Thus, only fine bore feeding tubes should be used and the cuff pressure regularly checked (see Chapters 11 and 22, Swallowing and Nutritional Assessment and Management of Patients with Tracheostomies). This complication may be suspected if the patient is coughing on swallowing saliva or eating. The diagnosis is confirmed endoscopically and repaired by an open procedure.

Difficult decannulation

This problem is largely addressed by following an appropriate weaning protocol with each patient. See Chapter 14, Decannulation for further details.

Tracheocutaneous fistula

In long-term tracheostomies there may be complete epithelialisation of the stomal tract. These stomas will not close off spontaneously after removal of the tube. It is necessary in these patients to formally excise the stoma and to close the wound in layers, interposing the strap muscles between the skin and the trachea. This will prevent puckering of the scar, as the skin cannot adhere to the anterior tracheal wall.

Laryngotracheal stenosis

As mentioned above damage to the 1st tracheal ring and the cricoid cartilage is the chief culprit but infection and pressure necrosis can also play a part. The surgical strategies for dealing with these problems are beyond the scope of this text.

Tracheostomy scar

Unsightly scars are usually the result of the skin attaching to the anterior tracheal wall. This results in a puckered scar that moves on swallowing. This can be excised and the underlying strap muscles are mobilised and apposed in the midline beneath the skin, effectively preventing the skin reattaching to the tracheal wall.

ACKNOWLEDGEMENT

Many thanks to Mike Biggs for his expertise in taking and processing the photographs for this chapter at such short notice.

REFERENCES

1. Bradley PJ. Management of the obstructed airway and tracheostomy. In: Kerr AG, Booth JB (eds). *Scott-Brown's Otolaryngology*, 6th edn. London: Butterworth-Heinemann, 1997; 5(7): 1–19.

2. Howard DJ. Emergency and elective airway procedures: Tracheostomy, cricothy-roidotomy and their variants. In: McGregor IA, Howard DJ (eds). *Rob & Smith's Operative Surgery Head and Neck*, Part 1, 4th edn. Oxford: Butterworth-Heinemann, 1992; 1: 27–44.

3. Hoffman LA. Timing of tracheostomy: What is the best approach? *Resp Care* 1994; 39: 378–385.

4. Jones RM. Influence of coexisting disease. In: Kirk RM, Mansfield AO, Cochrane J (eds). *Clinical Surgery in General RCS Course Manual*, 2nd edn. London: Churchill Livingstone, 1996; 6: 77.

5. Mehta AB. Haematological assessment and blood component therapy. In: Kirk RM, Mansfield AO, Cochrane J (eds). *Clinical Surgery in General RCS Course Manual*, 2nd edn. London: Churchill Livingstone, 1996; 7: 87.

6. Goldstraw P. The chest wall, lungs, pleura and diaphragm. In: Burnand KG, Young AE (eds). *The New Aird's Companion in Surgical Studies*. Edinburgh: Churchill Livingstone, 1996; 31: 730.

7. Myers EN. Technique and complications of tracheotomy in adults. In: Myers EN, Johnson JT, Murry T (eds). *Tracheotomy Airway Management, Communication, and Swallowing*. San Diego: Singular Publishing Group Inc., 1998; 15–32.

8. Rogers ML, Nickalls RWD, Brackenbury ET, Salama FD, Beattie MG, Perks AGB. Airway fire during tracheostomy: Prevention strategies for surgeons and anaes-thetists. *Annals of RCS of England* 2001; 83(6): 376–380.

9. Widmann WD. Technique for changing tracheostomy tubes in the early post-operative patient. *Crit Care Med* 1974; 2(5): 277–278.

10. Richardson J, Smith BP. Replacement of tracheostomy tubes. *Crit Care Med* 1974; 2(5): 519.

11. Tracheostomy. In: Roland NJ, McRae RDR, McCombe AW (eds). *Key Topics in Otolaryngology*, 2nd edn. Oxford: BIOS Scientific Publishers Limited, 2001; 336–339.

PERCUTANEOUS DILATATIONAL TRACHEOSTOMY

Jasmine Patel and Basil Matta

Percutaneous dilatational tracheostomy (PDT) is defined as the placement of a tracheostomy tube with the help of commercially available sets. It is an elective procedure frequently performed in the intensive care unit (ICU). Its popularity has partly been due to the procedure being more readily available with less restraints from theatre availability, accessing surgeons, cost and time involved in co-ordinating patient transfer compared to a standard surgical tracheostomy (SST).

Modern PDT was described in 1955[1] and in 1969.[2] PDT using serial dilators was introduced by Pasquale Ciaglia in 1985.[3] The dilating tracheostomy forceps were developed in 1989[4] and further by Griggs in 1990[5] who introduced the use of a guidewire. The most commonly used PDT kits are available from Cook including the single tapered tracheal dilator (Blue Rhino) developed by Ciaglia.

PDT – INDICATIONS AND BENEFITS

The benefits of a PDT over long-term translaryngeal intubation are the same as that of a SST.[6] Translaryngeal intubation for more than 10 days increases the risk of vocal cord paralysis, glottic and subglottic stenosis, infections, tracheomalacia, tracheal dilation and long-term tracheal stenosis. The decision to convert a translaryngeal tube to a tracheostomy tube in the ICU has to be individualised because though it has advantages, a PDT is an invasive procedure not without risks.

Critically ill patients predicted to require prolonged intubation (defined as between 7–21 days in various studies) for mechanical ventilation and weaning benefit from PDT. In the right patient, it is better to carry out a PDT early in the stage of the ICU stay rather than late. The other indications for PDT are similar to those for a SST, for example patients with depressed or absent pharyngeal and laryngeal reflexes who cannot protect their airway. A tracheostomy facilitates better pulmonary toilet, nursing care, feeding and promotes patient mobility and an early return of speech as against a translaryngeal tube. The anatomical dead space, with a tracheostomy, is reduced by 70–100 ml and as the airway resistance decreases, weaning is facilitated.

PRE-REQUISITES AND CONTRAINDICATIONS FOR PDT

PDT necessitates the administration of adequate pain relief, sedation and neuromuscular blockade to the already intubated and mechanically ventilated patient. Due to this a PDT cannot be used for emergency airway management as in supraglottis or orofacial trauma. The medical staff available in the hospital have to be trained and experienced in airway management, PDT, chest drain insertion, bronchoscopy and a SST in case the PDT fails or is complicated. Patients under the age of 16 years (some intensivist's quote the figure 12 years) are unsuitable candidates for the procedure.

Obvious deformities of the airway, previous scars from surgeries like a tracheostomy or a sternotomy, neck oedema, gross obesity, a mass (for example a goitre) or a tumour in the neck make it difficult to easily palpate the local landmarks like the cricoid cartilage. In these situations it is advisable to opt for a SST. Obvious blood vessels under the skin, inflammation and/or rash at the operation site are also contraindications to a PDT.

Inability to optimally extend the patient's neck due to cervical spine trauma or arthritis, the presence of a short neck or due to severe kyphosis is a contraindication to a PDT. PDT has to be delayed if a patient is haemodynamically unstable. Carrying out a PDT on a patient with a known difficult airway much depends on the operators opinion and experience.

An uncorrectable bleeding diathesis is an obvious risk for uncontrollable haemorrhage during the procedure.

COMPARISON BETWEEN PDT AND SST

As against a SST, transportation of critically ill patients away from the ICU environment to the operation theatre is avoided during a PDT. This reduces the threats imposed on the safe management of lines, monitors and any other life support systems required by the patient. In a prospective study of 125 critically ill patients who were transported from the ICU, one-thirds suffered from at least one mishap, from cardiac lead failure to vasoactive drug disconnection.[7] Additional costs on account of theatre personnel and anaesthesia are cut down because of PDT[8–11] and better resource management is possible.

A percutaneous tracheostomy can be carried out completely in as little as 15 min in experienced hands as against a SST, which takes at least 30 min.[8–10,12]

PDT utilises the smallest possible tracheostomy tube size and stoma size, which allows adequate ventilation and access for suctioning. This minimal size decreases haemorrhage, avoids damage to large blood vessels and the oozing accompanying the procedure is taken care of by the snugly fitting tracheostomy tube. As less tissue is exposed to contamination and as the procedure needs only a small incision, there are less opportunities for subsequent tissue reaction and infection.[12]

PDT reduces the time between decision to operate and the actual procedure itself from four days to one day as against a SST.[13]

The complication rates of PDT compare favourably to those of SST.[12,14] Post-decannulation stomal closure is quicker and a smaller scar is formed post-PDT as against a SST.[12,15]

PRE-PROCEDURE PATIENT PREPARATION

Before actually embarking upon the procedure, the operator (OP) has to confirm the suitability of the anatomy of the patient's neck. This is done with the patient's head and neck in an extended position. The medical staff will discuss the procedure with the patient and/or the family. These discussions will include a description, the necessity for and complications associated to the procedure. A written consent will also be obtained prior to the procedure, according to the respective hospital policy.

Nasogastric feed is stopped at least 2 h before the planned time of PDT and the stomach contents emptied just before the actual procedure to prevent aspiration into the airway.

For the procedure, the patient is administered 100% oxygen; adequate analgesia, sedation and muscle relaxation are also ensured. The ventilator settings for frequency, tidal volume and maximum airway pressure are adjusted to compensate for the air leak during the procedure. A positive end-expiratory pressure of 5–10 cmH$_2$O is recommended. Continuous oximetry and monitoring of all other vital parameters is essential during the procedure. The intracerebral pressure is also closely monitored wherever need be.

The optimal neck position is obtained by placing firm towel rolls between the patient's shoulder blades and an additional pillow or two under the neck as preferred by the airway manager (AM).

The AM introduces a bronchoscope so as to view the trachea just beyond the tip of the translaryngeal tube. The transillumination at the operation site provided by the bronchoscope light source can guide the OP to choose the correct site for an incision, in addition of course to the other surface landmarks. The fixation tapes of the translaryngeal tube are untied, the cuff is deflated and the tube is withdrawn until transillumination is obtained at the selected operation site. The cuff is then carefully reinflated to the original volume. The tip of the bronchoscope is withdrawn so that it lies just within the translaryngeal tube and can yet visualise beyond, this prevents any damage to the bronchoscope that can be caused by the operator's needle.

Simultaneously, the OP prepares the operation site, cleaning it with chlorhexidine and then draping it. The landmark structures like the thyroid notch, cricoid cartilage and the tracheal rings are palpated to define the proper location for the intended tracheostomy placement and the transillumination confirmed at the right site. The ultimate tube placement is made at the level of the first and the second tracheal cartilages or between the second and the third tracheal cartilages whenever possible. Ten to 15 ml of 1% Lidocaine with 1:200,000 adrenaline is then injected as a local anaesthetic. The PDT kit is then opened and the cuff of the appropriate sized tracheostomy tube is checked for any leakages.

PROCEDURE

The following is a description of the PDT using the Ciaglia et al. technique of serial dilation.[16]

A 2–3 mm midline subcricoid transverse incision is made on the skin at the pre-selected site. A pair of curved mosquito forceps can be used for blunt dissection vertically and transversely down to the pre-tracheal fascia. With the tip of the little finger, the front of the trachea is dissected in the midline, free of any tissues and then the intercartilaginous area is felt. If the isthmus of the thyroid is present, it is displaced away from the intercartilaginous area to be punctured.

The introducer needle with its catheter, attached to a saline filled syringe for continuous suction, is directed in the trachea – midline, posterior and caudad. This is guided by the bronchoscopic view and any paramedian insertion of the needle corrected by a repeated attempt. Entrance of the needle in the tracheal air column is also verified by aspiration on the syringe resulting in an air bubble return. The AM should confirm that the introducer needle is not in the Murphy's eye of the translaryngeal tube by looking at the movement of the needle with very slight sliding movements of the tube. The introducer needle is then slowly withdrawn while advancing the catheter over it for several millimetres in the trachea, checking with the AM bronchoscopic view.

Once the needle and the syringe have been completely removed, the wire guide (metal) is advanced several centimetres into the trachea. The catheter is then withdrawn completely while maintaining the wire guide position within the tracheal lumen. Maintaining the wire guide position at the skin level mark on the wire guide, the lubricated introducing dilator (dark blue) is advanced over the wire guide to dilate the initial access site into the trachea using a slight twisting motion. This dilator is then removed while maintaining the wire guide in the position with the skin level mark on it at its proper level. Maintaining safe positioning marks of the wire guide, guiding catheter and dilators during the dilating procedure, prevents trauma to the posterior tracheal wall.

Following the direction of the arrow on the guiding catheter (white) and keeping the end of the guiding catheter with the safety ridge towards the patient, it is advanced over the wire guide up to its skin level mark. The guiding catheter and the wire guide are inserted as a unit into the trachea until the safety ridge on the guiding catheter is at the skin level. The proximal end of the guiding catheter is aligned at the mark on the proximal portion of the wire guide. This will assure that the distal end of the guiding catheter is properly positioned back on the wire guide preventing possible trauma to the posterior wall of the trachea during subsequent manipulations.

The serial dilators (light blue) are then lubricated generously and serial dilation is begun at the access site into the trachea. This is accomplished by first advancing the smallest curved blue dilator over the wire guide/guiding catheter assembly. To properly align the dilator on the wire guide/guiding catheter assembly, the proximal end of the dilator is positioned at the single positioning mark on the guiding catheter (white). This positions the distal tip of the dilator at the safety ridge on the guiding catheter. Visually maintaining these safety positions, these three as a unit are advanced with a twisting motion, to the skin level mark on the blue dilator. The dilating assembly is advanced and pulled back several times, while twisting, to perform effective dilatation of the tracheal entrance site. The first or smallest blue dilator is then removed, leaving the guidewire/guiding catheter assembly in position again.

This dilation of the tracheotomy is continued with the use of dilators of increasing sizes. The tracheal entrance site is slightly over-dilated to a size appropriate for the passage of the tracheostomy tube of choice; over-dilation allows easy passage of the balloon portion of the tube into the trachea. Table 1 details the size of dilator to be used to over-dilate the stoma according to size of tracheostomy tube to be inserted.

The tracheostomy tube to be inserted is pre-loaded on the appropriate size blue dilator by first lubricating the surface of the dilator. The lubricated tube with the balloon deflated is positioned onto the dilator so that its tip is

Table 1: Size of dilator to achieve over inflation according to size of tracheostomy tube

Inner diameter of tube (mm)	6	7	8	9	9.3
Appropriate dilator for initial over-dilatation (Fr)	24	28	32	36	38

approximately 2 cm from the distal tip of the dilator. This system is now advanced over the guiding catheter assembly to the safety ridge and then further advanced, again as a unit, into the trachea. As soon as the deflated balloon enters the trachea, the blue dilator, guiding catheter and the guide wire are removed. For inserting dual cannula tracheostomy tube, the inner cannula is removed prior to insertion and then the procedure is carried out as above. The tracheostomy tube is advanced to its flange. If using a dual cannula tube, the inner cannula is inserted at this point. Now the tube is connected to the ventilator, the balloon cuff inflated and the translaryngeal tube is removed after confirming ventilation through the newly inserted tube. The AM has a look down the trachea through the tracheostomy tube using the bronchoscope, looking for areas of injury if any to the posterior tracheal wall and suctioning out any blood.

The tracheostomy tube is fixed with sutures and/or tapes and a proper dressing is placed at the skin wound site. The patient is relieved of the neck extension and the head end of the bed is elevated to 30–40 degrees for an hour. A post-procedure chest radiograph is needed to confirm the correct placement of the tube and to rule out complications like a pneumothorax. The pre-procedure ventilator settings are dialled in and the patient is administered analgesics as required.

COMPLICATIONS OF PDT[17]

Operator experience and the technique used affect the outcome of PDT. A learning curve exists for any of the techniques used in PDT. The present limited evidence suggests that PDT using the wire-guided serial dilatation is safe with a similar, or even lower, rate of complications (0–5%) as compared to SST. Deviation from the technique advised for the particular kit can lead to complications.

The incidence of most of the complications of PDT described below has been dramatically reduced, as supervision of the entire procedure by a fibreoptic bronchoscope has become routine. It has been reported that without a bronchoscope a potentially lethal initial needle puncture would have remained completely unnoticed.[19] Some reports state that endoscopy was performed only after a problem had occurred. Bronchoscopy then identified a tracheal tear or mucosal flap only after the PDT.

Life threatening injury to the posterior tracheal wall has not been reported since the regular use of bronchoscopy throughout PDT procedure. Bronchoscopy prolongs the procedure time minimally and needs expertise especially when used without a videoscope but is strongly advocated. Temporary loss of minute ventilation due to bronchoscopy and the creation of the stoma itself is usually not a great problem.

Erythema at the PDT site occurs in approximately 50% of cases. This is a cutaneous reaction to dilation and pressure of the tracheostomy tube and does not need antibiotics. Wound infection needing antibiotic treatment occurs in 0–3% cases. Sticking to a sterile procedure technique is the best prevention for wound infection. There is no place for prophylactic antibiotics except in patients with a high risk for endocarditis. Bacteraemia does occur post-procedure, but clinically evident sepsis is very rare.[20]

Minor haemorrhage or ooze is also one of the commonest complications of a PDT, occurs in 0–3% of cases. It usually stops with pressure and the tamponading effect of the firmly fitting serial dilator or the tracheostomy tube itself.[12]

Peri-procedure oozing can be tackled with local injections of lignocaine and adrenaline. If bleeding has occurred during the procedure, the tube should be changed the first time no earlier than 5–7 days after the PDT is performed. Minor bleeding occurring during changes of the tube also responds to local pressure.

Major haemorrhage rarely occurs during PDT. It can be due to improper patient selection or injury to blood vessels like the innominate artery, though fatal injury to a large artery is extremely rare. A low placed PDT increases the risk of major bleeding due to vessel erosion. The tip of an incorrectly fitting tube can cause pressure necrosis of the anterior tracheal wall and lead to bleeding.

The incidence of improper placement of the needle and the tracheostomy tube itself have now been greatly reduced with the routine use of bronchoscopic guidance during PDT. An experienced bronchoscopist avoid accidental extubation and damage to the tip of the bronchoscope during PDT. The incidence of an initial paramedian placement of the introducer needle is about 18% (especially in the obese) and this can be quickly corrected under visualisation through the bronchoscope. Perforation of the translaryngeal tube, passage of the introducer needle through the Murphy's eye, paratracheal tube placement and oesophageal perforation have all been minimised due to the use of bronchoscopy during PDT.[12,21,22] Without the use of fibreoptic bronchoscopy the incidence of paratracheal insertion of the tracheostomy tube is 0–6%. Paratracheal tube placement can be due to kinking of the guide wire anterior to a calcified tracheal cartilage. The stiffer guide wire now available within the kits aims to prevent this.

Mucosal obstruction of the tip of the tracheostomy tube can occur when the bronchoscope is not used.[23–25] The tip of the tube could get blocked due to a tortuous trachea.

The incidence of both subcutaneous emphysema and pneumothorax during PDT is 0–4% without the use of a bronchoscope. PDT when directed through the first or second tracheal interspace should be relatively safe. The lower the tube inserted within the neck, the higher the risk. Tension pneumothorax after PDT at the suprasternal notch has been reported.[26] Subcutaneous emphysema and pneumomediastinum can also occur due to dissection of the paratracheal soft tissue through stoma by the pressurised air from the ventilator. A tight seal around the PDT might prevent this.

Cardiac dysrhythmias occur during the procedure in 0.3% cases; these are mainly due to the underlying physical condition of the patient or due to the use of an anaesthetic agent.

Procedure failure needing SST occurs in 1% of all the attempts at performing a PDT. In the meta-analysis by Moe et al.[18] this was either due to failure of the dilating instrument to reach the trachea in oedematous necks, inexperienced operator or calcified tracheal cartilages hindering the path of the dilator.

Accidental decannulation of the tracheostomy tube can occur in 0–2% of cases. Three to 12 month follow-up tracheoscopies reveal minor changes like swelling or scar. Stomal granulations occur in a minor percentage of all patients undergoing PDTs. Patients present with cough to the follow-up clinics. These can be treated with local silver nitrate solution or microlaryngoscopical laser therapy.

Tracheal stenosis is a late complication of tracheostomy. The incidence quoted in various studies ranges from 3.7 to 18%, depending on the length of the follow-up.[14,26–28] Tracheomalacia after PDT has not been reported, perhaps due to the inadequate time periods for the follow-up.

Tracheal ring fracture, necrosis and deep mucosal ulcerations are highly common with PDT without bronchoscopic guidance.[29] The confounding factors are the translaryngeal tube itself and proper management of the tracheostomy. Regular cuff pressure monitoring and cuff deflation as soon as the patient is ready for it might help to prevent some of the damage.

After decannulation the stoma usually closes spontaneously within 3 to 9 days. An epithelialised channel can persist in patients who have had the tracheostomy for long periods. Long-term placement of a tracheostomy tube increases the risk of development of a tracheo-cutaneous fistula after tube removal.

In these cases a surgical review may be required for formal closure. Unsightly scars are a problem for only a small proportion of patients.

The overall mortality from PDT is about 0.4%. Meta-analysis reported fatalities were due to paratracheal insertion of the tracheostomy tube, accidental decannulation due to use of a short tube in a patient with an obese neck, an inability to maintain airway pressures during dilatation of stoma in a patient with adult respiratory distress syndrome and cardiac dysrhythmia (unrelated to the procedure).[19]

Conclusion

A tracheostomy is one of the commonest procedures carried out on the critically ill patient. If a prolonged stay on the ventilator is anticipated, there is a great benefit in converting a translaryngeal tube to a tracheostomy. There is enough evidence in literature to support the safe routine ICU use of PDT under the guidance of a fibreoptic bronchoscope in carefully selected patients. A learning curve exists and complications are rare in experienced hands. The complications of a PDT are comparable to, if not superior to, those of a SST. Thorough training under supervision is the key to performing PDT with the least possible complications.

REFERENCES

1. Shelden CH, Pudenz RH, Freshwater DB, et al. New method for tracheotomy. *J Neurosurg* 1955; 12: 428–431.
2. Toy FJ, Weinstein JD. A percutaneous tracheostomy device. *Surgery* 1969; 65: 384–389.
3. Ciaglia P, Firsching R, Syniec C. Elective percutaneous dilatational tracheostomy. A new simple bedside procedure; preliminary report. *Chest* 1985; 87: 715–719.
4. Schachner A, Ovil Y, Sidi J, et al. Percutaneous tracheostomy: A new method. *Crit Care Med* 1989; 17: 1052–1056.
5. Griggs WM, Worthley LIG, Gilligan JE, et al. A simple percutaneous tracheostomy technique. *Surg Gynecol Obstet* 1990; 170: 543–545.
6. Susanto I. Percutaneous tracheostomy in the ICU. Chest-PCCU; Lesson 22/ Volume 13.
7. Smith I, Fleming S, Cernaianu A. Mishaps during transport from the intensive care unit. *Crit Care Med* 1990; 18: 278–281.
8. Hill BB, Zweng TN, Maley RH, et al. Percutaneous dilational tracheostomy: Report of 356 cases. *J Trauma* 1996; 41: 238–244.
9. Cobean R, Beals M, Moss C, et al. Percutaneous dilational tracheostomy. *Arch Surg* 1996; 131: 265–271.
10. Fernandez L, Norwood S, Roettger R, et al. Bedside percutaneous tracheostomy with bronchoscopic guidance in critically ill patients. *Arch Surg* 1996; 131: 129–132.

11. Barba CA, Angood PB, Kauder DR, et al. Bronchoscopic guidance makes percutaneous tracheostomy a safe, cost-effective, and easy-to-teach procedure. *Surgery* 1995; 118: 879–883.

12. Friedman Y, Fildes J, Mizock B, et al. Comparison of percutaneous and surgical tracheostomies. *Chest* 1996; 110: 480–485.

13. Friedman Y. Indications, timing, techniques, and complications of tracheostomy in the critically ill patient. *Curr Opin Crit Care* 1996; 2: 47–53.

14. Hazard P, Jones C, Benitone J. Comparative clinical trial of standard operative tracheostomy with percutaneous tracheostomy. *Crit Care Med* 1991; 19: 1018–1024.

15. Fischler MP, Kuhn M, Cantieni R, et al. Late outcome of percutaneous dilational tracheostomy in intensive care patients. *Inten Care Med* 1995; 21: 475–481.

16. Ciaglia P. Tracheostomy: *Instructions for Use.* Europe: William Cook.

17. Ciaglia P, Graniero K. Percutaneous dilatational tracheostomy. Results and long term follow-up. *Chest* 1992; 101: 464–467.

18. Moe K, Stoeckli S, Schmid S, Weymuller E. Percutaneous tracheostomy: A comprehensive evaluation. *Annals of Oto Rhino Laryngo* 1999; 108: 384–391.

19. Winkler W-B, Karnik R, Seelman O, Havlicek J, Slany J. Bedside percutaneous tracheostomy with endoscopic guidance: Experience with 71 ICU patients. *Intensive Care Med* 1994; 20: 476–479.

20. Teoh N, Parr MJA, Finfer SR. Bacteraemia following percutaneous dilational tracheostomy. *Anaesth Inten Care* 1997; 25: 354–357.

21. Masterson GR, Smurthwaite GJ. A complication of percutaneous tracheostomy. *Anaesthesia* 1994; 49: 452–453.

22. Hill SA. An unusual complication of percutaneous tracheostomy. *Anaesthesia* 1995; 50: 469–470.

23. Sun KO. Obstruction of tracheostomy tube by tracheal wall after percutaneous tracheostomy. *Anaesthesia* 1996; 51: 288.

24. Rigg CD. Percutaneous dilational tracheostomy: Malposition leading to delayed weaning. *Anaesthesia* 1995; 50: 724–725.

25. Sakabu SA, Levine JH, Trottier SJ, et al. Airway obstruction with percutaneous tracheostomy [letter]. *Chest* 1997; 111: 1468.

26. Marx WH, Ciaglia P, Graniero KD. Some important details in the technique of percutaneous dilatational tracheostomy via the modified Seldinger technique. *Chest* 1996; 110: 762–766.

27. Law RC, Carney AS, Manara AR. Long-term outcome after percutaneous dilational tracheostomy: Endoscopic and spirometric findings. *Anaesthesia* 1997; 52: 51–56.

28. Friedman Y, Mayer AD. Bedside percutaneous tracheostomy in critically ill patients. *Chest* 1993; 104: 532–535.

29. van Heurn LWE, Theunissen PHMH, Ramsay G, et al. Pathologic changes of the trachea after percutaneous dilatational tracheotomy. *Chest* 1996; 109: 1466–1469.

DIFFICULT AIRWAY

Rakesh Tandon

INTRODUCTION

In this day and age of advanced technology we still face a problem in anaesthesia – maintaining patent airway and placing a tracheal tube. Expertise in airway management is important in every medical specialty. Maintaining a patent airway is a vital aspect of providing adequate oxygenation and ventilation. Failure to do so for even a brief period can be disastrous. Difficult airway has major implications on morbidity and mortality as evidenced in various studies. The data from the American Closed Claim Study showed that difficult intubation claims accounted for 17% of total adverse respiratory claims, out of which 75% of these were preventable and 85% resulted in brain death.[1] The approach should be to improve the situation by use of predictors of difficult airway and introducing safe and effective techniques to manage the difficult airway.

The American Society of Anesthesiologists (ASA) practice guidelines were drawn by a consensus group and ratified by the house of delegates of the ASA.[2] The guidelines consist of explanatory text, a list of airway techniques along with the algorithm. There is a list of airway devices but in alphabetical order, which is not very helpful, but there is also no evidence for their ranking. There are also Canadian group guidelines based on consensus. They have evaluated and ranked the airway techniques that differ from the ASA.[3]

Incidence
The incidence of difficulty in intubation is said to be between 1.2 and 2.5%, about 1 in 65 patients. Of these the problems are predictable in 90% of the patients. Incidence of failed intubation in a general population is 0.05%, about 1 in 2,230.[4]

DEFINITIONS

A simple definition of the difficult airway is the clinical situation in which a practitioner experiences difficulty with adequate maintenance and/or protection of the airway. The definition introduced by ASA Task Force[5] on management of the difficult airway is 'the clinical situation in which a conventionally trained anaesthesiologist experiences difficulty with mask ventilation, difficulty with tracheal intubation or both'.

- Difficult mask ventilation occurs when it is not possible either to ventilate or to maintain oxygen saturation over 90% with application of 100% inspired oxygen in a patient who has oxygen saturation above 90%.
- Failed intubation is defined as the inability to place an endotracheal tube.
- Difficult intubation as defined by ASA Task Force is 'intubation requiring more than three attempts at laryngoscopy or taking longer than 10 min'. This definition is inappropriate because the experienced anaesthetist may identify a difficult intubation at the first attempt or within 30 s. To overcome problems of optimal or best attempt it is important to include:

1. Two years full-time conventional training in anaesthesia (experience).
2. Use of optimal sniffing position. ('Sniffing the morning air' (Fig. 1)).
3. Application of optimal external laryngeal manipulation.
4. One change in length of blade.
5. One change in the type of blade.

The difficult intubation might be defined on the following basis:

- Time taken to achieve intubation.
- Number of attempts.

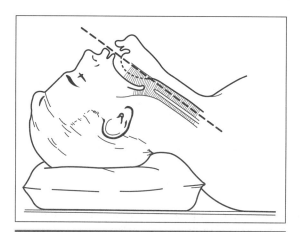

Fig. 1: The atlanto-occipital laryngeal axis (sniffing position).

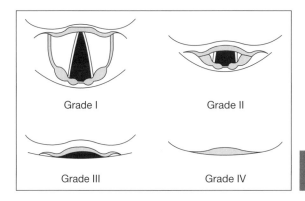

Fig. 2: Laryngoscopic grades.

- Change in the length and type of blade.
- View of the laryngeal structures seen at the laryngoscopy.
- Requirement for the airway equipment other than direct laryngoscopy to accomplish intubation.
- The prevalence of difficult direct laryngoscopy and difficult intubation will vary with the definition used. Difficult direct laryngoscopy means a Cormack and Lehane view of the larynx Grade III (epiglottis only) or Grade IV (no structure at all)[6] (Fig. 2).

PREDICTION OF DIFFICULT AIRWAY

Difficult or failed tracheal intubation is feared by all anaesthetists and this has resulted in many attempts to predict. Various methods of predicting airway difficulty have been studied but none of the tests performed singly or in combination, can achieve this ideally. Although the tests are not very sensitive they are essential to enable the anaesthetist to think about the airway and be prepared for the safe and effective management.[7]

The airway can be divided arbitrarily into three regions, i.e. the upper, middle and lower zones. These zones can be associated with difficult laryngoscopy, intubation and ventilation, respectively. Any of these three categories can cause a difficulty and the worse scenario is when there are problems with them all.

At the pre-operative visit, it is important to take full history, perform a general examination and specific airway assessment. The patient may volunteer information regarding previous difficulties with anaesthesia and these should be discussed in detail. Furthermore, the patient may produce a letter from a colleague highlighting the difficulty or carry a bracelet warning of the problem. Further details may be available from a NHS Website (supported by the Difficult Airway Society) held at St George's Hospital, London. This holds a register of airway difficulties that have occurred in such patients (www.uk-anaesthesia.co.uk).

The general examination of the patient may help identify systemic diseases or pathology that may be associated with the difficult airway such as obesity, scleroderma, rheumatoid arthritis, acromegaly etc. Hypoxia, hypercarbia, hypertension, tachycardia, altered mental status may suggest airway obstruction. Pattern of breathing can differentiate site and extent of obstruction. Change in voice may suggest pathology at the level of the glottis.

Direct laryngoscopy and intubation with a standard Mackintosh blade requires oral cavity, pharynx and larynx in the same axis (Fig. 1). This can be achieved when the patient is in supine sniffing position with neck slightly flexed and extension at atlanto-occipital joint, with adequate mouth opening and normal upper airway. These can be achieved when there is:

- Normal flexion.
- Normal extension of the atlas on the occiput.
- Normal temporal mandibular joint (TMJ).
- Normal forward movement of mandible and tongue.
- Normal upper airway anatomy.

Clinical examination and assessment of the airway is very important. Its purpose is to assess laryngoscopic access and ease of subsequent manoeuvres. Any gross abnormality of the face, mouth, nose and neck should be immediately apparent. The mouth, when open fully, should allow access to the patient's middle three fingers when held in the vertical plane. This distance varies from 4–6 cm and gives an indication of temporal mandibular joint mobility.

The normal anatomy of the oral cavity and pharynx should be examined with mouth open wide. This is Mallampati or Samsoon and Young modification test. The test determines the relative size of the tongue in relation to the size of the oral cavity. It is described as three classes and a fourth one is added by Samsoon and Young. High scores are caused mainly due to a large tongue or difficulty in opening mouth or extending head.

Inspection of the patient's open mouth
Inspection of the patient's mouth is done with the patient sitting upright with mouth widely open and the tongue fully extruded.

Classification of what is visible is described by Mallampati[8] (1985) (Fig. 3):

- Class I – soft palate, anterior and posterior faucial pillars and uvula.
- Class II – faucial pillars, soft palate and uvula.
- Class III – soft palate and base of uvula.

A further group was added by Samsoon and Young.[9]

- Class IV – soft palate not visible.

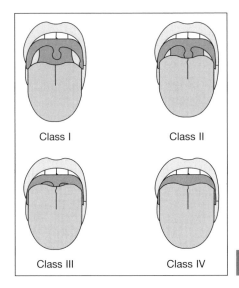

Class I

Class II

Class III

Class IV

Fig. 3: Mallampati classifications.

Thyromental distance is the distance between the tip of mandible and the anterior aspect of the thyroid cartilage which is normally 6.5 cm. A distance less than 6 cm may be associated with difficult intubation.[10]

The Sternomental distance between the tip of the mandible and sternal notch is normally 12.5 cm. Distance less than 12 cm may be associated with difficult airway.[11]

Wilson risk sum is the scoring system devised by Wilson,[12] which incorporates most of these tests. Five predicting factors (weight, head and neck movement, jaw movement, receding mandible, buck teeth) are scored individually on a 3-point scale (0–2). A total score of 2 or more is associated with an increased incidence of difficult intubation.

Radiological imaging of the neck and head in the neutral position and with the head extended can be of great assistance, e.g. illustrating a bamboo spine or atlanto-occipital restriction. However, this investigation is often performed when a difficult laryngoscopy or intubation occurs 'out of the blue'. When laryngopharyngeal pathology is present, a CT-scan can be extremely useful in demonstrating tracheal deviation and obstruction. In addition, the distal extension of a tumour within the airway can be delineated.

DIFFICULT INTUBATION IN ITU

Critically ill patients, by nature, are at risk of complications during manipulation of the airway, and may have a higher incidence of adverse reactions to anaesthesia-inducing drugs and muscle relaxants along with difficult airway. In critically ill patients, emergency tracheal intubation is associated with a significant frequency of major complications.[13] The patients requiring intubation in ITU should undergo an airway evaluation prior to anaesthesia to predict the nature and extent of possible problems. Most patients admitted to intensive care require some form of respiratory support. This is usually because of hypoxaemia, ventilatory failure or both. These patients are different from the normal elective surgery patient who are ambulatory and their airway can be assessed. Moreover these patients are supine in position, which increases the oedema of the oro-pharynx or had few intubations, which can make the normal airway difficult. Hypotension or hypovolaemia may occur due to haemorrhage or third space fluid loss, relative due to compensation, which may be exposed when there is a loss of vascular tone. The rapid sequence induction is not always appropriate in critical care patients. They are often drowsy, acidotic, hypotensive and dehydrated. Even a small amount of peripheral vasodilatation (with propofol) may expose intravascular dehydration and send the blood pressure spiralling downwards.

Familiarity with a difficult airway algorithm and various alternate techniques for endotracheal intubation is a mandatory requirement for all practitioners involved in airway management, and should be incorporated in critical care curricula.

Potential problems during intubation
- Incorrect positioning of endotracheal tube
- Hypotension
- Reduced intrinsic sympathetic drive
- Reduced cardiac output
- Severe hypoxaemia
- Regurgitation and aspiration of gastric contents
- Arrhythmias
- Electrolyte disturbances, especially hyperkalaemia after suxamethonium
- Inadequate familiarity with difficult airway trolley and equipment
- Nursing staff not familiar with equipment and also not trained in difficult airway.

The causes of difficulty in intubation

These may be:
- congenital
- anatomical
- acquired

Congenital causes include conditions such as:

- Pierre Robin syndrome
- Cystic hygroma
- Treacher–Collins syndrome
- Gargoylism
- Achondroplasia
- Marfan's syndrome.

Anatomical

Numerous anatomical features have been identified and most of these can be assessed by observation while talking to the patient at the pre-operative visit.

These include:

- excessive weight
- short muscular neck and a full set of teeth
- protruding incisors
- long high arched palate with long narrow mouth
- receding mandible
- large swellings in the neck, mouth or upper chest
- decreased distance between the occiput and the spinous process of C.1
- increase in posterior depth of the mandible
- increase in alveolar – mental distance requiring wide opening of the mandible.

Acquired

A relevant clinical history and physical examination will highlight the need for further investigation.

- Acute swelling in the neck due to trauma or post-operative bleeding.
- Restricted jaw opening.

This may be due to:

- Trismus associated with infection
- Fibrosis following infection, injury or radical cancer surgery/radiotherapy involving parotid or region of TMJ
- Rheumatoid arthritis or osteoarthritis affecting TMJ
- Mandibular fractures
- Restricted neck movement.

This may be limitation of flexion of the neck or extension of the atlanto-occipital joint:

- osteoarthritis of cervical spine
- scarring of the neck
- fusion of the cervical spine
- ankylosing spondylitis
- neck instability
  - intubation may be difficult if flexion of the neck is contraindicated because of cervical spine injury or severe rheumatoid arthritis
- radiotherapy to mouth may cause a 'wooden like' floor of mouth preventing displacement of the tongue at laryngoscopy.

Strategy for management of difficult airway

After the evaluation of the patient it is important to have a strategy, or combination of plans for successful management of the airway. The strategy of an individual practitioner will be influenced by the evaluation of the airway, the personal skills of the anaesthetist, available equipment and their competency. The particular concerns are at initial airway instrumentation and later when the patient is re-intubated or extubated. Strategy should always have primary plan to safeguard oxygenation. This should be followed by the use of an appropriate airway device and technique to insert it. A back-up plan should be considered to maintain oxygenation. This could include the use of another device, another means or abandoning the procedure.

The failed intubation drill described by Tunstell (1976) is of value in the fully anaesthetised patient. This includes continued cricoid pressure, head down with left lateral position, giving oxygen via intermittent positive pressure ventilation and using other airway devices.

The primary aim should be to oxygenate and consider:

- Anaesthesia of airway/laryngeal reflexes
- Ventilation during the intubation
- Technique and device
- Discuss with the patient and control the distress
- Plan extubation

Extubation

Difficult airway management is not complete without careful extubation of the patient. Therefore extubation of a patient who has been difficult to intubate should be performed with great care. There is always a possibility that the patient may need re-intubation, if there is a problem with extubation, and this may prove difficult or impossible. The patient should always be wide-awake, co-operative and able to maintain their airway and ventilation before extubation is considered. If there are any doubts about the airway, the safest way to perform extubation is to insert a bougie or guide wire through the endotracheal tube and extubate the patient over this. The endotracheal tube may then be re-introduced over the bougie if the patient requires re-intubation. Some bougies are specially made for this (the Cook Critical Care endotracheal tube changer bougie) and have ports to insufflate oxygen through during the tube change.

DIFFICULT AIRWAY SCENARIOS

A. Anticipated difficult airway

This is a scenario where the airway is already recognised to be difficult. In such a situation the prime importance is to secure and guarantee a patent airway while the patient is still awake.[4] The reason for this is that patients will help maintain the natural airway along with oxygenation with protective reflex and neurological status could be monitored.

Awake flexible fibreoptic intubation is a commonly used method in difficult airway, but there are certain limitations that include:

- Unco-operative patient
- Patients with stridor, laryngeal or tracheal lesion
- Massive bleeding
- Maxillary or facial trauma

B. Anticipated difficult airway but awake intubation is contraindicated

This is a scenario, which includes paediatric airway and some unco-operative adults. Anaesthesia may be conducted as a usual method but tracheal intubation can be done with the help of airway devices laryngeal mask airway (LMA), intubating laryngeal mask airway (ILMA) or fibreoptic intubation.

C. Unanticipated difficult airway can't intubate can ventilate

The patient in this situation was normally assessed but difficulty in intubation was recognised only after muscle relaxant was given. Ventilation is normally possible with bag and mask with an option to use other airway adjuncts like gum elastic bougie, LMA, ILMA or fibreoptic intubation.

D. Unanticipated difficult airway can't intubate can't ventilate

This is a difficult situation where it is important to maintain the ventilation. The ASA algorithm recommends use of airway adjuncts like LMA and Combitube to maintain the ventilation. If the ventilation is possible then the options are based on the kind of muscle relaxant used, if short then wake up of the patient is a good choice which could be followed by awake fibreoptic intubation. If a long acting muscle relaxant has been used then use of LMA assisted fibreoptic intubation can be used. But an emergency jet ventilation kit should be available for transtracheal ventilation.

USE OF AIRWAY TECHNOLOGY FOR DIFFICULT AIRWAY

The technological advances in airway have assisted the anaesthetist when dealing with the difficult airway. In the last few years, a number of new airway devices have become available. In addition to these devices, modifications of well-known techniques have also been suggested.

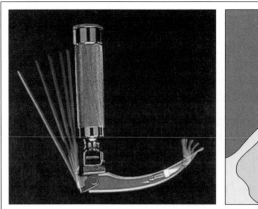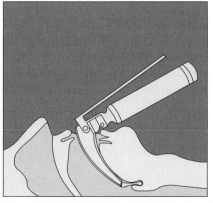

Fig. 4: McCoy laryngoscope.

The McCoy laryngoscope

Over the years many laryngoscopes have been developed in view to overcome problems of difficult airway. This McCoy laryngoscope appears to be the most popular and useful when dealing with difficult airway.[14] This device is a modified Mackintosh blade with a hinged distal tip (Fig. 4), activated by a lever attached to the laryngoscope handle. This improves the view at laryngoscopy significantly, particularly when the head is maintained in the neutral position, e.g. cervical spine pathology, and its role in dealing with the victims of trauma is now firmly established. McCoy laryngoscope is very useful especially for the Cormack and Lehane Grade 3 and 4 laryngoscopic views.[15] Furthermore it has some potential advantages as it requires reduced force to expose the laryngeal inlet and thus potential reduction in haemodynamic response to laryngoscopy, both of which may have further advantages when dealing with the head or cervical spine injury.

Cricoid pressure

The Sellicks manoeuvre described 40 years ago has been the mainstay for rapid sequence intubation and component of UK anaesthetic practice. Traditionally 44 N (Newton = Force) force has been applied but there is now good evidence that a force of 30 N is sufficient to prevent gastric regurgitation without causing any demonstrable airway obstruction particularly, since intragastric pressures rarely exceed 25 mmHg.[16] Two hands should be used (one supporting the posterior spine) if a cervical fracture is suspected. Nasogastric tubes should be left in situ as their presence improves the efficacy of cricoid pressure and simultaneously allows gastric 'venting'.

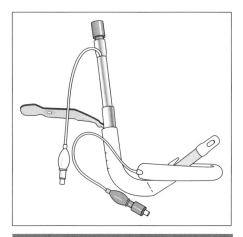

Fig. 5: The intubating laryngeal mask airway (ILMA).

The intubating laryngeal mask airway (ILMA)

The ILMA (Fig. 5) was introduced into clinical practice in 1997 following numerous clinical trials involving 1,110 patients.[17] The success rate of blind intubation via the device after two attempts is 88% in 'routine' cases. Successful intubation in a variety of difficult airway scenarios, including awake intubation, has been described, with the overall success rate in the 377 patients reported being approximately 98%.[18] The use of the ILMA by the novice operator has also been investigated with conflicting reports as to its suitability for emergency intubation in this setting.

The device is now established in UK anaesthetic practice and included in many published difficult airway algorithms around the world.[19–21] The development of ILMA is followed by the few reports the LMA being used as an intubating conduit. ILMA is a rigid metal tube with a guiding handle and is anatomically curved to fit the airway. A standard laryngeal mask head is attached distally and an epiglottic elevator bar replaces the grill seen with the standard LMA. It is available in sizes 3, 4 and 5 and comes with its own carefully designed 8 mm tracheal tube which is both flexible and has a uniquely shaped tip. To assist extubation of the LMA there is an introducer which fits on the tube.

The ILMA is easy to insert, more so than the LMA in inexperienced hands, and in particular, when the neck has to be maintained in the neutral position. There are numerous reports of the ILMA being used successfully in known difficult airway situations, both elective and unexpected. Of all the blind techniques for gaining entry into the trachea, the ILMA represents one of the least traumatic. The device has also been successfully used for awake intubation, both blindly and with the use of the fibrescope or illuminating stylet. The device represents a simple solution to gain access to the trachea when prediction of airway is difficult.[22]

Proseal laryngeal mask airway
Proseal LMA is the recent addition to the laryngeal mask devices. It is a modified, conventional LMA with an extra, independent lumen running from its tip in parallel with the standard airway lumen. In addition, there is a posterior cuff, which is inflated with the same pilot balloon as the conventional cuff. The advantages of the Proseal are its ability to independently 'vent' oesophageal contents and significantly improved airway sealing pressures. Recent work has shown that the device is easy to insert and that airway pressures of between 35–40 cmH$_2$O are common. A further advantage appears to be the ease with which a gastric tube can be passed whilst maintaining high pressure IPPV.

Combitube
The Combitube airway device is a double lumen tube available in two sizes 37 F and 41 F that is passed blindly into the mouth and oesophagus. It allows ventilation of the patient's lungs whether the tube enters the oesophagus or trachea. There are eight supraglottic 'tracheal' apertures and a single distal 'oesophageal' aperture. A large volume pharyngeal cuff (85–100 ml) and a small volume distal cuff (12–15 ml) are used to create seals so that the device may function correctly. Each cuff has an independent pilot balloon. The Combitube is positioned by opening the mouth and manually lifting the jaw. Pre-bending the device into a 'hockey stick' configuration aids placement. A laryngoscope is not necessary and, if correctly inserted, no fixation is required.[23]

Cuffed oropharyngeal airway (COPA)
This device is a modification of the Guedel oropharyngeal airway. It has a distal inflatable cuff and a proximal standard 15 mm connector. Four sizes are available (8, 9, 10, and 11) each colour coded and representing the length of the COPA in centimetres. The device has some distinct advantages as it could be used solo and in combination with fibreoptic intubation of trachea. IPPV using the COPA is possible with airway pressures up to 20 cmH$_2$O. The device can be used by non-anaesthetic staff in a resuscitation setting. It is similar to the Guedel airway with the ease in which it can be inserted (with apparently a minimal learning curve) this makes it an attractive addition to bag and mask ventilation in this group.[24]

Lighted stylets
The technique of the lightwand intubation evolved originally from the surgical usage. The principle of the technique is that a stylet with the distal light

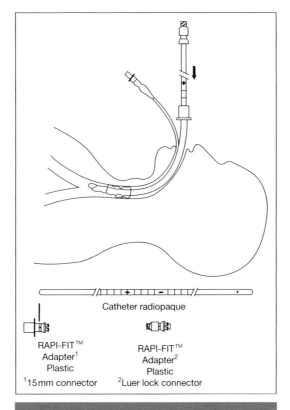

Catheter radiopaque

RAPI-FIT™
Adapter[1]
Plastic
[1]15mm connector

RAPI-FIT™
Adapter[2]
Plastic
[2]Luer lock connector

Fig. 6: Airway exchange catheters.

bulb is placed through a tracheal tube, bent into a suitable curve and placed blindly into the pharynx. If the device enters the oesophagus a poor, diffuse light source is seen.[25] However, upon entering the larynx, a distinct and clear source of light is identified transilluminating the cricothyroid membrane. The metal guide wire of the stylet is then withdrawn and the tracheal tube advanced blindly over the stylet into the trachea.[26] The Trachlight might be considered to be the modern lighted stylet, which is described, in an excellent review.

Airway exchange catheters
Airway exchange catheters are very much similar to intubating stylets; these are usually longer to allow exchange of the endotracheal tube while the catheter is still in the trachea (Fig. 6). These also come with central channel, which can be used for insufflation of oxygen. Some can be adapted to allow jet ventilation through the central channel. These could be used very easily in intensive care set-up, as it needs shorter learning time. Moreover allow

changing endotracheal tube with continued oxygenation in patients with a history of difficult intubation.

Fibreoptic intubation

The technique of fibreoptic intubation remains the main stay of management of difficult airway.[27,28] The anaesthetist who has mastered the technique of fibreoptic intubation oral or nasal will meet few airways, which cannot be managed. If there is a case of recognised airway difficulty for mask ventilation and intubation the airway patency should be secured and guaranteed while the patient remains awake. But fibreoptic intubation has limitations when there is massive bleeding, maxillary/mandibular fracture, glottic obstruction and unco-operative patient.

Summary

This chapter is devoted to management of the difficult airway and tries to give a modern perspective on some aspects of difficult airway. Preparation for patients with difficult airways includes gathering all of the equipment desired into a location that is easy to reach, such as in a difficult airway trolley. Preparation also includes practice since all of the devices designed to assist the practioner in intubating the trachea in patients with difficult airways require mastery of the associated technique to guarantee success. Adequate practice to allow mastery in non-emergency settings is essential. There will be patients in whom one technique may be more successful than another. Thus the practitioner must have more than one option available for managing the difficult airway.

Airway problems result in significant morbidity, mortality, and cost. By identifying which patient will have a difficult airway, having a well-thought-out management plan and disaster back-up plan, and by developing and improving our technical skills, we may improve the quality of care administered.

REFERENCES

1. Cheyney FW, Posner KL, Caplan RA. Adverse respiratory events infrequently leading to malpractice suits. A closed claims analysis. *Anaesthesiology* 1991; 75: 932–939.
2. http:www.asahq.org/practice/diff_airway/difficult.html.
3. Crosby ET, Cooper RM, Douglas MJ, Doyle DJ, Hung OR, Labrecque P, Muir H, Murphy MF, Preston RP, Rose DK, Roy L. The unanticipated difficult airway with recommendations for management (review). *Can J Anaesth* 1998; 45: 757–776.
4. Benumof JL. Management of the difficult airway: With special emphasis on awake tracheal intubation. *Anaesthesiology* 1991; 75: 1087–1110.

5. Caplan RA, et al. Practice guidelines for management of difficult airway. A report by the American society of Anaesthesiologist Task Force on the management of the difficult airway. *Anaesthesiology* 1993; 78: 597–602.

6. Cormack RS, Lehane J. Difficult tracheal intubation in obsterics. *Anaesthesia* 1984; 39: 1105–1111.

7. Yentis SM. Predicting difficult intubation-worthwhile exercise or pointless ritual. *Anaesthesia* 2002; 57: 105–109.

8. Mallampati SR, Gatt SP, Gugino LD, et al. A clinical sign to predict difficult tracheal intubation: Prospective study. *Can Anaesth Soc J* 1985; 32: 429–434.

9. Samsoon GLT, Young JRB. Difficult tracheal intubation: A retrospective study. *Anaesthesia* 1987; 42: 487–490.

10. Patil UV, Stehling LC, Zauder HL. Predicting the difficulty of tracheal intubation utilising an intubation guide. *Anesthesiol Rev* 1983; 10: 32.

11. Savva D. Prediction of difficult tracheal intubation. *Br J Anaesth* 1994; 73: 149.

12. Wilson ME. Predicting difficult intubation. *Br J Anaesth* 1993; 71: 333–334.

13. Schwartz DE, Wiener-Kronish JP. Management of the difficult airway. *Clin Chest Med* 1991 (Sep); 12(3): 483–495.

14. McCoy EP, Mirakhur RK. The levering laryngoscope. *Anaesthesia* 1993; 48: 516–519.

15. Gabbott DA. Laryngoscopy using the McCoy laryngoscope after application of a cervical collar. *Anaesthesia* 1996; 51: 812–814.

16. Vanner RG, Asai T. Safe use of cricoid pressure. *Anaesthesia* 1999; 54: 1–3.

17. Brain AI, Verghese C, Addey EV, Kapila A, Brimacombe J. The intubating laryngeal mask. II. A preliminary clinical report of a new means of intubating the trachea. *Br J Anaesth* 1997; 79: 704–709.

18. Baskett PJF, Parr MJ, Nolan JP. The intubating laryngeal mask. Results of a multicentre trial with experience of 500 cases. *Anaesthesia* 1998; 53: 1174–1179.

19. Benumof JL. Laryngeal mask airway and the ASA difficult airway algorithm (review). *Anaesthesiology* 1996; 84(3): 686–689.

20. Silk JM, Hill HM, Calder I. Difficult intubation and laryngeal mask. *Eur J Anesthesiol* 1991; (suppl 4): 47–51.

21. Frappier J, Guenoun T, Journois D, Philippe H, et al. Airway management using the intubating laryngeal mask airway for the morbidly obese patient. *Anesth Analg* 2003 (May); 96(5): 1510–1515.

22. Caponas G. Intubating laryngeal mask airway. *Anaesth Intens Care* 2002 (Oct); 30(5): 551–569.

23. Oczenski W, Krenn H, Dahaba AA, et al. Complications following the use of the Combitube, tracheal tube and laryngeal mask airway. *Anaesthesia* 1999; 54: 1161–1165.

24. Rees SGO, Gabbott DA. Use of the cuffed oropharyngeal airway for manual ventilation by non anaesthetists. *Anaesthesia* 1999; 54: 1089–1093.

25. Davis L, Cook-Sather SD, Schreiner MS. Lighted stylet tracheal intubation: A review. *Anesth Anal* 2000; 90(3): 745–756.

26. Hung OR, Pytka S, Morris I, Murphy M, Steward RD. Lightwand intubation in patients with difficult airway. *Can J Anaesthesia* 1995; 42(9): 826–830.

27. Taylor PA, Tower RM. The broncho-fiberscope as aid to endobroncheal intubation. *Br J Anaesth* 1972; 44: 611–612.
28. Conyers AB, Wallace DH, Muliders DS. Use of fibreoptic bronchoscope for nasotracheal intubation: A case report. *Can Anaesth Soc J* 1972; 19: 654–656.
29. Benumof JL. Management of the difficult airway: With especial emphasis on awake tracheal intubation. *Anaesthesiology* 1991; 75: 1087–1110.

TRACHEOSTOMY TUBES

Claudia Russell

INTRODUCTION

Increasingly tracheostomies are being used for the long-term management of a wide variety of conditions.

This chapter will discuss the components and functions of tracheostomy tubes currently available in the UK and offer information on how to select the most appropriate tube. This chapter will also identify the associated complications of the use of an inappropriate tube.

In order to select the correct tube for each patient it is important that the initial and ongoing indication for the tracheostomy is considered and understood. This will clarify the required clinical function which the tube will be expected to comply with.

Functions of a tracheostomy include:

- to allow prolonged positive pressure ventilation
- to protect from aspiration
- to bypass an upper airway obstruction
- to allow access to aspirate secretions

THE TRACHEOSTOMY TUBE

The ideal tracheostomy tube should be rigid enough to maintain an airway and yet flexible to limit tissue damage and maximise patient comfort.[1]

The tube shape is designed to allow correct entry angle into the trachea to facilitate ventilation and clearance of secretions (Fig. 1). A tracheostomy tube entering the trachea at an incorrect angle may endanger the positioning for safe ventilation via the tracheostomy. It may also cause irritation and trauma to the tracheal mucosa. The tracheostomy tube is arc shaped, which is referred to as the Jackson Curve.[1]

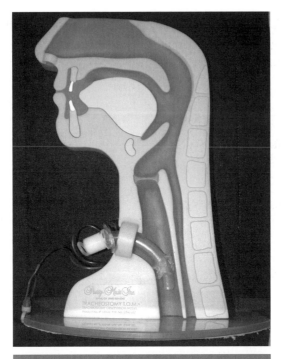

Fig. 1: Tracheostomy tube correctly positioned in model.

Tracheostomy tubes are available in a variety of lengths and diameters and available with attachments to meet the needs of each patient. The tube sizes are often defined according to the age group they serve, i.e. neonate, paediatric and adult. The varying styles of tubes to be discussed include: cuffed, uncuffed, fenestrated, variable length, single lumen and double lumen tubes. The chapter will also briefly discuss the specialist tubes available for the small minority of patients where a tube from the standard range is not suitable.

Parts of a tracheostomy tube

(See Figure 2: Fenestrated cuffed tube, Tracoe Twist, Kapitex)

1. *Outer cannula* – This is the main body of the tube which passes into the trachea. The stated size of the tube will often, but not always, refer to the inner diameter of this outer cannula.
2. *Inner cannula* – An inner cannula is a removable tube which passes into the outer cannula and can be removed/replaced to promote a clear airway.

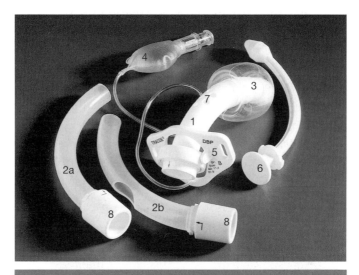

Fig. 2: Fenestrated cuffed tube (courtesy of Kapitex).

These are narrower and slightly longer than the outer cannula which prevents the build up of secretions at the end of the outer tube. They are secured in place by turning the hub until it is 'locked' in place or by pushing until a 'click' is felt.

Inner cannula are available in re-usable, disposable, plain (2a) and fenestrated (2b) styles. Fenestrated inner cannula are often coloured to ensure easy identification prior to suction or ventilation.

3. *Cuff* – A balloon at the distal end of the tube which, when inflated, can provide a seal between the tube and tracheal wall. The cuff can be deflated, as on insertion, or inflated to protect from aspiration and allow positive pressure ventilation.

4. *Pilot balloon* – An external balloon connected by an inflation line to the internal cuff. When the internal cuff is inflated the pilot balloon is also inflated, and vice versa.

5. *Flange/neck plate* – The neck plate supports the main tube structure, preventing it from descending into the trachea and allowing the tube to be secured with tapes/ties/sutures. The tube code, size or type is often demonstrated on the neck plate.

   Most neck plates in adult size tubes are a straight strip, however neonatal and some paediatric tubes have an angled neck plate to accommodate the shorter, developing neck.

   Other variations include adjustable flange tubes (Fig. 3) which allow variable tube lengths to be used. These may be useful for patients with larger necks or increased pre-tracheal space.

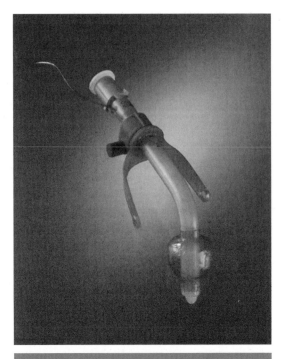

Fig. 3: Adjustable flanged tube (courtesy of Portex).

Certain tubes have a swivel neck plate which rotates on two planes and promotes easier dressing and wound care (see Figure 2).

6. *Introducer/obturator* – A bevel tipped shaft, which is placed inside the outer cannula of the tube during tube insertion. It provides a smooth rounded dilating tip, which will reduce the trauma of tube insertion. It is removed once the tube has been inserted to allow air entry and exit and assessment of correct tube placement. An introducer/obturator is supplied with the majority of adult tubes and some paediatric and neonatal tubes.

7. *Fenestrations* – Single or multiple holes are positioned on the superior curvature of the shaft.
Fenestrations permit airflow through these holes, which in addition to the air flow around the tube, allows the patient to speak and cough more effectively.

8. *15 mm adaptor* – In order to allow attachment to ventilation equipment, the majority of tracheostomy tubes used in the hospital setting will have a universally sized 15 mm hub to allow attachment to ventilators, re-breath bags, humidification circuits and closed circuit suction units. Whenever clinical stability allows, the patient may be changed to a tube with a flush finish to the neck shape to improve the cosmetic appearance of the tube.

TRACHEOSTOMY TUBE ACCESSORIES

Speaking valve

These are one-way valves which can be placed on the exposed (distal) end of the tracheostomy tube when the patient is clinically suitable to attempt phonation (speaking) trials. With the valve in place the patient will inhale through the tracheostomy and as they exhale, the valve is forced shut and air has to pass around the tube, passing through the vocal cords and then exiting through the nose and mouth. Medical agreement must be gained to support the suitability for cuff deflation and patency of the upper airway for speaking valve trials.

To allow successful use of the speaking valve the tube must be an appropriate size and type to allow adequate air passage through and/or around the tube.

Most speaking valves are used with patients who are self ventilating. Passy Muir has developed a range of speaking valves (see Figure 4), the aqua valve being suitable for use within the ventilator circuit with both adults and children.

Occlusion cap

This is a solid piece of plastic which is placed on the end of a 15 mm tracheostomy tube. It blocks all airflow via the tracheostomy and is used as a tool in the end stages of weaning a patient from their tracheostomy tube. It can be

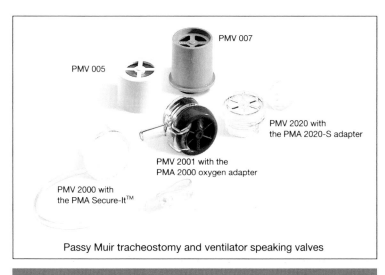

PMV 007

PMV 005

PMV 2020 with
the PMA 2020-S adapter

PMV 2001 with the
PMA 2000 oxygen adapter

PMV 2000 with
the PMA Secure-It™

Passy Muir tracheostomy and ventilator speaking valves

Fig. 4: Passy Muir valves (courtesy of Kapitex).

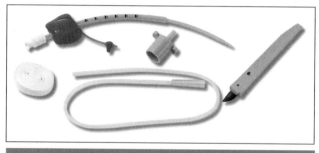

Fig. 5: Minitrach (courtesy of Portex).

easily removed if the patient needs suctioning or has become fatigued by the increased respiratory workload.

Disconnection wedge

This wedge facilitates the disconnection of a circuit, occlusion cap or speaking valve from the tracheostomy tube.

Minitracheostomy (Fig. 5)

This 16 Fg single lumen PVC tube is most commonly used to provide an airway in the emergency situation until the patient improves or a more permanent airway can be established. The tube is sometimes used at the end stages of weaning, although due to its longer length (92 mm) compared to a standard tracheostomy tube, patients can report irritation from the tube.

TUBE SELECTION

The properties of a tracheostomy tube are selected to best suit the individual patient's anatomy and clinical needs. The age, height and weight of the patient will give an indication of the size of a tracheostomy. The aim of the tracheostomy tube is to allow adequate airflow without causing complications associated with the placement of too large a tracheostomy tube.

It is recommended that the external diameter of the tracheostomy tube is no larger than two-thirds to three-quarters of the tracheal lumen.[1,2] This will reduce the contact on the tracheal walls which can cause damage from repeated shearing forces. Other criteria will include the depth of tissue between skin and trachea which affects the required length of the proximal aspect of the tube (neck plate to curve). A longer tube may be indicated for patients with an enlarged thyroid or in the obese. A tube that is too short or lies at the wrong angle will hold the risk of misplacement, a potentially fatal complication in the early stages following a tracheostomy.[1] In certain instances a longer tube length may be needed, e.g. tracheal malacia, stenosis or obesity in order to provide safe ventilation.[1]

TYPES OF TRACHEOSTOMY TUBE

Cuffed tube

The initial tube inserted at time of tracheostomy should be a cuffed tube. It provides a safe airway until a patient is weaned from the ventilator, the wound site has stabilised and the patient can control his/her own secretions.

The cuff or balloon at the distal end of the tube can be inflated or deflated depending on the patient's needs. Most modern tubes have a barrel shaped cuff which has a high volume with a low pressure. This allows a wider distribution of pressure on the tracheal wall and aims to reduce the incidence of tracheal ulceration, necrosis and/or stenosis at the cuff site. A complication of a cuffed tube is an impaired swallow action due to the anchorage on the larynx by the inflated cuff. This anchorage can inhibit laryngeal elevation which thus limits the protection of the tracheo bronchial tree from aspirated secretions. The majority of patients with an inflated cuff will be kept 'nil by mouth' (NBM) and alternative methods of feeding will need to be established. For more information (see Chapters 11 and 22, Swallowing and Nutritional Assessment and Management of Patients with Tracheostomies)

A cuff pressure manometer (Fig. 6) should be used to measure the cuff pressure being exerted on the tracheal wall. The recommended limits to minimise damage to the trachea are 15–25 cmH$_2$O (10–18 mmHg),[1] which is clearly indicated on the dial of the manometer.

Tracheal capillary pressure lies between 20 and 30 mmHg. It suffers impairment at 22 mmHg and total obstruction at 37 mmHg.[1] Complications of continued cuff over inflation (see Figure 7) include tracheal stenosis, tracheal malacia, and tracheosophageal or tracheoinominate fistula, desensitisation of the larynx and potential loss of the cough reflex.[1]

If a cuff pressure above the recommended limit is required for a patient in order to provide an adequate seal then a tube of a larger diameter may be indicated. This may necessitate a surgical revision of the tracheostomy to allow the atraumatic insertion of a larger tube.

There are variations within the range of cuffed tubes. For a patient with a high risk of aspiration a specialist tube may be required which offers additional protection.

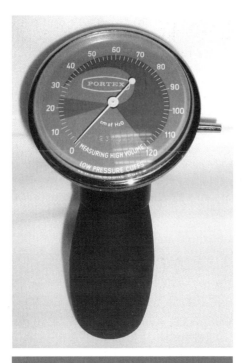

Fig. 6: Cuff pressure manometer.

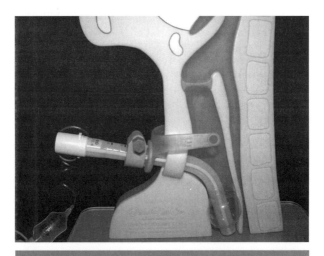

Fig. 7: Cuff over inflation demonstrated on model.

Table 1a: Indications for a cuffed tube

- Risk of aspiration
- Newly formed stoma (adult)
- Positive pressure ventilation
- Unstable condition

Table 1b: Contra-indications for a cuffed tube

- Child less than 12 years of age
- Significant risk of tracheal tissue damage from cuff

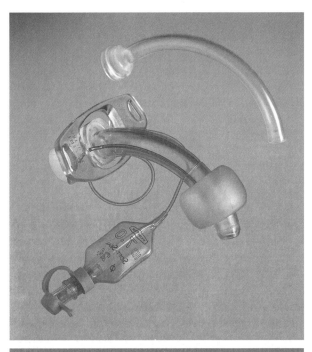

Fig. 8: Plain cuffed tube with inner tube (courtesy of Portex).

In the paediatric and neonatal patient, it is unusual to have a cuffed tube due to the risk of tracheal damage of the developing tracheal membranes.[3] Children under the age of 12 years have a narrow trachea particularly around the cricoid ring and therefore air leaks are minimal.[4] This enables an uncuffed

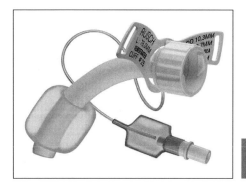

Fig. 9: Tracheofix (courtesy of Rüsch).

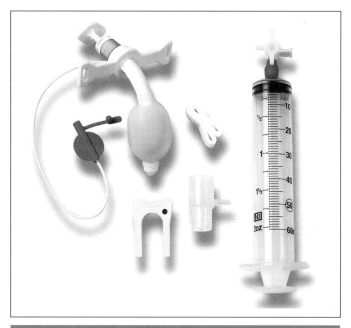

Fig. 10: Fome-Cuf (courtesy of Portex).

tube to be used effectively and a cuffed tube is seldom required (Table 1a, 1b).[5]

The majority of patients are managed with a 'standard' cuffed tube as shown in Figures 8 and 9. However there are occasions where a customised or specialised cuffed tube is necessary to maintain a safe airway. The following are a selection currently available in the UK.

Specialist cuffed tubes

Foam cuffs
A foam cuff spontaneously inflates on insertion and will then conform to the patients trachea, while remaining consistently inflated, therefore eliminating the risk of overinflation. Due to the spontaneous inflation of the cuff the use of a standard speaking valve or occlusion cap are contra-indicated. These tubes are available with a 'talk attachment'.

E.g. Fome-Cuf, Bivona (Fig. 10).

Tight to shaft cuff
Tight to shaft tubes have a cuff which when deflated has the profile of an uncuffed tube. This allows a less traumatic tube insertion and withdrawal compared to a standard cuffed tube.

E.g. TTS™, Bivona (Fig. 11).

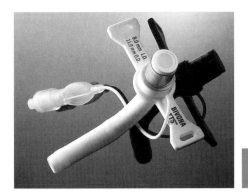

Fig. 11: Tight to shaft (courtesy of Portex).

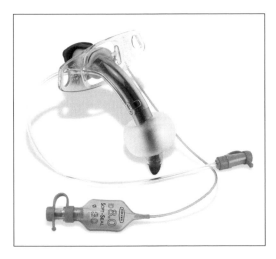

Fig. 12: Suctionaid (courtesy of Portex).

Suction ports

The cuff minimises but does not necessarily prevent aspiration.[1] The suction port above the cuff allows regular removal of secretions thereby reducing the risk of aspiration and also the associated infection risks.

E.g. Blueline Ultra Suctionaid™ Portex (Fig. 12).

Tracheosoft™ EVAC Mallinckrodt.

Double cuffs

Double cuffed tubes use the alternation of the cuff inflation to allow pressure relief on high risk tracheal mucosa, e.g. tracheomalacia.

E.g. Double cuff, Portex.

Lanz™ system

This cuff system automatically controls and limits cuff pressure for the entire duration of intubation.

E.g. Tracheosoft Lanz™, Mallinckrodt.

Cuffed talking tubes

Where a patient cannot tolerate the use of a speaking valve and/or cuff deflation alternative tubes may be used. These tubes have an additional airflow line attached to the outer cannula. It will deliver air from an external source above the cuff which can then pass through the vocal cords to potentially allow phonation.

E.g. Fome-Cuf® tracheostomy tube with talk attachment Bivona, Aire-Cuf® tracheostomy tube with talk attachment Bivona, Vocalaid Portex (Fig. 13) and TracheoSoft Pitt™ Mallinckrodt.

Uncuffed tubes

Indications for an uncuffed tube

An uncuffed or cuffless tube refers to a tube which does not have a cuff at the distal end of the tube (Figs 14–16). This type of tube is useful when the patient no longer needs positive pressure ventilation and has no significant aspiration risk and has tolerated the cuff being deflated continually. The tracheostomy is still required for access to chest secretions or to bypass an upper airway obstruction. These tubes can be recognised by the absence of a pilot balloon (Table 2a, 2b).

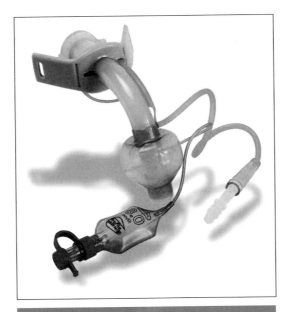

Fig. 13: Vocalaid (courtesy of Portex).

Uncuffed tubes are available in most adult (Figs 14–16), paediatric (Figs 17, 18) and neonatal tubes (Fig. 19). Uncuffed tubes offer a variety of specifications: plain, fenestrated, with speaking valves attached and with or without a 15 mm hub.

Fenestrated tubes

Fenestrated tubes have a single or multiple holes on the outer curvature of the tube. If the tube has an inner cannula then the tube will be supplied with a plain and a fenestrated inner cannula.

Fenestrated tubes are available with or without a cuff. Cuffed fenestrated tubes (Fig. 2) are particularly useful when a stable patient is weaning from the tracheostomy and requires both periods of cuff inflation and also cuff deflation and a speaking valve. Uncuffed fenestrated tubes are used for patients who are no longer dependent on a cuffed tube. A patient with a small trachea or marginal respiratory status may benefit from a fenestrated tube.[6] The additional airflow through the fenestrations in the tube can

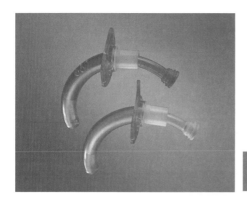

Fig. 14: Fenestrated uncuffed tube (courtesy of Portex).

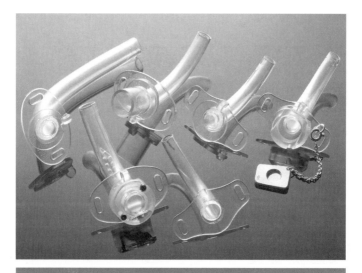

Fig. 15: Tracoecomfort range (courtesy of Kapitex).

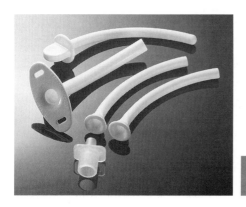

Fig. 16: Moores uncuffed tube (courtesy of Kapitex).

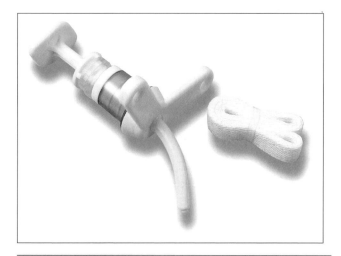

Fig. 17: Paediatric uncuffed tube (courtesy of Portex).

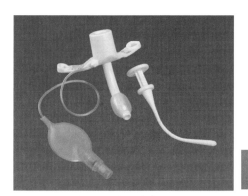

Fig. 18: Paediatric uncuffed tube (courtesy of Tyco Healthcare).

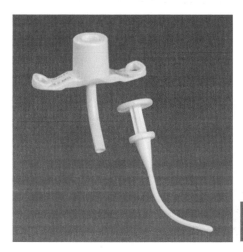

Fig. 19: Neonatal uncuffed tube (courtesy of Tyco Healthcare).

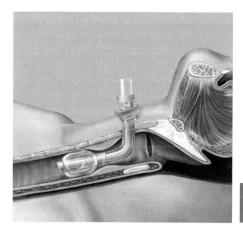

Fig. 20: XLT Distal (courtesy of Tyco Healthcare).

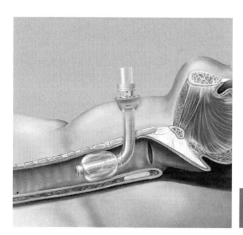

Fig. 21: XLT Proximal (courtesy of Tyco Healthcare).

Table 2a: Indications for an uncuffed tube

- Vocal cord palsy
- Head and neck tumour
- Respiratory insufficiency
- Neuromuscular disorders
- Paediatric or neonatal tracheostomy

Table 2b: Contra-indications for an uncuffed tube

- Dependent on positive pressure ventilation
- Significant risk of aspiration
- Newly formed tracheostomy

increase the tolerance of a speaking valve and/or occlusion cap thereby aiding weaning.

The accurate position and size of the holes will dictate the effectiveness of the tube for speech. It will also reduce the incidence of granulation tissue caused by the shearing of the holes at the anterior wall of the trachea.[7]

It is inadvisable to suction via a fenestrated single lumen tube as the suction catheter can pass through the fenestration and cause tracheal damage which will increase the risk of granulation tissue at the site of the fenestration. In a dual cannula system, the plain (unfenestrated) inner cannula should be inserted prior to suctioning to avoid this problem.

Fenestrated tubes are contra-indicated for use with patients requiring positive pressure ventilation as a significant air leakage through the outer cannula fenestrations may occur and compromise the effectiveness of the ventilation.

Extra long/adjustable flange

Standard tracheostomy tubes have a standard curve, referred to as the Jackson Curve. The standard tube lengths are 60–90 mm (adult), 39–45 mm (paediatric) and 30–36 mm (neo-natal). These tubes may not be safe for patients with an increased tracheocutaneous layer or an enlarged thyroid gland. For these patients, a standard length tube may not enter the trachea or enter at an angle which will make ventilation and clearance of secretions difficult. They may cause posterior wall erosion by resting on and/or shearing at the tracheal wall.[1]

The first known tube to offer greater flexibility for individual patients with a variety of depths and inclinations of the trachea was developed by Arthur Durham in 1872 and is known as the Durham 'lobster tail' tube.[8]

Adjustable flange tubes (Fig. 3 and 7) are often the first tube of choice for this group of patients in the intensive care setting and/or for short term use. These tubes are not recommended for home care as, due to the absence of a removable inner cannula, they are more prone to a build up of secretions which may lead to partial or complete tube occlusion.

In the home setting it is advisable to have a tube with an inner cannula system which can allow removal and cleaning of the inner cannula which facilitates a patent airway, e.g. Moores tube, Kapitex (Fig. 16) Tracoe XLT, Shiley (Figs 20, 21).

To ensure that the tube fits correctly several measurements may be required and also fibre optic nasoendoscopy and/or lateral neck radiograph to assess correct tube placement (Table 3).[1]

Table 3: Indications for an extra long tube

Increased distal length
- Tracheal obstruction, e.g. tumour growth
- Tracheomalacia
- Low level tracheal stenosis

Examples
- Moore, Boston Medical (uncuffed silastic tube which can be trimmed to fit an individual patient) (Fig. 16)
- Tracoe Comfort™ Extra Long, Bivona (an uncuffed tube range which can be plain or fenestrated)
- Traceosoft™ XLT Distal, cuffed, uncuffed (Fig. 20)

Increased proximal length
- Increased pre-tracheal space from obesity or oedema
- Enlarged thyroid
- Kyphoidosis[CLC]
- To allow easier wound care around stoma

Examples
- Traceosoft™ XLT/Shiley (Fig. 21)
- Adjustable flange tube, Portex (Fig. 3)

Adult single lumen tubes

A single lumen tube has only one cannula that stays in situ throughout its use. The alternative to this is a tube system that has an inner cannula. It is recommended that, where possible, all adult tubes have an inner cannula present. This system allows regular removal and cleaning (or replacing) of the inner cannula to prevent the build up of secretions. This reduces the risk of tube occlusion necessitating an urgent tube change and the risks associated to this.

Single lumen tubes made of silicone or a mixture of silicone and PVC have an increased resistance to secretions adhering to the tube (Figs 10, 11).

Double lumen tubes/inner cannula tube systems
(Figs 1, 2, 8, 9, 12, 14–16, 20–21)

The first inner cannula system was designed by Martin in 1730 who identified the discomfort and risk involved with regular tube removal for cleaning.[8] It is recommended that all patients, particularly on the general ward have a tube system with an inner cannula. However with the fast turn over of intensive care beds, the patient is often ready to leave intensive care before the first tube change. Considering this, it is advisable, unless contra-indicated, that a tube system with an inner cannula should be used from tracheostomy formation, so as to help prevent tube occlusion.

The use of an inner cannula will assist the cleaning of the tube, particularly if the patient has copious secretions. This reduces the risk of tube occlusion and the frequency of tube changes which causes the patient discomfort and trauma to the stoma site.

The presence of an inner cannula will reduce the lumen by approximately 1 to 1.5 mm. Patients with known respiratory pathology may not tolerate the increased respiratory effort and this should be considered when selecting a tube type for these patients.[9]

Neonatal and paediatric tubes

A tracheostomy tube for an infant or child must offer patency, flexibility and comfort. The appropriate size, shape of tube shaft and neck plate and the material it is made from needs to be considered while deciding which tube to use.

These ranges of tubes are from 2.5 to 5.5 mm in internal diameter and have lengths from 30–36 mm (neonates) and 39–56 mm (paediatrics). The age and weight will be a guide for the surgeon when choosing the size of tube (Table 4). As the child grows and develops their respiratory requirements will also grow. The ENT surgeon will follow these children and if the child still requires a tracheostomy, they will determine whether an increase in tube size may be indicated. The recommendations, as for the adult tracheostomy is to have the outer diameter of the tube no larger than two-thirds the diameter of the trachea. A smaller tube may not offer sufficient airflow and a larger tube may cause granulation tissue and limit the success of speech development.

Table 4: Tracheostomy tube sizes according to age and tracheal transverse diameter[11]

Age	Trachea (transverse diameter, mm)	Inner diameter tracheostomy tube, mm
Pre-term–1 month	5	2.5–3.0
1–6 months	5–6	3.5
6–18 months	6–7	4.0
18 months–3 years	7–8	4.5
3–6 years	8–9	5.0
6–9 years	9–10	5.5
9–12 years	10–13	6.0
12–14 years	13	7.0

Due to the small size of the tracheostomy tube lumen a paediatric tube (Figs 17–18) and neo-natal tube (Fig. 19) will not have an inner cannula. To avoid a build up of secretions causing respiratory difficulties, the tube should be changed every week.[1] To help prevent the build up of secretions, a silicone tube (Fig. 17) is recommended as it allows mucus to pass more effectively through the tube and reduce the adherence of secretions and bacteria to the tube surface.[1] Silicone is an inert material which reduces the likelihood of skin irritation, it offers greater comfort and due to its non-adherent surface, allows easier removal.

The ideal length of a paediatric tube is recommended to be 1 cm above the carina, this position can be checked using a small diameter paediatric flexible endoscope.[10]

Due to the delicate developing tracheal tissue and the narrow cricoid ring a cuffed tube (Fig. 18) is not recommended and seldom necessary.

WHAT ARE TUBES MADE OF?

The development of medical grade plastics and silicones has allowed a wider range of functions for tracheostomy tubes in line with medical advances. This together with increased knowledge, has led to a decrease in tracheostomy related complications.

The various materials used to manufacture tracheostomy tubes include silver, plastics, polyurethane and silicone. The materials most commonly used today are the light weight medical grade plastics as they can offer greater comfort, variation of styles and functions. They are also more cost effective for short-term use.

Choice of material for the tracheostomy tube

Selecting the most appropriate tube for each patient will include consideration of the tube material. This will contribute to both the effectiveness and comfort of the tube. The tube is required to be rigid yet flexible so as to provide adequate respiratory support, while also being a comfortable tube for the patient. It should be checked whether each patient has a known allergy to any of the products used to make the tube.

Polyvinylchloride (PVC)

This medical grade plastic is the most cost effective material for the short-term tube and is used on the widest range of products. This material allows the tube to be flexible yet maintains its shape. It is also thermosensitive to adjust to body temperature.[12] It is more prone to the retention of bacteria and is therefore disposable/single use.

Silicone

Silicone is a soft material with the unique characteristic of reducing the adherence of secretions and bacteria to the tube by promoting the easier passage of mucus.[1]

Although single patient use it can be sterilised and therefore cost effective in long-term use.[13]

E.g. Bivona range (Figs 10, 11, 17).

Siliconised polyvinylchloride (PVC)

PVC is a thermosensitive material with sufficient rigidity for effective intubation which also can conform to the individual patient's upper respiratory tract at body temperature thereby promoting patient comfort.

E.g. Portex Blueline Ultra (Figs 8, 14).

Silver

Silver tubes are usually made from 92.8% silver, copper and phosphorus (trace) with silver plating.[14] This mix is required to strengthen the tube although a pure silver tube would be less liable to the chemical erosion to which various alloys appear prone.[14] A review of the literature includes the comment that silver tubes can fracture with prolonged use. Recommendations are that the tube should be replaced after 5 years.[13]

E.g. Negus, Chevalier Jackson and Alderhey.

Silastic

Silastic is a medical grade silicone rubber which can offer comfort and flexibility but may lack sufficient rigidity for particular clinical requirements.

E.g. Kapitex, Moores (Fig. 16).

Armoured tubes

These tubes have embedded within the main shaft of the tube, a spiral or rings of stainless steel which assists in keeping the shape of the tube. This prevents kinking or compression of the tube.

E.g. Rusch, Tracheoflex (Fig. 22)

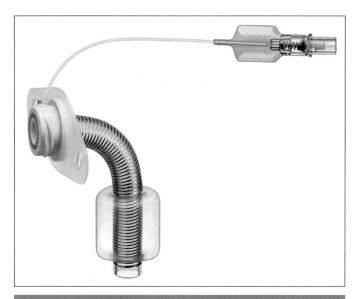

Fig. 22: Tracheoflex armoured tube (courtesy of Rüsch).

COMPLICATIONS OF A TRACHEOSTOMY TUBE

The aim of a tracheostomy is to provide the necessary clinical function with the minimal risk of complications to the patient due to the tracheostomy and/or tube. The meticulous care and close monitoring of these patients should identify early signs of complications arising from the tracheostomy and/or the tube.

Regardless of the clinical requirements of the tracheostomy, the body often treats the tube as a foreign body. This can lead to adverse effects (Tables 5a, 5b, 6, 7) which can often be related to the material and manufacturing process.[14]

Choosing the right tube

The width of the tube should be guided by the height, age and weight of the patient and in particular the diameter of the patient's trachea. The tube is recommended to be no larger than two-thirds the diameter of the trachea. This will allow adequate ventilation and minimise tissue abrasion from the shearing effect of the tube.

The initial tube size is likely to be determined in theatre or in the intensive care unit by the clinician performing the tracheostomy. The correct placement of the tube can be confirmed with a chest X-ray. This should be between 6–20 mm above the carina to prevent mucosal damage and coughing.[1]

Table 5a: Complications of a tracheostomy tube

- Tracheal ulceration and necrosis
- Tracheal stenosis (narrowing)
- Tracheo-oesophageal fistula
- Tracheo-onimate artery fistula and haemorrhage
- Stoma ulceration and breakdown
- Overgranulation tissue
- Tracheal irritation and coughing
- Discomfort
- Cosmetic appearance

Table 5b: Complications caused by tube length

Too long
- Trauma caused by the tube tip or suction catheter catching the carina
- Collapsed lung due to unilateral ventilation caused by tracheostomy tube entering bronchi
- Patient discomfort
- Convulsive or excessive coughing due to irritation of the carina

Too short
- Tube displacement, loss of tracheostomy tract, respiratory arrest and/or death
- Tube displacement causing ventilation into pre-tracheal space leading to surgical emphysema
- Ulceration and/or erosion of the posterior tracheal wall, from poorly positioned tube within trachea
- Ineffective ventilation from a poorly positioned/angled tube within the trachea

The correct length of tube will ensure safe entry into the trachea and will reduce the risk of tube misplacement with patient movement.

Selecting a tracheostomy tube

When selecting tubes it is important to evaluate the effectiveness of the current tube and its suitability for its required use.

Some of the questions worth asking to assist the selection of the most appropriate tube include:

- Does the current tube support sufficient ventilation and clearance of secretions?

Table 6: Complications caused by tube width

Too wide
- Tracheal ulceration
- Tracheal necrosis
- Granulation tissue caused by the shearing effect of the tube against the tracheal wall
- Discomfort
- Difficulty in swallowing
- Inability to tolerate speaking valve
- Stoma site stenosis
- Difficult tube changes
- Subcutaneous emphysema (a collection of air caused by shearing and tearing of the tracheal wall)
- Tracheosophageal fistula caused by the tube and/or cuff pressing against the posterior wall of the trachea

Too narrow
- Inadequate ventilation
- Increased respiratory effort
- Ventilator indicates leakage via nose and mouth
- Ineffective clearance of secretions
- Increased risk of aspiration from an inadequately sized tube and cuff (while maintaining recommended cuff pressures)

Table 7: Complications from cuffs

Over inflated cuff (Fig. 7)
- Tracheal mucosa ischaemia causing ulceration and erosion
- Tracheoesophageal fistula, caused by cuff pressing the posterior tracheal wall
- Tracheoinnominate fistulae, necrosis of the tracheal mucosa and artery wall, this can lead to a potentially fatal bleed
- Laryngotracheal stenosis
- Difficulty in swallowing

Under inflated cuff
- Insufficient seal for ventilation
- Aspiration of saliva and gastric contents into the tracheo-bronchial tree

- Has the initial indication for the tracheostomy changed or been resolved?
- Does the tube size allow for weaning trials/speaking valve use?
- Have there been incidences of difficulty in suctioning below the level of the tube and/or breathing difficulties?
- Does the patient still require a tube with a 15 mm connector?
- Has the patient complained of discomfort from the tube?
- Is the patient concerned about the appearance of the tracheostomy tube?
- What tube range is available and are the carers are familiar with it?
- Which tube style is most suitable for the patient to care for?
- Does the tube range have the necessary accessories/adaptations?
- Which is the most cost effective tube type and material for the patient?

Once these questions have been asked the team can refer to the available tube ranges from various manufacturers. If the current tube does not fulfil the clinical needs or potential for rehabilitation a change in size or type may be indicated.

When changing tube manufacturer or style, you must compare and match the outer diameter measurements to allow the tube to be passed with minimal trauma. The size of a tracheostomy tube will often refer to its inner diameter and so depending on the presence of an inner cannula and the thickness of the tube wall, the outer diameter measurements will differ.

Tables 8–13 indicate the dimensions and availability of some of the tube styles from the manufacturers of tracheostomy tubes currently available in the UK.

Summary

Today's healthcare offers an ever improving range of treatment options supported by medical, surgical, pharmacological and technological advances. Tracheostomies are increasingly utilised in support of this ever increasing range of treatments for all age groups. There have been many different types of tracheostomy tubes developed to best meet the diverse needs of these patient groups. However, the balance between survival and quality of life must be carefully considered and an individualised treatment plan will aim to facilitate and balance patient survival with their quality of life.

The aim is to provide the most appropriate tracheostomy tube to offer flexibility and comfort by providing a safe airway and facilitating rehabilitation while reducing the incidence of tracheostomy related complication.

REFERENCES

1. Myers E, Johnson J, Murry T. *Tracheotomy: Airway management, communication and swallowing.* San Diego: Singular, 1998.

2. Dikeman KJ, Kazandjian MS. *Communication and Swallowing Management of Tracheostomised and Ventilator Dependent Adults.* San Diego: Singular, 1997.

3. Deutsch ES. Early tracheostomy tube change in children. *Arch Otolarygol Head Nec Surg* 1998; 124: 1237–1238.

4. St. George's Healthcare NHS Trust. *Guidelines for the Care of Patients with Tracheostomy Tubes.* London: St. George's NHS Trust, 2000.

5. Mallinckrodt Medical. *A Parents Guide to Pediatric Tracheostomy Home Care.* Mallinckrodt Medical, 1999.

6. Hussey JD, Bishop MJ. Pressures required to move gas through the native airway in the presence of a fenestrated vs. a nonfenestrated tracheostomy tube. *Chest* 1996; 110: 494–497.

7. Siddarth P, Mazzella L. Granuloma associated with fenestrated tracheostomy tubes. *Am J Surg* 1985; 150(2): 279–280.

8. Weir N. *Otolaryngology: An Illustrated History.* London: Butterworths, 1990.

9. Docherty B. Tracheostomy management for patients in general ward settings. *Prof Nurs* 2002; 18(2): 100–104.

10. Bleile KM. *The Care of Children with Long-term Tracheostomies.* San Diego: Singular, 1993.

11. Wyatt ME, Bailey CM, Whiteside JC. Update on paediatric tracheostomy tubes. *Laryngol Otol* 1999; 113: 35–40.

12. Tippett DC. *Tracheostomy and Ventilator Dependency.* New York; Thieme, 2000.

13. Okafor BC. Fracture of tracheostomy tubes: Pathogenesis and prevention. *Laryngol Otol* 1983; 97: 771–774.

14. Ayshford CA, Walsh RM, Proops DW. Corrosion of a silver Negus tracheostomy tube. *Laryngol Otol* 1999; 113: 68–69.

APPENDIX

Table 8: Adult tubes: Tracheostomy tubes with inner cannula

Shiley, Mallinckrodt	Size		4	6		8				10
	O.D. (mm)		9.4	10.8		12.2				13.8
	I.D. (mm)		5.0	6.4		7.6				8.9
	Length (mm)		65	76		81				81

Tracoe Twist, Kapitex	Size	4	5	6	7		8	9		10
	O.D. (mm)	7.2	8.6	9.2	10.4		11.4	12.5		13.8
	I.D. (mm)	4.0	5.0	6.0	7.0		8.0	9.0		10.0
	Length (mm)	56	66	72	74		76	78		80

Blueline Ultra, Portex	Size		6	7	7.5	8	8.5	9	10
	O.D. (mm)		9.2	10.5	11.3	11.9	12.6	13.3	14.0
	I.D. (mm)		5.0	5.5	6.0	6.5	7.0	7.5	8.5
	Length (mm)		64.5	70.0	73.0	75.5	78.0	81.0	87.5

Dimensions listed include outer diameter (O.D.), inner diameter of inner cannula (I.D.) and length (L) and are stated in mm.

Table 9: Adult tubes: Uncuffed tracheostomy tubes with inner cannula

Tracoe Comfort, Kapitex

Size	3	4	5	6	7	8	9	10
O.D. (mm)	6.4	7.3	8.7	10.0	10.5	11.3	12.6	13.7
I.D. (mm)								
Length (mm)	46	55	57	60	65	70	75	85

Silver Negus, Kapitex

Size	20 Fg	22 Fg	24 Fg	26 Fg	28 Fg	30 Fg	32 Fg	34 Fg	36 Fg	38 Fg	40 Fg
O.D. (mm)	6.7	7.3	8.0	8.2	9.0	10.1	10.3	11.0	12.2	12.4	13.0
I.D. (mm)											
Length (mm)	56	60	62	64	68	72	74	76	82	86	90

Table 10: Adult tubes: Single lumen tubes

Fome-Cuf™, TTS™, Aire-Cuf™, Bivona

Size	5.0	6.0	7.0	8.0	9.0	9.5
O.D. (mm)	7.3	8.7	10.0	11.0	12.3	13.3
I.D. (mm)						
Length (mm)	60	70	80	88	98	98

Blueline, Portex

Size	5.0	6.0	7.0	7.5	8.0	9.0	10
O.D (mm)	6.9	8.3	9.7	10.4	11	12.4	13.7
I.D (mm)							
Length (mm)	50	55	65	71	76	89.9	100.7

Blueline Ultra, Portex

Size	6	7	7.5	8	8.5	9	10
O.D. (mm)	9.2	10.5	11.3	11.9	12.6	13.3	14.0
I.D. (mm)	6.0	7.0	7.5	8.0	8.5	9.0	10.0
Length (mm)	64.5	70.0	73.0	75.5	78.0	81.0	87.5

Mini-Trach, Portex

Size	4.0
O.D (mm)	5.4
I.D (mm)	4.0
Length (mm)	92

Table 11: Adult tubes: Longer length tracheostomy tubes

Adjustable flange, Portex

Size	6	7	8	9	10
O.D. (mm)	8.3	9.6	11.0	12.4	13.7
I.D. (mm)	6.0	7.0	8.0	9.0	10.0
Length (mm)	70–90	77–100	90–110	100–120	110–130

Comments:
Single lumen only
Cuffed and uncuffed

Hyperflex™, adjustable neck flange, Bivona

Size	6	7	8	9
O.D. (mm)	8.7	10.0	11.0	12.3
I.D. (mm)	6.0	7.0	8.0	9.0
Length (mm)	110	120	130	140

Comments:
Available with Aire-Cuf®, or Tight to Shaft, TTS™

XLT, Shiley

Size	5	6	7	8
O.D. (mm)	9.6	11.0	12.3	13.3
I.D. (mm)	5.0	6.0	7.0	8.0
Length (mm)	90	95	100	105

Comments:
Cuffed and uncuffed
Increase can be either at proximal or distal end of shaft

Moore, Boston Medical

Size	6	8
O.D. (mm)	11.0	12.0
Length (mm)	115	115

Comments:
Uncuffed only
Can be trimmed to fit

Tracoe Comfort, Extra Long, Kapitex

Size	5	6	7	8	9	10
O.D. (mm)	8.7	10.0	10.5	11.3	12.6	13.7
Length (mm)	92	95	100	105	110	115

Comments:
Uncuffed only
Increased proximal length only

Table 12: Paediatric tube ranges

	2.5	3.0	3.5	4.0	4.5	5.0	5.5	6.0	6.5	7.0
Paediatric tube-PED, Shiley										
Size (I.D.) mm		3.0	3.5	4.0	4.5	5.0	5.5			
O.D. (mm)		4.5	5.2	5.9	6.5	7.1	7.7			
Length (mm)		39	40	41	42	44	46			
Cuffed Paediatric tube-PDC, Shiley										
Size (I.D.) mm				4.0	4.5	5.0	5.5			
O.D. (mm)				5.9	6.5	7.1	7.7			
Length (mm)				41	42	44	46			
Long Tube-PDL (uncuffed), PLC (cuffed), Shiley										
Size (I.D.) mm						5.0	5.5	6.0	6.5	
O.D. (mm)						7.1	7.7	8.3	9.0	
Length (mm)						50	52	54	56	
GOS Pattern, Rüsch										
Size (I.D.) mm		3.0	3.5	4.0	4.5	5.0	5.5	6.0		7.0
O.D. (mm)		4.5	5.0	6.0	6.7	7.5	8.0	8.7		10.7
Length (mm)										
Paediatric, Portex with clear angled 15 mm connector										
Size (I.D.) mm	2.5	3.0	3.5	4.0	4.5	5.0	5.5			
O.D. (mm)	4.5	5.2	5.8	6.5	7.1	7.7	8.3			
Length (mm)	30	36	40	44	48	50	52			
Blueline, Portex with and without 15 mm connector										
Size (I.D.) mm		3.0	3.5	4.0	4.5	5.0		6.0		7.0
O.D. (mm)		4.2	4.9	5.5	6.2	6.9		8.3		9.7
Length (mm)		35	39	43	46	50		55		65
Fome-Cuf®, Aire-Cuf®, TTS™ cuffed and uncuffed tubes, Bivona										
Size (I.D.) mm	2.5	3.0	3.5	4.0	4.5	5.0	5.5			
O.D. (mm)	4.0	4.7	5.3	6.0	6.7	7.3	8.0			
Length (mm)	38	39	40	41	42	44	46			
Uncuffed adjustable neck flange tube, Bivona										
Size (I.D.) mm	2.5	3.0	3.5	4.0	4.5	5.0	5.5			
O.D. (mm)	4.0	4.7	5.3	6.0	6.7	7.3	8.0			
Length (mm)	55	60	65	70	75	80	85			
Equivalent Jackson size	00	0	1	2		3	4			
Equivalent French gauge (Fg) size	13	15	16	18	19	21	23			

Table 13: Neonatal Tracheostomy tubes

NEO, Shiley	**Size** (I.D.) mm	**3**	**3.5**	**4.0**	**4.5**
	O.D. (mm)	4.5	5.2	5.9	6.5
	Length (mm)	30	32	34	36
Neonatal with 15 mm connector, Portex	**Size** (I.D.) mm	**2.5**	**3.0**	**3.5**	
	O.D. (mm)	4.5	5.2	5.8	
	Length (mm)	30	32	34	
Uncuffed and FlexTend Plus™, Bivona	**Size** (I.D.) mm	**2.5**	**3.0**	**3.5**	**4.0**
	O.D. (mm)	4.0	4.7	5.3	6.0
	Length (mm)	30	32	34	36
Fome-Cuf®, Aire-Cuf®, TTS™ cuffed tubes, Bivona	**Size** (I.D.) mm	**2.5**	**3.0**	**3.5**	**4.0**
	O.D. (mm)	4.0	4.7	5.3	6.0
	Length (mm)	30	32	34	36
Equivalent Jackson size		**00**	**0**	**1**	

TRACHEOSTOMY MANAGEMENT IN THE INTENSIVE CARE UNIT

Lisa Hooper

INTRODUCTION

The initial management of a patient on an intensive care unit (ICU), involves a series of interventions that aim to stabilise and then optimise their physiological state. Mechanical ventilation is a commonly utilised intervention to support a patient's respiratory function. The second phase in ICU management focuses on weaning the patient from the artificial supportive mechanisms. The principle role of tracheostomy in the ICU is to expedite the weaning process in patients requiring prolonged mechanical ventilation and those predicted to be at risk of persistent pulmonary aspiration. Tracheostomy formation facilitates weaning primarily by allowing increased level of patient activity and mobility. In this chapter we will explore the physiological consequences of mechanical ventilation and the role of tracheostomy in ICU management.

AIMS

- Discuss the use of mechanical ventilation
- Outline the indications, benefits and disadvantages of tracheostomy for the ICU patient
- Review the physiological impact on respiratory function (of ICU management)
- Review of the issues governing the choice of tracheostomy tube in ICU
- Outline key issues within respiratory management of tracheostomy patient
- Look at the complications associated with tracheostomy on ICU
- Overview the evidence on weaning from mechanical ventilation
- Explore the role of speaking valve, Passy Muir, in weaning
- Review the role of the physiotherapist

MECHANICAL VENTILATION

Mechanical ventilation is perhaps the most universally employed intervention in ICU management. This intervention is highly effective however, it incurs complications and weaning can be problematic. On the ICU the principle indication for tracheostomy formation is to facilitate weaning from mechanical ventilation. It is therefore important to review the role of mechanical ventilation.

Assisted ventilation refers to application of intermittent positive pressure to an airway. The pressure gradient from the airway to the alveoli results in inspiratory flow. When the driving force of pressure drops, the effects of elastic recoil of the lungs and gravity on the chest wall reverse the pressure gradient resulting in an expiratory flow.

The purpose of mechanical ventilation is to correct the effects of respiratory compromise by optimising oxygen delivery and CO_2 clearance.

Indications

Acute respiratory failure is the most common indication for mechanical ventilation on the ICU. Respiratory failure describes a state of deficient gas exchange resulting in a decreased arterial oxygen concentration, hypoxaemia, and retention of CO_2 hypercapnia. Hypoxaemia being the most dangerous and any patient with a PaO_2 <8 kPa while on supplemental oxygen therapy should be urgently reviewed for supportive ventilation. There are two types of respiratory failure (Table 1), which can present singularly or in combination:

- *Type I (Hypoxaemia)* is due to significant ventilation perfusion mismatch and increased intrapulmonary shunt, in the presence of a normal respiratory drive. Hypoxaemia stimulates reflex lungs and chemoreceptors which may increase ventilatory drive and thereby decrease the alveolar and arterial pCO_2. This type of failure is commonly the result of atelectasis, pulmonary collapse/consolidation and pulmonary oedema. All can be complications of: thoracic and abdominal surgery, prolonged anaesthesia, prolonged immobility, mechanical ventilation, pain, respiratory infection, aspiration and tracheostomy patients. Hypoxaemia is responsive to oxygen therapy if measures to decrease the shunt utilising physiotherapy and minimising the pulmonary oedema.
- *Type II (Ventilatory)* is due to decrease in overall ventilation. Thus the patient is both hypoxaemic and hypercapnic. This type of failure can be the result of central drive problems (head injury, cerebral bleed/tumour, opiates, anaesthetic drugs) neuromuscular weakness (spinal cord injury, myopathies, Guillain–Barre syndrome, myasthenia gravis) resistance to ventilation (respiratory tract obstruction, obesity, bronchospasm, kyphoscoliosis) and pulmonary disease (emphysema, chronic obstructive pulmonary disease,

Table 1: Respiratory failure Type I and II

Respiratory failure

Type I or Hypoxaemic
Defined
    Normal or slightly decreased alveolar and arterial pCO_2
    Decreased alveolar and arterial pO_2
    Poor ventilation/perfusion match or increased intrapulmonary shunt

Precursor
    Atelectasis, segmental collapse, consolidation pulmonary oedema

Interventions
    Oxygen therapy, fluid management and physiotherapy

Type II or Ventilatory
Defined
    Increased alveolar and arterial pCO_2
    Decreased alveolar and arterial pO_2
    Decreased in minute ventilation and/or increased alveolar dead space

Precursor
    Decrease in central respiratory drive
    Neuromuscular weakness – respiratory muscles
    Increase in resistance to ventilation
    Increase in alveolar dead space

Intervention
    Oxygen therapy and urgent assessment for ventilation support

adult respiratory distress syndrome). Oxygen therapy is of little benefit without some form of ventilatory support.

Indications for tracheostomy

Elective tracheostomy formation in the ICU is an increasingly common procedure in the management of patients who are predicted to have difficulty in weaning from mechanical ventilatory support. Initially a patient's airway is secured via translaryngeal intubation. The presence of a translaryngeal tube incurs soft tissue changes, the extent and severity of which are principally related to the length of time the tube remains in situ. Those having a delayed emergence from coma, cranial nerve dysfunction, high spinal cord injuries, significant neuromuscular weakness or chronic lung pathology are all typical ICU patient groups requiring tracheostomy insertion due to prolonged ventilatory support. Other indications include the provision of airway protection from serial pulmonary aspiration in patients with predictable dysphagia or in those having previously failed a trial extubation.

Table 2: Indications for tracheostomy in the ICU

Indications for tracheostomy	ICU patient groups
Facilitate prolonged assisted ventilation	Coma • Major head injury • Cerebral bleed/infarct/lesion • Encephalitis High spinal cord injury Neuromuscular disorder • Guillain–Barre syndrome • Critical care polyneuropathy Chronic obstructive pulmonary disease
Inability to prevent pulmonary aspiration	Posterior fossa/infratentorial lesions • Cerebellum/brain stem • Basilar/posterior cerebral artery Cranial nerve dysfunction
Upper airway obstruction	Maxillofacial surgery or trauma Congenital malformation Facilitate upper cervical surgery Vocal cord paralysis

Tracheostomy is also required when the upper airway is known to be obstructed most commonly seen in ICU as a direct consequence of maxillofacial surgery and trauma (Table 2).

Benefits of tracheostomy for the ICU patient

- Secures the airway below the level of the larynx – spares the larynx from direct injury.
- Allows the patient to be more active – sedatives used to decrease patients stress with translaryngeal tubes can be removed.[1]
- Allows increased patient mobility – secure airway for movement in bed, chair, stand and walk.
- Shortens the ventilatory weaning process – increased patient activity and mobility.
- Improves patient comfort – removes potentially noxious stimulus from the oral cavity, salivary glands, pharynx and larynx.
- Facilitates care given – practitioners have positive perceptions of tracheostomy and link them with rehabilitation, whereas they hold negative perceptions of translaryngeal airways in their patients.[2]
- Enhances verbal communication – patient can now mouth words.

- Permits return of speech – intermittent cuff deflation and speaking valve in the ventilatory circuit. Can improve hearing with return of pressure to upper respiratory tract.
- Facilitates swallow and may allow a return to oral nutrition.
- Psychological benefit to patient and visitors.

The disadvantages of a tracheostomy for the ICU patient

- Surgical intervention with risk of complications
- Bacterial airway colonisation – usually pre dates the tracheostomy but will often persist until after decannulation
- Risk of tube displacement – with increased patient mobility
- Risk of tracheal erosion from the cuff, fenestrations or shaft of the tube resulting in stenosis or malacia
- Scarring

Timing of tracheostomy formation

Much has been written on the timing of tracheostomy with more favourable outcomes in early rather than later. Prolonged translaryngeal intubation has been associated with acute laryngeal oedema, ulceration, granulation and scar tissue formation in up to 65% of patients reviewed on extubation.[3,4] However a high rate of spontaneous healing post extubation of laryngeal lesions has been demonstrated.[3,5] Acute laryngeal pathology does not accurately predict evolution of chronic lesions. Despite this a limit of 10–14 days on translaryngeal intubation is supported in test series.[6] Whited prospectively found a 12% incidence of laryngeal stenosis in patients intubated for 11 days or more which dropped to only 2% in those remaining intubated for less than 6 days.[7] Independent variables associated with prolonged ventilation and need for tracheostomy include: presence nosocomial pneumonia, previous failed extubation trial, Glasgow Coma Scale <8 and those with high cervical spinal injury. Patients requiring tracheostomy due to aspiration risk include neurological patients with cranial nerve deficits and those sustaining infratentorial lesions.[8]

Benefits of early formation include reduced mechanical ventilation requirements, days in ICU and risk of hospital acquired pneumonia.

IMPACT OF ICU MANAGEMENT ON RESPIRATORY FUNCTION

Elective tracheostomy occurs most commonly in the second stage of ICU management. Typically this means the patient will already have physiological consequences of mechanical ventilation and enforced immobility for a period of 3–14 days prior to instituting the tracheostomy.

Consequences of immobility and the supine position on respiratory function:

- The gravitational effect on the chest wall in the supine ICU patient decreases inspiratory excursion and lowers the resting position at end of expiration. This reduction in the transverse diameter of the chest wall results in a decrease in functional residual capacity (FRC). Reduction in residual volume allows airways to narrow which increases the resistance to inspiratory flow and promotes alveolar emptying.
- In supine position, gravity acts on the abdominal contents displacing the diaphragm to a resting position higher in the chest cavity. Furthermore the abdominal contents behave as fluid, creating a hydrostatic pressure greatest in the dependent areas. This results in a sinusoidal like displacement and resistance across the diaphragm. On inspiration the contracting diaphragm moves unequally with greater movement in the uppermost aspect. This asymmetrical movement potentiates an increased transpleural pressure anteriorly, which creates a traction force on the anterior lung. The differential opening force on the airways determines inspiratory volume greatest in the upper and mid sections with less to dependant areas. The region with optimal ventilation is in the mid section. This is due to the gravity-induced atelectasis in the dependant areas and the uppermost areas continuously held open. Over time this pattern becomes more acute with progressive collapse and under ventilation in the dependant regions. In this situation blood passing through the dependant pulmonary circuit will return to left side of the heart deoxygenated, increasing the shunt. The effect of abdomen on respiratory function is exacerbated in the obese, those with distended abdomen or obstructed gastro-intestinal tract. These changes further decrease the FRC, which leads to alveolar collapse. Persistent posterio-basalar collapse is associated with recurrent consolidation, pleural effusion and risks being a source septicaemia (Fig. 1).
- Supine positioning results in a decrease of 700–800 ml in FRC with sedation/paralysis contributing to a further 300–500 ml loss.[9] In this situation FRC can approach residual lung volume. As FRC is directly related to lung compliance and inversely related to airway resistance, decrease in FRC can result in airway closure in dependent lung regions and lead to hypoxaemia.
- Immobility induces progressive muscle weakness and atrophy. Critical care polyneuropathy is sensori-motor denervation specifically found in ICU patients.[10] This has a significant impact on weaning and predisposes tracheostomy formation.
- Gravity reconfigures the perfusion zones, in supine, so that the non-dependent area becomes Zone 2 and the dependent Zone 3 (see Chapter 1, Anatomy and Physiology of the Respiratory Tract).

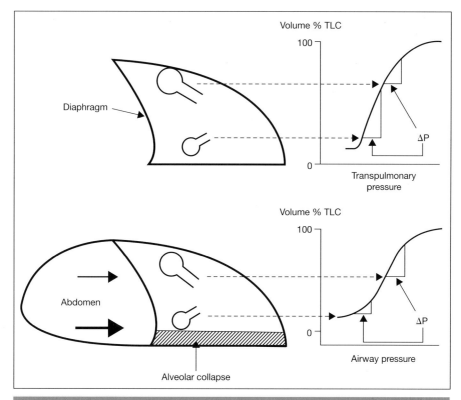

Fig. 1: Distribution of ventilation. (above) Spontaneous breathing. Gravitationally induced gradient of pleural pressure causes non-dependent alveoli to be exposed to larger transpulmonary (distending) pressure than dependent alveoli at end of expiration. Because dependent alveoli are situated on a steeper portion of the pressure-volume curve, they will receive a greater proportion of tidal volume when transpulmonary pressure difference increases by a given increment of pressure (ΔP) during spontaneous inspiration. (below) Controlled ventilation. When diaphragm is inactive, hydrostatic pressure generated by abdominal contents decreases regional compliance of dependent zones, so diverting more ventilation to non-dependent zones. This effect may be accentuated by collapse of alveoli in dependent zones. From Sykes K, Young D. Principles and practice series. In: Hahn CEW, Adams AP (eds). *Respiratory Support in Intensive Care*, 2nd edn. London: BMJ Publishing Group, 1990.

- The most significant effect is on regional ventilation. While supine, the lung is suspended from the anterior chest wall. This effects a traction force splinting open the airways uppermost alveoli and conversely collapsing the dependent areas. The decreased ventilation to this region contradicts the shift to greater perfusion in the dependent areas. The combined effect is to worsen ventilation perfusion match and thus respiratory effectiveness.

Mechanical ventilation is the application of intermittent positive pressure to an airway. Consequences to normal respiratory function include:

- Ventilation varies regionally within the lung based on airway resistance. With positive pressure driven ventilation, uppermost lung regions are preferentially ventilated as the airways/alveoli are splinted open with gravity.
- In the acute phase of ICU management patients are most commonly maintained in supine or a 15–30 degree lateral tilt. If position and controlled ventilation are maintained over days little variance in regional ventilation pattern occurs. As a result dependent lung areas become progressively less compliant and less recruited in ventilation. This is a natural evolution whereby collapsed alveoli have a traction effect on adjacent lung tissue predisposing further collapse. Once collapsed, atelectatic, an alveolus can require 30–40 cmH$_2$O to reinflate. As compliance of the dependent lung region decreases, the inspiratory pressure is transferred to the middle and uppermost lung regions. If left unchallenged, this potentiates progressive over-inflation of uppermost regions with the risk of baro/volume trauma.
- High levels of inspired oxygen concentration and decreased FRC are associated with atelectasis formation, which is directly related to shunt and can result in hypoxaemia.[9]
- Cilary dysfunction is associated with sub-optimal humidity, oxygen therapy, trauma from tracheal tubes and cuff, repeated suction and significant sputum load. This situation is potentiated with artificial airways and assisted ventilation.
- Mucus production at approximately 100 ml/day is exacerbated as a consequence of oxygen therapy, irritation from the tracheal tubes and repeated suction. Furthermore there is the immunoactivated response to foreign matter such as aspirate, infection and the tube itself. This results in increased secretion volume and consistency which can precipitate airway obstruction.
- Aspiration is potentiated in 86% of supine ventilated tracheostomy patients.[11–15] This is magnified in those with head injury or infratentorial lesions which are associated with cranial nerve dysfunction. Furthermore these neuro patients may be 'silent aspirators' – where the protective cough reflex is absent.[16] Aspiration results in serial pulmonary infections, colonisation, sputum load, increased physiological demand, extending the wean process and potentiating infiltration septicaemia.

The tracheostomy bypasses the upper airway. This can bring about the following consequences:

- Decrease in the anatomical dead space by 60–70 ml. This has not been found to be clinically significant during assisted ventilation but must be overcome before successful weaning and tube removal.[17]

- Loss of intrinsic positive end expiratory pressure (PEEP) normally mediated by glottic activity – usually equivalent to $4\,cmH_2O$. This decreases alveolar ventilation, FRC and compliance. This predisposes alveolar collapse or atelectasis. This is particularly significant in chronic obstructive pulmonary disease (COPD) patients who utilise increased intrinsic PEEP as a compensatory strategy for pulmonary dysfunction.[18] Early use of speaking valve during ventilatory weaning can be beneficial as it imitates the patient's normal respiratory dynamics.
- Inability to cough which is mediated by glottic closure. Initial difficulty in achieving the required inspiratory effort to 85–90% of total lung capacity which is $2.3 \pm 0.5\,l$.[19] There is a steep increase in work of breathing when high flow rates meet the static resistance of the tracheostomy tube. A tracheostomy tube has no mechanism to gate the expiratory flow and build intrathoracic pressure in order to effectively clear secretions.
- Tracheostomy tubes decrease the work of breathing as compared to an endotracheal tube of the same inner diameter.[20]

Strategies to prevent/reduce these consequences include:

- Early tracheostomy formation in anticipated ventilator dependant patients to facilitate mobility and weaning.
- Appropriate sized tracheostomy tube for patients respiratory demand.[21]
- PEEP incorporated as integral part of the ventilation strategy with the therapeutic level titrated on evolving respiratory dynamics.
- Early encouragement of spontaneous ventilatory effort within the assisted ventilation strategy.
- Minimise ventilatory pressure drops with in-line suction circuits and nebuliser kits.[22]
- Appropriate humidification system – warm water bath systems for those patients with predicted sputum load, colonised respiratory infection, prolonged ventilation or high flow support. Patients in ICU with tracheostomies have many if not all of the listed indicators.[23]
- Respiratory physiotherapy.
- Encourage active participation in weaning strategy.
- Early rehabilitation, in particular mobilisation, is integral part of the weaning process.
- Position patient to stimulate spontaneous activity and transfer to chair (recliner) daily to optimise regional ventilation and decrease aspiration.[24]
- Begin early speaking valve trials on conscious patients still requiring assisted ventilation as part of the weaning strategy.

TRACHEOSTOMY TUBE SELECTION

Tracheostomies in the ICU are principally indicated in patients with persistent respiratory failure necessitating ventilatory support and as an adjunct to the weaning process.

Therefore the choice of tube should be principally defined by the impact the tube has on ventilatory flow and work of breathing. The resistance of any tube is described by Poiseuille law which relates the pressure drop across a tube to be inversely proportional to the fourth power of the radius in the presence of laminar flow. As the mechanical resistance attributable to the tracheostomy is an inversely related function of the inner diameter of the tube, the largest tube that is anatomically viable should be chosen. For adults a tube with an inner lumen size 8–10 mm has been recommended as it is thought to deliver the nearest approximation to the ventilatory flow of the normal upper respiratory tract.[21]

Several authors have commented on the disparity of tracheostomy tube sizes and the actual internal diameter of the tube.[20,21,25] This may be clinically significant when the insertion of the appropriate inner cannula reduces the internal airway diameter by 1.5 mm of the parent tube. Unsurprisingly removal of the inner cannula has been shown to decrease tube resistance and work of breathing.[25] However removal is at the cost of the protection afforded by the inner tube. The outer diameter of tubes manufacturers and styles also varies and must be considered prior to tube selection (see Chapter 6, Tracheostomy Tubes).

In adults the use of tracheostomy tubes with inner cannula are advocated to decrease the risk of obstruction from blood, mucus and sputum.[26] The function of a removable inner tube is to facilitate lavage of the inner lumen and thereby ensure the maintenance of a clear airway. By allowing frequent cleaning the inevitable sputum build up within a tube is reduced along with the risk of obstruction and the patency of the tube is prolonged.[27,28] In the event of acute tube obstruction having the capacity to remove an inner cannula, thereby immediately resolving the respiratory distress while maintaining a patent airway, is of considerable clinical worth. Such a situation with an unlined tube may result in a tube change, which is never ideal in a critical situation and is often only routinely performed by certain members of the team. Sputum adherence within the tube has a significant impact on increases to airflow resistance, morbidity and mortality.[29] Other variables on tube choice that effect resistance are radius of curvature, roughness of inner lumen and length of tube.[30] The most significant determinant of resistance remains the dimensions of the inner lumen.

Cuffed tracheostomy tubes

The function of the cuff is to form an effective seal with the tracheal mucosa while exerting minimal compression force. Ischaemic damage results when the cuff pressure exceeds that of the capillary perfusion pressure thought to be 20–30 mmHg.[31] Modern materials have resulted in the evolution of high-volume low-pressure cuffs (HVLP) adopted by most systems although some variance in compliance is still found.[32,33] However over inflation of the cuff creates a high pressure situation which must be avoided. Regular 8–12 hourly monitoring of cuff pressures, longer cuffs and insertion of an appropriately large tracheostomy tube which requires only moderate inflation of the cuff to provide a seal is advocated.[31,34,35]

Cuff inflation techniques

Various methods are advocated to establish optimal cuff inflation but with poor consensus. Historically tracheal cuffs were progressively inflated just to the point that air leak was prevented. Cessation of the leak was determined by auscultation above the cuff while the patient received positive pressure ventilation. This method of cuff inflation establishing a seal within the trachea is termed the *'just seal' pressure* or the *minimum occlusion pressure*. With the adoption of HVLP cuffs the assumption that the occlusion pressure was below the capillary perfusion is found to be unreliable.[36–39] The use of a pressure manometer is advocated in conjunction with a HVLP cuffed tube.

Once the cuff is inflated its pressure against the tracheal wall varies according to the airway pressure acting upon it.[37] When the peak airway pressure exceeds cuff pressure the inferior aspect of the cuff is compressed against the tube. This compression displaces volume laterally and raises the pressure within the cuff proportionally, which maintains the integrity of the seal.[38] As peak pressure falls, the cuff returns to the resting pressure 20–30 mmHg. This cycle of changing cuff pressure should allow for capillary refill resulting in less potential tracheal damage. Due to the linear relationship, peak cuff inflation pressures greater than 25 mmHg or peak airway pressure greater than 35 mmHg can be used to identify those patients at greater risk.[37,39]

RESPIRATORY ASSESSMENT OF THE TRACHEOSTOMY PATIENT ON ICU

The basis of effective intervention is the accurate assessment of the patient's current situation and how it is evolving. On the ICU there is a plethora of objective data monitored in real time available to the practitioner. However it is as important to analyse the trend of the data in order to make proactive rather than reactive strategies to management. This is particularly essential in weaning tracheostomy patients from mechanical ventilation. The following is a systems based approach to respiratory assessment.

Central nervous system

- Is the patient conscious/rousable/unconscious/sedated and does this vary – this is measured most commonly by the Glasgow Coma Scale. The respiratory centre in the brain stem is part of the reticular formation which governs cerebral arousal. Lack of CNS activation depresses respiratory function and on ICU maybe due to: intracranial pressure, cerebral vasospasm, opiates, respiratory or metabolic dysfunction and infection. Intervention should aim to reverse the abnormality and then use stimulatory positioning and early rehabilitation.
- Pain directly inhibits respiratory function and must be effectively addressed without sedating.
- Psychological stress with loss of speech, fear, frustration and psychological withdrawal. All patients face a degree of reactive depression.[42]

Respiratory system

- Ventilatory support – what artificial support is being used and how much spontaneous respiratory activity is the patient achieving? If assisted ventilation is used, what is the mode and where is its effect on the patient? Are there mandatory breaths (SIMV, BiPAP), continuous pressure (CPAP, PEEP) and or patient triggered pressure support on every breath (PSV). The goal of weaning is to remove this assistance as the patient recovers their normal function.
- Tracheostomy tube – size, type and cuff are important as previously discussed. Check that the tube sits perpendicular to the neck and is flush to the skin as misalignment can easily occur by the dragging of ill positioned or supported ventilatory equipment.
- Physiological objective markers: respiratory rate (mandatory and spontaneous) tidal and minute volume, peak airway pressures and lung compliance. Of these the most sensitive to deterioration is respiratory rate.
- Oxygen support coupled with arterial blood gas analysis and pulse oximetry to determine it effectiveness.
- Chest movement – is it symmetrical (asymmetrical may be due to sputum plugging or rarely a pneumothorax)? Increased or excessive work of breathing is reflected in high spontaneous respiratory rate, shallow depth, use of accessory muscles, indrawing intercostals, paradoxical abdominal movement, ventilator patient mismatch tachycardia and patient distress. All of which indicates fatigue or respiratory failure. This should prompt cessation of weaning trial and clearance of any sputum load.
- Sputum load – tracheostomy patients in ICU are invariably bacterially colonised resulting in significant sputum load that requires efficient humidification, regular secretion removal (manual techniques and suctioning),

and patient mobilisation for regional ventilation. Note quantity, viscosity, colour and culture results and amend interventions accordingly.

- Humidification – due to bacterial colonisation the majority of ICU tracheostomy patients require a heated system. If sputum load increases in quantity or viscosity add saline nebulisers, increase patient mobility and frequency of respiratory clearance.

- Aspiration – neuro patients on ICU can silently aspirate and those with NG feeding, and/or mechanical ventilation all pre-dispose to pulmonary aspiration. Ensure cuff inflated effectively, and position greater than 60 degrees upright.

- Airway reflexes – return of reflex cough when the trachea is stimulated by suction or sputum is an objective step in recovery. Abdominal and intercostal strength can be assessed in the volume exchanged during a cough. Remembering that tracheostomy patients cough less effectively as the open airway cannot gate the expiratory flow and allow build pressure. Early use of a speaking valve facilitates coughing by returning function to the upper respiratory tract.

- Respiratory capacity – pre-existing dysfunction i.e. deformities, pulmonary disease neuromuscular disorder, disuse atrophy experienced by bed bound patients.[10]

- Auscultation – breath sounds are proportional to tidal volume so for accurate review the patient should be stimulated to take deep breaths in an upright position. Are the sounds symmetrical, diminished, increased or absent? Abnormal sounds include crepitations, wheezes, bronchial (if in the periphery), pleural rubs, cuff leaks and ventilator equipment. Tracheostomy patients are prone to basilar collapse and consolidation due to the drop in FRC, relative immobility and central bacterial colonisation. This will remain until they are extubated although use of speaking valve, early intensive rehabilitation and regular sputum clearance are effective.

- Chest X-rays are useful but findings may be delayed by up to 48 h and thus aspiration is best diagnosed on clinical assessment rather than on radiograph. Sudden changes in ventilation merit X-ray as part of assessment. Some authors suggest that a lateral film may be useful to check tube alignment within the trachea, position of fenestrations and tube tip and carina positioning.

Cardiovascular system

- Cardiovascular stability – assessment of heart rate and rhythm, central venous pressure, pulmonary artery wedge pressure, blood pressure and cardiac function need to be stable and within a therapeutic range. Any adverse reaction to intervention should be noted. A common risk involves vagal stimulation by the tracheostomy tube due to ventilator equipment traction or when changing inner tubes and suctioning.

- Mechanical ventilation increases the pressure on the pulmonary vascular circuit, especially if PEEP/CPAP are implemented. Prolonged immobility associated with ventilatory assistance causes a shift in fluid back to the thorax and a delayed systemic vascular response necessitating a graduated program of positioning and mobilsation to upright.

Renal system

- Renal function has a direct effect on the respiratory system in terms of acid base balance and fluid management. Note urine output, fluid balance and renal function markers.

COMPLICATIONS OF TRACHEOSTOMY IN ICU

Some of the early complications with tracheostomy formation are discussed (Fig. 2a–2l).

Cuff failure to form a seal

Failure to seal is detected by audible air leak into the upper respiratory tract (Fig. 2a). With positive pressure ventilation any leak is easily audible as it bubbles through the secretions in the larynx, however in the self ventilating patient use of a stethoscope positioned over the larynx is required. Once the appropriate sized tube is inserted head neck alignment and the traction forces imposed by the ventilation equipment pose significant risk to the tube position and cuff pressure. Cuff pressure is highest if the patient's head and neck are in a rotated position, less so if flexed or extended and conversely pressure is minimally affected when in neutral alignment.[35] Traction forces of unsupported ventilation equipment results in obvious tube torsion and potentiates tube occlusion or displacement (Fig. 2b). Thus if cuff fails to seal check alignment, support ventilation equipment, consider a larger tube but do not over inflate the cuff. Complications of an over inflated cuff include compression of the tube (Fig. 2c), dilatation of trachea (Fig. 2d) and risk of ulceration of the tracheal wall exacerbated by the presence of a nasogastric tube (Fig. 2e).

Subcutaneous emphysema (Fig. 2f)

Seen in the early post-operative period is detected by crepitus over the neck and radiating out over the chest wall. This may be caused by poor cuff seal, tube alignment, partial tube displacement or where tube fenestrations are

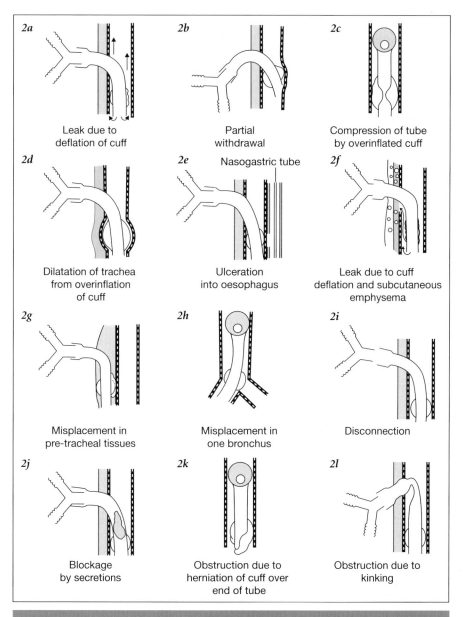

Fig. 2: Some complications of tracheostomy. From Sykes K, Young D. Principles and practice series. In: Hahn CEW, Adams AP (eds). *Respiratory Support in Intensive Care*, 2nd edition. London: BMJ Publishing Group, 1990.

positioned outside the trachea in a patient with mechanically assisted ventilation. It may also be caused by coughing against a tightly packed stomal dressing. Ensure tube position and cuff is optimal, chest X-ray to check for pneumothorax and mark extent of emphysema. The body will reabsorb the air over a matter of days.

Accidental tube displacement

Unsupported ventilation tubing can cause a traction force sufficient to displace the tube. Head, neck and tube alignment is critical in the first 72 h and from then risk is greatest during: rolling, coughing, being hoisted or sitting. If the tube is partially displaced (Fig. 2b), tube proud of neck but chest expansion and auscultation confirm tube still within trachea, then deflate cuff reposition tube and reseal cuff. If chest fails to expand with ventilation, auscultation reveals absent tracheal breath sounds and the tube is not obstructed with sputum then tube is in a false passage and is compressing the trachea. This is a medical emergency, remove tube and prepare for reintubation – initially use a bougie to railroad a new tracheostomy tube failing that intubate with a translaryngeal tube. Tube misplacement can also occur, in particular in the early post-operative period, those with a large neck and/or agitated (Fig. 2g). This can be prevented by the selection of an appropriate tube and a secure method of maintaining tube position. Adversely a tube which is too long may extend past the carina and enter into one bronchus leading to unilateral ventilation (Fig. 2h), management of this includes the withdrawal of the tube to approximately 1–2 cm from the carina.

Self extubation

Any patient on ICU is at potential risk to self extubate due to significant levels of anxiety, frustration and sleep deprivation. This group may experience metabolic disturbances and acute reactive depression that may include hallucinations. Those with cognitive dysfunction or in post traumatic amnesic states post major head injury are at great risk. Information, reassurance psychological support, early speaking valve and communication aids and appropriate medication may include night sedation, anti-depressants and anti-psychotics. Extubation management follows the same guide as accidental tube displacement. Disconnection from ventilator systems may also occur (Fig. 2i).

Airway obstruction

This may be due to sputum or blood and is most common as a progressive encrusting of the inner surface of tracheostomy tubes (Fig. 2j). Removable inner cannula, appropriate humidification, regular sputum clearance and early mobility are effective in offsetting this risk. Tubes without inner cannula should be changed regularly and at the first sign of crust formation. Signs of tube obstruction are those of increased work of breathing, stridor and can have increased resistance to passage of suction catheter. The airway may be obstructed as a result of poor alignment of the tube within trachea. This is usually obvious from the orientation of the tube to the neck. The cuff can be herniated (Fig. 2k) over the inferior pole of the tube and will require changing. Tube failure of excessive pressure from the tracheal wall and surrounding tissues may also cause the tube to kink (Fig. 2l), this may be managed by the use of an armoured tube (see Chapter 6, Tracheostomy Tubes).

A standard set of equipment and documentation needs to be easily accessible within the patient area at all times (Table 3).

Table 3: Equipment for tracheostomy patient in ICU

Emergency
- Tracheostomy tubes – 1 × same size and 1 × size smaller
- Tracheal dilators
- Bougie
- Stitch cutters
- Ambu bag + PEEP valve + catheter mount
- Syringe
- Stethoscope

Therapeutic
- Humidification – heated system or heat and moisture exchanger
- Nebuliser kit – in-line with ventilation circuit
- Suction – in-line with ventilation circuit, appropriate size
- Spare unfenestrated inner cannula
- Cuff pressure manometer
- Stoma dressing – Lyofoam
- Tube ribbons or holders

Documentation – Daily observation chart: Airway
- Type of tube and size
- Fenestrated or unfenestrated system
- Percutaneous or surgical insertion and date
- Cuff pressure check 8–12 hourly – observation and manometer
- Inner cannula reviewed and cleaned
- Suction frequency and sputum load

WEANING THE TRACHEOSTOMY PATIENT ON ICU

Weaning is one of medicines conundrums; much is written, even more is postulated much less is agreed. What is accepted is that mechanical ventilation is associated with significant morbidity, mortality and cost.[44] Furthermore that although the mortality rate peaks in the first 10 days, it then remains constant for every day that mechanical ventilation is continued.[45] A useful indicator was found to be percentage of total ventilation days that are spent on weaning. In a Spanish review it was found that as high as 41% of total ventilation time was spent on weaning.[45] As there is a positive relationship between the number of days spent in weaning and the amount of daily input by the multiprofessional team, any reduction in mechanical ventilation days has a direct effect on reducing cost and increasing ICU capacity. This supports the role of tracheostomy in safe and expeditious weaning.

When sourcing evidence to guide practice it is important to recognise the term weaning describes two different events. The American College of Chest Physicians Consensus Conference on Mechanical Ventilation holds weaning to be the process of gradual reduction of ventilatory support and its replacement with spontaneous ventilation.[46] This involves modes of ventilation and their manipulation being assessed for effectiveness. Whereas other authors consider weaning to be the act of liberation from mechanical ventilation and this is to be determined by the timely recognition of recovery from respiratory failure. In particular, the ability to recognise respiratory recovery and act upon it is more pivotal to success than manipulation of ventilation strategies.[47] However to wean successfully a unified pragmatic approach is non-negotiable.

Tracheostomy patients on an ICU form a heterogeneous group so that implementing a uniform weaning strategy is not practical. Within this group there will be those who wean off mechanical ventilation in days, 1–2 weeks or longer than a month. All groups have particular needs but the philosophy of a weaning program incorporating periods of work and rest while avoiding fatigue can be successfully applied to all.[48]

Weaning should begin as soon as the patient's condition has been stabilised.[47] Early reintroduction of spontaneous respiratory effort has been shown to be beneficial. By encouraging early respiratory muscle activity the disuse atrophy associated with immobility and mechanical ventilation can be lessened.[48]

There are a plethora of suggested predictors for successful weaning however on review none are recommended for formal use.[44,49] The authors felt that the predictors failed in that practitioners had already screened the patients before selecting those to begin weaning trials. What is recommended is a daily trial of spontaneous breathing.[44–47,49] Of interest is the group of tracheostomy patients that require prolonged ventilation, greater than 21 days, who are locked into graduated weaning protocols have been shown to benefit from use of Yang's Rapid Shallow Breathing Index. This allowed patients to accelerate the weaning steps thus decreasing ventilator days.[50–52]

Modes of ventilation used in weaning

Synchronised intermittent mandatory ventilation (SIMV)

The ventilator delivers a pre-set number of mandatory breaths the goal of which is to synchronise these with the patient's respiratory effort. The volume of each mandatory breath is identical but the inspiratory pressure required to deliver it will vary depending on the patient's response. This is volume cycled but pressure limited ventilation. By setting the mandatory breaths/minute the ventilator calculates a window of time within which the patient should trigger a breath. If the patient does initiate a breath the ventilator will deliver the mandatory volume. If the window of time is nearing an end without patient involvement then the mandatory breath is delivered. If the patient tries to breathe out against the incoming flow the result will be a sharp increase in the peak airway pressure experienced by the patient. The patient can breathe between the mandatory cycles but maybe too weak to achieve initially so PEEP and pressure support ventilation (PSV) are added to assist.

Biphasic positive airway pressure (BiPAP)

BiPAP is a pressure cycled ventilation. The ventilator delivers a set number of breaths by alternating between a high pressure (inspiratory pressure) and a lower pressure (PEEP). The patient can initiate at any point in the ventilatory cycle. However lung compliance determines the tidal volume. The tidal volumes could vary significantly for a tracheostomy patient with significant sputum load and would need to be monitored. PSV is usually added to BiPAP to support the patient's respiratory effort. Patients can be fully weaned using BiPAP, as the mandatory rate is reduced and the pressure difference narrows BiPAP becomes CPAP.

Positive end expiratory pressure (PEEP)

PEEP acts as a mechanical gate to expiratory flow. PEEP maintains a greater than atmospheric pressure within the patient's airways at end of expiration and increases the patient's residual lung volume or FRC. In splinting the airways at the end of expiration, the work of inspiration is decreased and alveolar ventilation is potentiated. This is beneficial as one of the consequences of tracheostomy formation is to decrease the normal physiological PEEP.

Pressure support ventilation (PSV) or assisted spontaneous breathing (ASB)

This is pressure assistance that is triggered by the patient's inspiratory effort to deliver volume until a pre-set maximal pressure is reached and then it shuts off. Low level PSV can be used to overcome the work of breathing associated with the tracheostomy tube and ventilator circuit. By decreasing the respiratory work the patient can rest comfortably between weaning trials.[49] PSV is often combined with CPAP as the step down from mandatory to spontaneous ventilation strategies.

Continuous positive airway pressure (CPAP)

This is a high flow delivery system with an expiratory gate. CPAP increases FRC and decreases the work of breathing, both beneficial to the tracheostomy patient on ICU. This is often the last step down to unsupported ventilation. This is passive support and the patient must have a functional respiratory drive.

The evidence on the choice of specific ventilator mode used in the progressive removal of mechanical support does not support the use of SIMV.[44,49] However it was noted that despite new modes being available the older modes were most commonly used.[45] What is important is a program that moves from mechanical ventilation to spontaneous supported and then unsupported, mediated by the result of a daily trial of spontaneous breathing. As the capacity for spontaneous ventilation returns the choice of supportive ventilation needs to be comfortable to the patient and effective at offsetting the work of breathing.[47] In the tracheostomy patient the work of breathing is dependant on tube size, muscle strength/endurance and minute ventilation. The greater the minute ventilation the greater the resistance to flow through the tube and the work needed to overcome this. CPAP and PSV have been shown to be effective in patients with moderate minute ventilation however automatic tube compensation (ATC) is more effective in patients with high ventilatory demand such as COPD.[53]

Protocol directed weaning

The most effective component to successful weaning is the implementation of a weaning protocol that is respiratory therapist or nurse lead rather than physician directed.[44,46,47,49,51,52]

The protocols driven by respiratory therapists or nurses incorporate daily screen of the patient's respiratory function, a spontaneous breathing trial with a systematic reduction in ventilatory support. Implementation of protocols consistently results in significantly shorter weaning durations with comparable or improved outcomes to controls. It is interesting to note that varying the protocol content did not appreciably alter the weaning outcome.[46] Rather the beneficial effect is derived from the team having a unified and systematic approach to weaning and where the gatekeepers are those professionals most consistently involved with the patient. Wall charts displaying weaning progress are a beneficial adjunct to engage and inform the patient. Furthermore wall charts help to co-ordinate the input of the many professionals involved ensuring the patient has a balance between activity and rest.

Spontaneous breathing trial must involve patient triggered ventilation but is valid when performed while breathing on CPAP, on PSV or freely with a tracheostomy mask. The trial must involve a step down in support for a period of 30 min to 2 h. Measures sensitive to wean trial failure reflect a >15% change from baseline values in respiratory rate, heart rate, pulse oximetry <90% or paradoxical breathing pattern with accessory respiratory muscle activity. The most sensitive measure is respiratory rate and pattern.[54] Non-invasive capnography can also be used.[52] Failure of the trial should result in:

- Patient returned to a comfortable well monitored mode of assisted ventilation
- Consideration and optimisation of all remediable factors – patient position, retained secretions/sputum load, pain, sedation, electrolyte derangement, bronchospasm sleep deprivation, etc.
- Review rehabilitation and mobility program
- Repeat trial daily and reassure patient

Protocols should be derived by the multi-professional team utilising published evidence but addressing the specific needs of the patients involved, the clinical preferences and the resources available.[47]

Speaking valve – role in weaning

Tracheostomy patients have a diminished laryngeal abductor and adductor reflex activity which is reinstated on return of airflow through the larynx.[55,56] Thus normal laryngeal function depends on afferent feed forward provided by airflow.

Recurrent aspiration has been found in up to 86% of tracheostomy patients on mechanical ventilation.[11,12] This risk is greatest in the head injury patients and those with posterior fossa lesions due to the associated cranial nerve dysfunction.[8] Not only will they serial aspirate but silently aspirate due to the motor sensory dysfunction.[16] Failure to detect liquid and particulates around the glottis resulting in aspiration has been linked to desensitisation of the larynx.[57,58] Persistent aspiration and bacterial colonisation result in pulmonary infection and recurrent lobar collapse and consolidation which in turn potentiates systemic infiltration and pleural effusion.

A speaking valve is a simple device that uses a one-way valve that allows inspiration via the tracheostomy and then on closing forces air to exit via the patent upper airway. This one-way valve must only be used with an uncuffed tube or a cuffed tube which allows adequate airflow around the deflated cuff (see Chapter 12, Communication).

The Passy Muir is compatible with both mechanical ventilation and external CPAP units, being positioned between the inline suction unit and the rest of the ventilation circuit. This allows for suctioning of the trachea during speaking valve use without having to interrupt the circuit. See Table 4 for an overview of the use Passy Muir speaking valve.

Benefits of the use of a one-way valve for the acute tracheostomised, ventilator dependant patient, is derived by the return of normal upper respiratory

Table 4: Patient using Passy Muir speaking valve while ventilator dependant and progressing onto an external CPAP circuit

Indication
- Patient is conscious, medically stable and maybe mouthing
- Oxygen demand 60% or less
- Tracheostomy >48 h post formation
- Requires multi-professional team agreement
- Is respiratory retraining so must be part of the weaning program

Procedure
- Explain the role and benefits of speaking valve – use models
- Explain it will feel different: throat sore, nose runs, a lot of coughing and an initial increase in respiratory work but will be easier over time and with each trial
- Position is supported sitting with normal head neck alignment or lying in the case of spinal injuries
- Turn off apnoea ventilation mode
- Increase assist to ventilation to offset the expected inspiratory leak – suggest increase PSV (5 cmH$_2$O, decreasing inspiratory trigger value) or increasing CPAP (if only on CPAP) to the next stronger valve
- Clear central airway of secretions and check inner cannula is clean
- Ask patient to clear oro-pharynx – encourage spitting
- Deflate trache cuff at end of inspiration – to suspend supracuff secretions with expiratory flow
- Suction via trache tube
- Connect speaking valve to the inline suction in the ventilator circuit – allows patient to cough and be suctioned during the trial
- Encourage coughing to clear sputum from mouth and trachea
- Encourage patient active breath control – modifying ventilation assist to optimise: respiratory rate, chest expansion, inspiratory leak and SaO$_2$
- Encourage speech

Speaking valve in situ
- Monitor for signs of respiratory fatigue/distress = worsening: respiratory rate, chest expansion, heart rate, inspiratory leak and SaO$_2$

Table 4 (continued)

- Monitor signs of aspiration – bubbling in larynx, unable to clear larynx with coughing, wet/drowning voice increased work of breathing
- Encourage deep breathing, coughing and communication
- Swallow assessment by Speech and Language Therapists when speaking valve regime tolerated for >1 h

Termination
- Increasing work of breathing or persistent laryngeal secretions
- Remove speaking valve from circuit
- Inflate trache cuff – minimal leak technique then check with manometer
- Clear trachea of secretions, ensure inner cannula is clean and encourage inspiratory holds to recruit alveoli
- Reset ventilation support back to original level
- Monitor respiratory function – if beneficial, repeat speaking valve as part of weaning strategy
- Document outcome: duration, ventilation assist required, presence and content of speech, aspiration risk and assessment of respiratory function

function which can shorten the weaning process. Communication, return of a functional cough, re-establishing airway protection reflexes, olfaction, increased FRC, respiratory muscle retraining and stimulation for return of swallow are all associated benefits of speaking valve use as part of the weaning strategy.[59–62] Communication is often positive for the patient and families/loved ones and where possible they should be included in the session.

ROLE OF PHYSIOTHERAPY

The role of physiotherapy in respiratory management of the ICU patient is well established.[63] However it is in the management of a tracheostomy patient that the full scope of that role is realised. With knowledge of respiratory function, neuro-muscular capacity, weaning and rehabilitation; the physiotherapist is essential in the decision and timing of tracheostomy insertion to the patient's eventual discharge.

Initially the physiotherapist assesses the tracheostomy patient for the respiratory complications of: mechanical ventilation, immobility, retained secretions, pulmonary consolidation and acute/progressive atelectasis. In the sedated patient the physiotherapist will advise on therapeutic positions, including prone, for optimising regional ventilation and secretion drainage as part of the teams daily management. The physiotherapist will utilise specific manual techniques to the chest wall and manual hyperinflation, if appropriate, as adjuncts in mobilising secretions and recruiting alveoli. Advice on humidification, review of soft tissue length and joint range are also part of the early physiotherapy management.

As sedation is withdrawn the physiotherapist will collaborate in the formation and implementation of the weaning program from mechanical ventilation. Daily screening of respiratory capacity and weaning protocols by physiotherapists and nursing staff has been shown to decrease time spent to wean.[46,47,51,52]

The physiotherapist will structure an appropriate exercise regime and facilitate early mobilisation as an integral part of the weaning process in order to optimise respiratory recovery.

Working alongside Speech and Language Therapists, the early use of speaking valve in ventilator dependant patients has a dynamic role in weaning. This gain is titrated against the increased respiratory load and aspiration risk associated with early implementation.

In recognition that all tracheostomy patients on ICU will be clinically depressed at some point, the physiotherapist seeks to actively engage the patient with their own rehabilitation, weaning strategy and promotion of functional activity. This strategy extends to the family and loved ones, with the consent of the patient. Wall charts displaying weaning progress both in terms of ventilatory assistance, spontaneous respiratory drive, activity and rest has been found to be an effective tool to inform professionals and actively engage the patient.

A few patients will be successfully extubated while still on ICU but more commonly the tracheostomy tube weaning will be done on the acute wards, rehabilitation units or specialist centres. The physiotherapist will advise on the optimal placement of the tracheostomy patient.

Conclusions

Tracheostomy is an increasingly utilised adjunct in the ICU management of patients predicted to have difficulty in weaning from mechanical ventilation and those at risk of serial pulmonary aspiration. Effective tracheostomy management must involve the multi-professional team in a co-ordinated approach before the point of formation and extends to beyond decannulation. Weaning is achieved through jointly derived protocols that integrate active involvement by the patient and the promotion of mobilisation. There is an emerging role for early speaking valve with ventilator dependant patients as part of the weaning program.

The greatest blocks to ventilatory weaning are related to poor spontaneous respiratory capacity, immobility and depression. The prevalence and consequences of silent aspiration found in the majority of tracheostomy patients presents significant risk to morbidity and mortality. Management must exploit the benefits associated with tracheostomy while minimising the potential risks. The good news is that the complications associated with tracheostomy patients in the ICU are responsive to therapeutic intervention.

REFERENCES

1. Kollef MH, Levy NT, Ahrens TS, Schaiff R, Pretice D, Sherman G. The use of continuous IV sedation is associated with prolongation of mechanical ventilation. *Crit Care Med* 1989; 17: 671–677.
2. Astrachan DI, Kirchner JC, Goodwin WR Jr. Prolonged intubation vs. tracheostomy: Complications, practical and psychological considerations. *Laryngoscope* 1988 (Nov); 98(11): 1165–1169.
3. Colice GL, Stukel TA, Dain B. Laryngeal complication of prolonged intubation. *Chest* 1989; 96: 877–884.
4. Kastanos N, Miro RE, Perez AM. A laryngo-tracheal injury due to endotracheal intubation: Incidence, evolution and predisposing factors: A prospective and long-term study. *Crit Care Med* 1983; 11: 362–367.
5. Pecora DV. Prolonged endotracheal intubation. *Chest* 1982; 82: 130.
6. Heffner JE. Timing of tracheostomy in ventilator-dependent patients. *Clinics in Chest Medicine* 1991; 12(3): 611–625.
7. Whited RE. A prospective study of laryngotracheal sequelae in long-term intubation. *Laryngoscope* 1984; 94: 367–377.
8. Qureshi AI, Suarez JI, Parekh PD, Bhardwaj A. Prediction and timing of tracheostomy in patients with infratentorial lesions requiring mechanical ventilatory support. *Crit Care Med* 2000 (May); 28(5): 1383–1387.
9. Sykes K, Young JD. Principles and practice series. In: Hahn CEW, Adams AP (eds). *Respiratory Support in Intensive Care*, 2nd edn. London: BMJ Publishing Group, 1999.
10. Coakley JH, Nagendraan K, Yarwood GD, Honavara M, Hinds CJ. Patterns of neurophysiological abnormality in prolonged critical illness. *Intens Care Med* 1998; 24(8): 801–807.
11. Nash M. Swallowing problems in the tracheotomized patient. *Otolaryngol Clin North Am* 1988; 21: 701.
12. Mackay LE, Morgan AS, Berstein BA. Swallowing disorders in severe brain injury: Risk factors affecting return to oral intake. *Arch Phys Med Rehabil* 1999; 80: 365–371.
13. Treloar DM, Stechmiller J. Pulmonary aspiration in tube fed patients with artificial airways. *Heart Lung* 1984; 13: 667–671.
14. Cameron JL, Suidema G. Aspiration pneumonia: Magnitude and frequency of the problem. *JAMA* 1972; 219: 1194.
15. DeVita MA, Spierwe-Runback L. Swallowing disorders in patients with prolonged orotracheal intubation or tracheostomy tubes. *Crit Care Med* 1990; 18: 1328–1330.
16. Elpern EH, Scott MG, Petro L, Reis M. Pulmonary aspiration in mechanically ventilated patients with tracheostomies. *Chest* 1994; 105: 563–566.
17. Berlauk JF. Prolonged endotracheal intubation vs. tracheostomy. *Crit Care Med* 1986; 14: 742–745.

18. Tami TA, Chu F, Wildes TO. Pulmonary oedema and acute upper airway obstruction. *Laryngoscope* 1988; 95: 506–509.
19. Bach JR, Saporito LR. Criteria for extubation and tracheostomy tube removal for patients with ventilatory failure. A different approach to weaning. *Chest* 1996; 110: 1566–1571.
20. Davis K Jr, Campbell RS, Johannigman JA, Valente JF, Branson RD. Changes in respiratory mechanics after tracheostomy. *Arch Surg* 1999; 134: 59–62.
21. Mullins JB, Templer JW, Kong J, Davis WE, Hinson J Jr. Airway resistance and work of breathing in tracheostomy tubes. *Laryngoscope* 1993; 103(12): 1367–1372.
22. Maggiore SM, Iacobone E, Zito G, Antonelli M, Proietti R. Closed versus open suctioning techniques. *Minerva Anastesiol* 2002 (May); 68(5): 360–364.
23. Martin C, Perrin G, Gevaudan MJ, Saux P, Goin F. Heat and moisture exchangers and vaporizing humidifiers in the intensive care unit. *Chest* 1990 (Jan); 97(1): 144–149.
24. Tolep K, Getch CL, Criner G. Swallowing dysfunction in patients receiving prolonged mechanical ventilation. *Chest* 1996; 109: 167–172.
25. Cowan T, Op'T Holt TB, Gegenheimer C, Izenberg S, Kulkarni P. Effect of inner cannula removal on the work of breathing imposed by tracheostomy tubes: A bench study. *Resp Care* 2001; 46(5): 460–465.
26. Stock MC, Woodward GC, Sharpiro BA, Cane RD, Lewis V, Pecaro B. Perioperative complications of elective tracheostomy in critically ill patients. *Crit Care Med* 1986; 14: 861–863.
27. Johnson JT, Wagner RL, Sigler BA. Disposable inner cannula trachesotomy tube: A prospective trial. *Otolaryngol Head Neck Surg* 1988; 99: 83–84.
28. Myers EN, Carrau RL. Early complications of tracheostomy. *Clinics in Chest Med* 1991; 12(3): 589–595.
29. Wright PE, Marini JJ, Bernard GR. In vitro versus in vivo comparison of endotracheal airflow resistance. *Am Rev Respir Dis* 1989; 140: 10–16.
30. Siddharth P, Mazzearella L. Granuloma associated with fenestrated tracheostomy tubes. *Am J Surg* 1985; 150: 279–280.
31. Crimlisk JT, Horn MH, Wilson DJ, Marino B. Artificial airways: A survey of cuff management practices. *Heart Lung* 1996 (May–Jun); 25(3): 225–235.
32. Asai T, Shingu K. Leakage of fluid around high volume, low pressure cuffs apparatus: A comparison of four tracheal tubes. *Anaesthesia* 2001 (Jan); 56(5): 38–42.
33. Bernherd WN, Yost L, Joynes D, Cothalis S, Turndorf H. Intracuff pressures in endotracheal and tracheostomy tubes. Related cuff physical characteristics. *Chest* 1985 (Jun); 87(6): 702–705.
34. Wood DE, Mathisen DJ. Late complications of tracheostomy. *Clinics in Chest Medicine* 1991; 12(3): 597–609.
35. Brimacombe J, Kellar C, Giampalmo M, Sparr HJ, Berry A. Direct measurement of mucosal pressures exerted by cuff and non-cuff portions of tracheal tubes with different cuff volumes and head and neck positions. *Br J Anaesth* 1999 (May); 82(5): 663–665.
36. Ganner C. The accurate measurement of endotracheal tube cuff pressure. *Br J Nurs* 2001 (Sep 27–Oct 10); 10(17): 1127–1134.

37. Guyton DC, Barlow MR, Besselievre TR. Influence of airway pressure on minimum occlusive endotracheal tube cuff prerssure. *Crit Care Med* 1997 (Jan); 25(1): 91–94.

38. Crawley BE, Cross DE. Tracheal cuff. A review and dynamic pressure study. *Anaesthesia* 1975; 30(1): 4–11.

39. Inada T, Ueusugi F, Kawachi S, Inada K. The tracheal tube with a high volume, low-pressure cuff at various airway inflation pressures. *Eur J Anaesthesiol* 1998 (Nov); 15(6): 629–632.

40. Hussey JD, Bishop MJ. Pressures required to move gas through the native airway in the presence of a fenestrated vs. a nonfenestrated tracheostomy tube. *Chest* 1996 (Aug); 110(2): 494–497.

41. Heffner JE, Miller KS, Sahn SA. Tracheostomy in the intensive care unit. Part 2: Complications. *Chest* 1986 (Sep); 90(3): 430–436.

42. Heffner JE. Care of the intensive care unit patient with a tracheostomy. *Probl Anesth* 1988; 2: 269–274.

43. Richard I, Giraud M, Perrouin-Verbe B, Hiance D, de la Greve IM, Mathe JF. Laryngotracheal stenosis after intubation or tracheostomy in patients with neurological disease. *Arch Phys Med Rehabil* 1996 (May); 77(5): 493–496.

44. Meade MO, Guyatt GH, Cook DJ. Weaning from mechanical ventilation: The evidence from clinical research. *Resp Care* 2001 (Dec); 46(12): 1408–1415.

45. Esteban A, Alia I, Ibanez J, Benito S, Tobin MJ. Modes of mechanical ventilation and weaning. A national survey of Spanish hospitals. The Spanish Lung Failure Collaborative Group. *Chest* 1994 (Oct); 106(4): 1188–1193.

46. Kollef MH, Sharpario SD, Silver P, St John RE, Prentice D, Sauer S, Ahrens TS, Shannon W, Baker-Clinkscale D. A randomized, controlled trial of protocol-directed versus physician-directed weaning from mechanical ventilation. *Crit Care Med* 1997 (Apr); 25(4): 567–574.

47. Ely EW, Meade MO, Haponik EF, Kollef MH, Guatt GH, Stoller JK. Mechanical ventilator weaning protocols driven by nonphysician health-care professionals: Evidence-base.

48. Bruton A, Conway J, Holgate ST. Weaning adults form mechanical ventilation: Current issues. *Physiotherapy* 1999; 85(12): 652–661.

49. Meade M, Guyatt G, Cook D, Griffith L, Sinuff T, Kergl C, Mancebo J, Esteban A, Epstein S. Predicting success in weaning from mechanical ventilation. *Chest* 2001 (Dec); 120(Suppl 6): 400S–424S.

50. Yang KL, Tobin MJ. A prospective study of indexes predicting the outcome of the outcome of trials of weaning from mechanical ventilation. *N Engl J Med* 1991; 324: 1445–1450.

51. Gluck EH, Corgian L. Predicting eventual success or failure to wean in patients receiving long-term mechanical ventilation. *Chest* 1996; 110: 1018–1024.

52. Scheinhorn DJ, Chao DC, Stearn-Hassenpflug M, Wallace WA. Outcomes in post-ICU mechanical ventilation. A therapist – Implemented weaning protocol. *Chest* 2001; 119: 236–242.

53. Haberthur C, Fabry B, Stocker R, Ritz R, Guttmann J. Additional inspiratory work of breathing imposed by tracheostomy tubes and non ideal ventilator properties in critically ill patients. *Intens Care Med* 1999; 25: 514–519.

54. Rumback MJ, Graves AE, Scott MP, Sporn GK, Walsh FW, McDowell Anderson WM, Goldman AL. Tracheostomy tube occlusion protocol predicts significant tracheal obstruction to air flow in patients requiring prolonged mechanical ventilation. *Crit Care Med* 1997; 25: 413–417.

55. Saski CT, Fukuda H, Kirchner JA. Laryngeal abductor activity in response to varying ventilatory resistance. *Trans Am Acad Opthalmol Otolargol* 1973; 77: 403–409.

56. Saski CT, Suzki M, Horiuchi M. The effect of tracheostomy on reflex laryngeal closure. *Laryngoscope* 1977; 87: 1428–1433.

57. Burgess GE, Cooper JR, Marino RJ. Laryngeal competence after tracheal extubation. *Anaestheiology* 1979; 51: 73–77.

58. Godwin JE, Heffner JE. Special critical considerations in tracheostomy management. *Clinics in Chest Medicine* 1991; 12(3): 573–583.

59. Lichtman SW, Birnbaum IL, Sanfilippo MR, Pellicone JT, Damon WJ, King ML. Effect of A tracheostomy speaking valve on secretions, arterial oxygenation, and olfaction: A quantitative evaluation. *J Speech Hear Res* 1995 (Jun); 38(3): 549–555.

60. Passy V. Passy-Muir tracheostomy speaking valve. *Otolaryngol Head Neck Surgery* 1986; 95: 247–248.

61. Dettelbach MA, Gross RD, Mahlmann S, Eibling DE. Effect of the Passy-Muir valve on aspiration in patients with tracheostomy. *Head & Neck* 1995; 17(4): 297–302.

62. Manzano JL, Lubillo S, Henriquez D, Martin JC, Perez MC, Wilson DJ. Verbal communication of ventilator-dependent patients. *Crit Care Med* 1993 (Apr); 21(4): 512–517.

63. Smith M, Ball V. *Cardiovascular/Respiratory Physiotherapy*. London: Mosby International Limited, 1998.

HUMIDIFICATION

Claudine Billau

The formation of a tracheostomy significantly alters the patient's respiratory physiology. In bypassing the upper respiratory tract, the patient is more susceptible to changes in humidity and there is a consequential change in the function of the respiratory mucosa. Understanding these changes is fundamental to managing these patients effectively (see Chapter 1, Anatomy and Physiology of the Respiratory Tract).

NORMAL MECHANISM OF HUMIDIFICATION

The upper respiratory system: the nose, pharynx, larynx and the trachea (Fig. 1), normally provides an effective system for conditioning inspired gases. As well as acting as a filter for foreign particles and microbes, the upper airway also warms and humidifies inspired gases so that the gas travelling beyond the carina enters the lower airways and the alveoli at body temperature and fully saturated with water vapour.[1] As inspired air enters the upper airway and passes over the nasal turbinates and conchae, gas flow becomes turbulent. This leads to an increase in the number of gas molecules coming into contact with the nasal mucosa. The nasal mucosa is highly vascular and is kept moist by a combination of secretions from mucous glands and direct transudation of fluid through cell walls.[1,2] The secreted mucus is hydroscopic and its viscosity varies depending on its glycoprotein content.[2,3] The turbulent gas flow results in an increasing efficiency in the warming and conditioning of inspired gases by turbulent convection. As the air is warmed, water from the mucosa evaporates and is transferred to the incoming gas.

In normal conditions, when the upper respiratory tract is normal, room air is inhaled at a temperature of around 20°C with a relative humidity of 50%. As it passes across the warmer and more humid mucosa the air becomes progressively warmer and more saturated. When the air reaches body temperature (37°C), it reaches 100% relative humidity. At this point the inspired gases

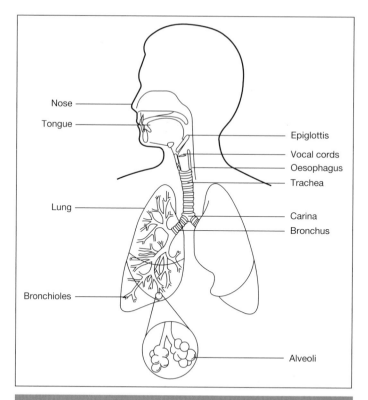

Nose

Tongue

Epiglottis

Vocal cords

Oesophagus

Trachea

Lung

Carina

Bronchus

Bronchioles

Alveoli

Fig. 1: Respiratory anatomy (courtesy of Mallinckrodt).

are said to have reached alveolar conditions. This point is known as the Isothermic Saturation Boundary (ISB).[3] Under normal conditions this point is approximately 5 cm below the carina. This point remains relatively constant, even with the extremes of environmental conditions.[3,4] However as the result of disease processes, or in the presence of a tracheostomy the ISB can be shifted downwards. This places the burden of heat and moisture exchange upon the lower respiratory tract, a job to which it is poorly suited. This burden is further increased by the delivery of cold, anhydrous medical gases, such as oxygen.[2-4] The loss of heat and moisture from the respiratory mucosa has the potential to lead to damage of the respiratory epithelium itself.[5]

Humidity is the amount of water vapour transported by air or other gases; it can be either absolute or relative. Absolute Humidity (AH), is the mass of water held by a volume of gas, where as Relative Humidity (RH) describes, as a percentage, the water vapour content compared to the maximum water vapour that could be held at that given temperature. When the water content is at its maximum, at a given temperature, the gas is saturated.[6] This occurs

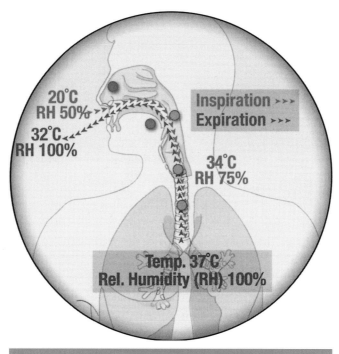

Fig. 2: Human air conditioning (courtesy of Tyco).

under normal conditions at the ISB. Appropriate conditioning of inspired gases is vital to facilitate oxygen exchange in the alveoli.

On expiration, heat is transferred from the alveolar gas at 37°C and 100% RH to the cooler upper respiratory mucosa. Air leaves the nose at approximately 32°C on expiration. As gases cool, their capacity to hold water vapour is reduced. It is at this point that condensation occurs. This in turns leads to a further cooling of the gases due to loss of latent heat of vaporisation.[7] This heat is then transferred back into the respiratory mucosa. The mucosa is thus rewarmed and rehydrated (see Figure 2). The maintenance of this warm and moist environment ensures optimal function of the respiratory tract and its epithelium. The nose and upper respiratory tract act as a counter current heat and moisture exchanger (HME), ensuring that inspired gases are conditioned and cleaned, while retaining heat and moisture on expiration.[8] Maintenance of the correct balance between temperature and relative humidity in the upper airway is important to maintain effective function.[9]

In the presence of a tracheostomy the upper respiratory tract is bypassed. This can lead to a shift in the ISB further down the respiratory tract. If the patient is receiving supplementary oxygen therapy the demands on the natural heat/moisture exchange system are further increased. In order to prevent the adverse effects of under humidification, artificial supplementation will be necessary. Over humidification is not without its dangers. Both issues will be considered.

CONSEQUENCES OF UNDER HUMIDIFICATION

Under humidification of inspired gases can result in changes in respiratory physiology and function. The changes that occur are the result of heat loss, moisture loss and altered pulmonary function.

Heat loss

Heat is lost, predominately from the mucosa, from the latent heat of vaporisation.[3,10] Some of this heat will be lost in the gases expired. In the absence of the upper respiratory tract and inspiration of dry gases the need for water to be vaporised from the respiratory mucosa is increased, so is the loss of heat from the body.[10,11] If this heat loss is excessive it may lead to a drop in body temperature. This in itself is hazardous, particularly in the critically ill, infants and young children.[10]

Moisture loss

In the presence of dry gas inspiration (with or without supplementary medical gases) the respiratory tract is at risk of considerable water loss. This loss of water may lead to dehydration of the ciliated mucosa. This leads to histological changes in the tracheobronchial mucosa (see Table 1 for histological changes).

Most importantly, this can lead to altered function of the mucociliary elevator. The tracheobronchial tree is lined with mucus secreting, ciliated epithelium. The cilia clear any debris collected by the mucous in a cephalad direction. The cilia have long finger like projections at the end of which are claw like structures. The cilia are bathed in low viscosity periciliary mucus.

Table 1: Histological lesions resulting from dry gas inspiration
a. Destruction of cilia and damage to mucous glands
b. Disorganisation and flattening of pseudostratified columnar epithelium and cuboidal epithelium
c. Disorganisation of basement membrane
d. Cytoplasmic and nuclear degeneration
e. Desquamation of cells
f. Mucosal ulceration
g. Reactive hyperaemia following damage

The cilial 'claws' extend through this layer and make contact with a mucus layer of higher viscosity. The claws grip the mucus and propel it and any debris proximally along the tracheobronchial tree. During the recovery stroke, the cilia pass through the periciliary mucus layer. If the layer is too shallow the cilia will stick to the viscid mucus without completing their beat.[5] This will directly affect the clearance of secretions from the tracheobronchial tree. Damage to the mucus secreting glands reduces mucus production and increases viscosity.[12] Reduced function of the mucociliary elevator leads to secretion retention and atelectasis.[3,12,13] Damage to the basement membrane and cells of the airway can lead to bronchiolar collapse and ultimately atelectasis.[13]

Pulmonary function
The downward shift of the ISB during the respiration of dry gases alters the pulmonary mechanics, causing hypoxemia. There is a fall in the functional residual capacity and static compliance with a rise in alveolar arterial oxygen tension difference. These changes are thought to reflect areas of atelectasis with intrapulmonary shunting.[13] Surfactant activity is impaired resulting in increased surface tension and gas exchange impairment.[13,14] Bronchoconstriction can also occur in some individuals.

EFFECTS OF OVER HUMIDIFICATION

Excessive artificial humidification of inspired gases may result in alteration of pulmonary function. If the temperature of inspired gas is above 37°C, with a relative humidity close to 100%, over humidification is possible.

Heat gain
If inspired gases are heated to above body temperature heat may be added to the respiratory system. Mucosal burning, leading to pulmonary oedema and airway stricture may result.[15] A rise in body temperature may also occur.

Moisture gain
Excessive humidification can lead to impaired efficiency of the mucociliary elevator. This may be the result of increased depth of periciliary mucus. This inhibits the cilial 'claws' from propelling the more viscid mucus cephalad. Retention of secretions may result.[5]

Pulmonary function
The ISB may move upward leading to changes in pulmonary function. This includes a reduction in residual capacity and in status compliance leading to atelectasis and arterial hypoxemia.[13,14] Surfactant activity may also be

decreased. This may be due to the inactivation or dilution of surfactant by excess water or by the inhibition of production as the result of atelectasis.[13,14]

ASSESSMENT OF EFFECTIVE HUMIDIFICATION

The effectiveness of humidification is subjective in day-to-day clinical practice. The use of a sputum score is simple and uses descriptors including volume, tenacity and colour as well as the presence and quantity of blood.[2,3,16] The tenacity of secretions can be a useful indicator and readily reassessed when suction is applied.[16]

Thin The suction catheter is clear of secretions following suctioning.

Moderate The suction catheter has secretions adhering to the sides after suctioning which are cleared easily by aspirating water through the catheter.

Thick The suction catheter has secretions adhering to the sides after suctioning which are not removed by aspirating water through the catheter.

This simple scale can be used to help decide the nature of humidification device required.

METHODS OF HUMIDIFICATION

Many different types of humidifiers are available to artificially humidify inspired gases. As well as the ability to deliver adequate levels of heat and moisture to the patient, a humidifier should be safe with no risk of malfunction, electrical hazard or microbiological contamination and possess the appropriate physical properties and are economical to use. The device should be easy to use, clean (if re-usable), and store (see Table 2).

Microbiological safety is of paramount importance, as the functions of the upper respiratory tract are bypassed and organisms are able to enter or leave

Table 2: The properties of an ideal humidifier

- Provision of adequate levels of humidification
- Maintenance of body temperature
- Safety
- Lack of microbiological risk to the patient
- Suitable physical properties
- Convenience
- Economy

the bronchial tree directly. In the case of the tracheostomy patient they may already be severely immunocompromised and thus more susceptible to infection from mircroorganisms. The humidifier used should pose no further microbiological hazard to the patient. Organisms should be unable to survive or multiply within the equipment itself or allow an increase in the incidence of colonisation within the breathing system.[17]

HUMIDIFICATION EQUIPMENT

Several types of humidifier are available. Their use will depend upon the individual needs and status of the patient and their ventilator requirements. Each humidifier will have its own individual properties that will influence the choice of the apparatus to be used.

Cold-Water Humidifiers

Bubble through units (Fig. 3)
Of the more simple humidifiers this is commonly used for supplying humidified medical gases. It comprises of a water reservoir, a diameter safety system (DISS) connector for attachment to a gas source (e.g., a flow metering device), a capillary tube that is submerged in the water reservoir, and an outlet for attachment to a delivery device (a tracheostomy mask).

A dry gas such as oxygen enters the humidifier through a DISS connector, travels down the capillary tubing, and exits via the tip, breaking up into many tiny bubbles. Humidification of the gas bubbles occurs as they rise to the surface of the water. Once at the surface, the gas bubbles burst and their water vapour content is released. Some devices have an open lumen at the end of the capillary tubing while others employ a diffuser tip to enhance the creation of small gas bubbles. Diffuser type humidifiers are more efficient than the capillary tube type of humidifiers because the diffuser has the capacity to create more gas bubbles, therefore allowing a greater surface area for water and

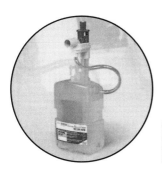

Fig. 3: Cold-water humidification (courtesy of Tyco).

gas interaction.[17] The efficiency of the bubble type humidifiers depends upon the surface area of the water and gas, the time available for the bubbles to remain in contact with the water, and the size of the bubbles. These factors are influenced by the gas flow through the unit (i.e., the higher the flow rate, the less time the bubbles has in contact with the water), the depth of water in the reservoir (i.e., with a deeper reservoir, the bubbles spend longer travelling through the water and therefore acquire greater water content), and the ambient temperature (i.e., the greater the ambient temperature, the lower the relative humidity leaving the device).[17,18] Room air can be entrained into the system so that the gas being delivered can reach room temperature and increase the amount of humidification delivered.[18] Efficiency of the device is related to the gas flow through it. Using a flow rate of approximately 5 l per minute humidification is thought to be at it greatest.[18] At flow rates above this, delivered humidity decreases as a result of the reduction in time the gas spends in contact with the reservoir water. The temperature will also be reduced.

Complications of cold-water humidifiers include:

- Microbiological colonisation of the reservoir water.[18] (Water reservoirs should be changed every 24 h to prevent infection.)
- High flow rates required to support some levels of oxygen therapy could reduce the levels of humidification achieved. They may also produce an aerosol, which could transport water-bred microbes from the humidifier or the delivery tubing.
- Leakage can occur from the equipment. Regular checks should be carried out to ensure that the reservoir chamber contains sufficient water at all times.
- Mobilisation of the patient can be limited as the equipment is not really portable.

Hot-Water Humidifier (Fig. 4)

These devices produce heated water vapour, using a variety of methods to provide a heat source. Many have submerged sources within a water reservoir, while others will employ an adjacent heat source or heating chambers or plates to vaporise part of the reservoir at a time. In theory they are the most versatile of humidifiers. The absolute humidity of inspired gases can be altered by changing the temperature in the water bath.[2,3,10] As the temperature increases so does the absolute humidity, saturating more vapour than is possible with the cold-water method.[3,4,19] This method of humidification may help to restore the isothermic boundary to a near normal position by producing sufficiently humidified gases at a normal physiological temperature and saturation.

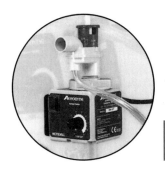

Fig. 4: Heated water humidification (courtesy of Tyco).

Complications of hot-water humidifiers include:

- Patient discomfort: the warmed gases delivered via tracheostomy mask can be uncomfortable and may need to be reduced.
- Excessive temperatures can lead to burning of the airways.
- 'Rain out': this occurs when water vapour cools along the length of the tubing and condenses. Care should be taken to ensure that the excess water is not accidentally introduced into the tracheostomy tube. Water traps introduced within the tubing, near the patient, make collection and disposal of this condensed water easier. Heated wires running the length of the tubing also help to minimise this problem.[13]
- Mobilisation of the patient will be limited. This type of equipment needs to be maintained in a static position. As the water within the reservoir is heated and spillage may lead to burning. Thermostatic control of temperature is also sensitive to movement.

Heat and Moisture exchangers

HME's (Fig. 5) are a group of humidification devices generically referred to as 'Artificial noses' or 'Swedish noses'. The term artificial nose comes from the similarity in function to the human nose. By definition, an artificial nose is a passively acting humidifier that collects the patient's expired heat and moisture and returns it during the following inspiration.[20] There are several types of artificial nose/HME. Although design may differ between devices the physical principals of conserving heat and moisture are common to all.

The four types of artificial nose/HME are:

- Heat and moisture exchanger (HME)
- Heat and moisture exchanging filter (HMEF)
- Hygroscopic heat and moisture exchanger (HHME)
- Hygroscopic heat and moisture exchanging filter (HHMEF)

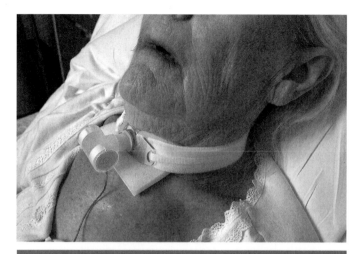

Fig. 5: Heat and moisture exchanger.

The HME is the simplest of these devices. An HME usually consists of a layered aluminium inset with or without the addition of a fibrous element. Aluminium exchanges temperature quickly, and during expiration condensation forms between the layers. The retained heat and moisture are returned during inspiration. In addition the fibrous element aids the retention of moisture and helps reduce the pooling of condensate in dependent areas of the device.[20]

The HMEF have a spun filter media, often with an increased surface area (the result of pleating). This is felt to attribute to its increased moisture retaining ability.

The HHME uses a paper or polypropylene inset treated with a hydroscopic chemical, usually calcium or lithium chloride, to enhance moisture conservation.

The HHMEF employs all of the previously mentioned elements.

The artificial nose has specific advantages over other methods of humidification. They are relatively inexpensive, simple to use and portable. As there is no cumbersome equipment attached to the patient using an artificial nose facilitation of mobility is greatly improved.

Complications of heat/moisture exchangers include:

- Patients who have established respiratory pathology productive of tenacious secretions or those with an acute respiratory tract infection or blood in their secretions may not be suitable for this type of humidification.
- They may become occluded by water and/or secretions.

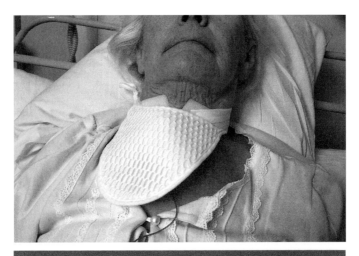

Fig. 6: Buchanan bib (stomal protectors).

STOMA PROTECTOR/TRACHEAL BIB

Patients with a long-term tracheostomy often use a stoma protector (Fig. 6) to aid humidification. A crude but useful device that is re-usable and easily cared for. It also offers a degree or cosmesis, as not only does it hide the tracheostomy but it also controls the flow of expectorated air or secretions. A moist piece of gauze can be used to similar effect and disposed of when soiled. Although these methods provide humidification they are insufficient during an acute phase or immediately following tracheostomy formation. In phases of acute infection an increase in humidification may be required.

The lower respiratory tract may adapt to provide greater heat and moisture exchange capabilities over time where the need for supplementary humidification may therefore be reduced. In these instances the stoma protector may be sufficient.

Careful observation of secretion viscosity will give an indication when a change in the nature of humidification is required.

NEBULISATION

Humidification provides the respiratory system with water vapour held in a gas source. The particular size is extremely small and not visible to the naked eye.[21] Nebulisation produces a mist saturated with water droplets. The water content is greater than that of humidified gas, and due to the particle size, penetrates further down the respiratory tree.[21] Nebulisation can increase

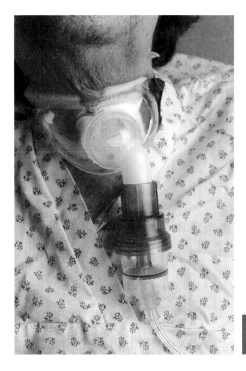

Fig. 7: Nebuliser and tracheostomy mask.

sputum clearance of those patients with chronically elevated sputum levels.[22,23] It is also used to administer medicines to peripheral areas of the lungs. Although it can be used to boost humidification it is not an alternative. Long-term, prolonged use can lead to fluid overload and increased airway resistance.[23] A nebuliser can be used in circuit or delivered via a tracheostomy mask (Fig. 7).

Summary

In a situation where the upper respiratory tract is bypassed the normal mechanisms of humidification and conditioning of inspired gases are compromised. This situation is further exacerbated if dry, anhydrous medical gases are used. To ensure that optimal respiratory function is maintained it is essential that humidification is provided. The clinician should be aware of the devices available to supplement humidification.

Appropriate assessment and criteria should be established before a choice of humidification is made. A patient's status should be continually reviewed and appropriate changes to the levels of humidification carried out in accordance with these findings.

Many hospitals and clinicians will have their individual preference for the type of humidification equipment available to their patients. Each type should be considered for its own merits and design abilities. The type/nature of the device used should primarily meet the clinical needs of the patient.

Care and observation of the equipment used is of vital importance, especially those with water reservoirs. These are susceptible to spillage and evaporation. Reservoirs should be re-filled or changed in accordance with the manufacturers or hospital guidelines.

The use of the portable methods, HME or stoma protector has great advantages. However the clinician should ensure that the device used is changed/cleaned regularly to prevent possible complications. Supplementary methods of humidification such as nebulisation should not be substituted for appropriate primary humidification.

Key Points

- Adequate humidification is essential to respiratory function.
- When a tracheostomy is formed the upper respiratory tract is bypassed. As the normal mechanisms of humidification will not be functioning it is essential that alternative methods of humidification be used.
- The clinician should make themselves aware of the methods of humidification available.
- Selection of the device used for humidification should meet the clinical needs of the individual patient. One type of humidification will not be appropriate for all patients.
- Frequent re-assessment of the patient's humidification requirements is essential, (sputum tenacity is one simple method).
- Nebulisation is not a substitute for adequate humidification.
- Humidification devices should be cared for and cleaned/changed regularly.

REFERENCES AND FURTHER READING

1. Shelly MP. Measurement of humidification. *Br J Inten Care* 1997; 9: 1–6.
2. Shelly MP, Lloyd GM, Park GR. A review of the mechanisms and methods of humidification of inspired gases. *Intens Care Med* 1998; 14: 1–9.
3. Shelly MP. *Basic Principles of Humidification. Humidification Handbook*. Sweden: Hudson, 2000.
4. Fowler S. A guide to humidification. *Nurs Times* 2000 (May).
5. Sleigh MA, Blake JR, Liron N. State of the art: The propulsion of mucus by cilia. *Am Rev Resp Dis* 1988; 137: 726–741.
6. Walker JEC, Wells RE, Merrill EW. Heat and water exchange in the respiratory tract. *Am J Med* 1961; 30: 259–267.

7. Nolan DM. Problems of inadequate humidification. *Prob Resp Care* 1991; 4: 413–417.
8. Forbes AR. Temperature, humidity and mucus flow in the intubated trachea. *Br J Anaesth* 1974; 46(1): 29–34.
9. Dery R, Pelletier J, Jacques A, Clavet M, Houde JJ. Humidity in anaesthesiology III: Heat and moisture patterns in the respiratory tract during anaesthesia with the semi-closed system. *Can Anaes Soc J* 1967; 14: 287–298.
10. Miyao H, Hirokawa T, Miyasaka K, Kawazoe T. Relative humidity, not absolute humidity, is of great importance when using a humidifier with a heating wire. *Crit Care Med* 1992; 20: 674–679.
11. Rashad K, Wilson K, Hunt HH, Graff TD, Benson DW. Effects of humidification of anaesthetic gases and static compliance. *Anesth Analg* 1967; 46(1): 27–33.
12. Conway JH, Holgate ST. Humidification for patients with chronic chest disease. *Prob Resp Care* 1991; 4: 463–467.
13. Jackson C, Webb AR. An evaluation of heat and moisture exchange performance of four ventilator circuit filters. *Intens Care Med* 1992; 18: 264–268.
14. Jackson C. Humidification in the upper respiratory tract: A physiological overview. *Intens Crit Care Nurs* 1996; 12: 27–32.
15. Klein EF, Graves SA. 'Hot pot' tracheitis. *Chest* 1974; 65: 225–226.
16. Suzukawa M, Usuda Y, Numata K. The effects of sputum characteristics of combining an unheated humidifier with heat-moisture exchanging filter. *Resp Care* 1989; 34: 967–984.
17. Darin J. The need for rational criteria for the unheated bubble humidifiers. *Resp Care* 1982; 27: 945–947.
18. Darin J, Braodwell J, MacDonell R. An evaluation of water vapour output from four brands of unheated, prefilled bubble humidifiers. *Resp Care* 1982; 27: 41–50.
19. Estey W. Subjective effects of dry versus humidified low flow oxygen. *Resp Care* 1990; 35: 1265–1266.
20. Cigada M, Elena A, Solca M, Damia G. The efficiency of twelve heat moisture exchangers: An in vitro evaluation. *Int Care World* 1990; 7: 98–101.
21. Graff TD, Benson DW. Systemic and pulmonary changes with inhaled humid atmospheres. *Anaesthesiology* 1969; 30: 199–207.
22. Conway JH, Fleming JS, Perring S, Holgate ST. Humidification as an adjunct to chest physiotherapy in aiding tracheobronchial clearance in patients with bronchiectasis. *Resp Med* 1992; 86: 109–114.
23. Modell JH, Moya F, Ruiz B. Blood gas and electrolyte during exposure to ultrasonic nebulised aerosols. *Br J Anaesth* 1968; 40: 20–26.

SUCTIONING

Claudine Billau

Tracheal suctioning is a necessary intervention in the management of a patient with a tracheostomy.

Maintaining this artificial airway is a crucial aspect of care. Appropriate suction will stimulate the cough reflex and prevent accumulation of secretions, which can block the tracheostomy.

The artificial airway created by the tracheostomy affects the normal function of the respiratory tract (see Chapter 1, Anatomy and Physiology of the Respiratory Tract). The normal actions of the ciliated membrane, the local immune system and the cough reflex are inhibited.[1] In addition, the drying effect of air on the tracheobronchial mucous membrane is also increased, as the normal warming; filtering action of the nose is bypassed. This in turn causes paralysis of the cilia,[2] and the mucociliary apparatus becomes less effective,[1] and the respiratory tract more vulnerable to opportunist organisms. Furthermore, the tracheostomy can result in an increase in mucus production,[3] a reduction in premyocytes and surfactant thereby influencing gaseous exchange and the elasticity of pulmonary tissue.[4,5] Coupled with an inability to expectorate this material, which is often tenacious,[2] removal of these secretions by suction from the tracheostomy tube forms a significant aspect of care of the airway.

The frequency of suction required will depend upon the individual patients need and should not be considered a routine procedure.[6] Given the serious nature of the potential consequences of suctioning, the health care professional (HCP) should base suction protocols on solid clinical research data, which indicates the safest, least traumatic suctioning technique.[6,7] The HCP should perform a thorough assessment of the patient before suction is undertaken.

ASSESSMENT PRIOR TO SUCTIONING

Patients need to be suctioned when they are unable to effectively clear their airway, i.e. 'A state in which an individual is unable to clear secretions or obstructions from the respiratory tract to maintain airway patency'.[7] The signs of ineffective airway clearance are shown in Table 1.

If any of the aforementioned signs are evident during general observation of the patient, a thorough assessment should then be made to establish if the need for suction is indicated. A stethoscope, pulse-oximetry and measurements of arterial blood gas levels (if available) will be useful when assessing the need for suction. Table 2 highlights the salient points to be noted when considering a patient for suction.

Table 1: Patient assessment to indicate suctioning

Signs	Reason
Abnormal breath sounds	Excessive inspiratory/expiratory sounds caused by secretions in or below the tracheostomy tube.
Irregular respiratory pattern	Breathing rate may be increased. Accessory muscle activity may be evident. Increased work of breathing.
Changes in secretions:	
• Quantity	Increase in production by presence of tracheostomy. Presence of 'foreign body', secondary infection.
• Tenacity	Due to inadequate humidification, secondary infection.
• Colour	Presence of blood. Colour changes related to infection.
Increase in coughing	Irritation caused by excess uncleared secretions. Irritation caused by tracheostomy movement.
Change in skin colour/ SaO$_2$	Clammy/cyanosed. Poor perfusion/oxygenation as a result of decreased respiratory efficiency.
Anxious appearance	Patient may appear distressed due to difficulties in breathing.

Table 2: Patient assessment

- Heart rate and rhythm
- Skin colour
- Respiratory rate and pattern
- Auscultation of chest
- Noisy and/or moist respirations?
- Alteration in the amount and consistency of secretions?
- Decrease in oxygen saturation?
- Increase in coughing (which may indicate ineffective airway clearance)?

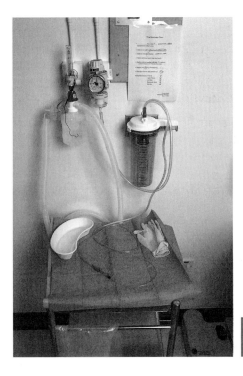

Fig. 1: Wall suction unit and oxygen delivery system.

Once assessment has established the need for suction to be carried out the HCP should ensure all relevant equipment is available at the bedside before proceeding.

Equipment needed to suction

- A functional suction unit (wall suction unit – Figure 1, portable suction unit – Figure 2)
- Sterile catheters
- Disposable gloves
- O_2 therapy – wall flow meter/portable bottle and tracheostomy mask (Fig. 1)
- Sterile water and bowl (labelled 'for cleaning suction tubing' with opening date)
- Yankeur suction catheter
- Protective eyewear/facemask

Selecting a suction catheter

Choosing the right size suction catheter is essential for safe and efficient suctioning. The external diameter of the suction catheter should not be greater than half of the internal diameter of the tracheostomy tube.[1,6,8] The formula for

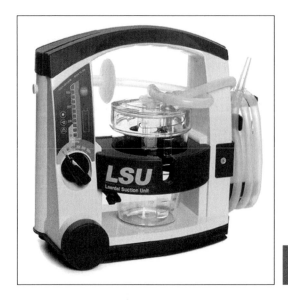

Fig. 2: Portable suction unit (courtesy of Laerdal).

choosing a catheter is as follows:

1. Divide the internal diameter (mm) of the tracheostomy tube by 2, this gives the external diameter (mm) of the catheter.
2. Multiply this by 3 (to obtain the French gauge): e.g., a size 8 tracheostomy tube.
3. $8 \div 2 = 4$ (external diameter) of catheter.
4. $4 \times 3 = 12$ (French gauge).
5. Therefore the appropriate catheter is a size 12.

See Table 3.

PRE-SUCTION PREPARATION

Suctioning can be a frightening and unpleasant experience for the patient. The HCP should give adequate explanation and reassurance before the procedure is undertaken. Where possible, consent should be gained. The procedure should be performed with confidence and speed.[6] The ideal suctioning technique is one in which maximum removal of secretions is achieved with the minimum of tissue damage and hypoxia.[7,9,10,11]

Before beginning the procedure the following infection control methods should be used:

- Hand hygiene; wash hands and wear disposable gloves.
- A plastic apron should be worn, both to protect your clothing and other patients that you may make subsequent contact with.

Table 3: Appropriate suction catheter size according to tracheostomy inner diameter

Tracheostomy tube		Suction catheter	
Internal diameter (mm)	French gauge (Fg)	French gauge (Fg)	External diameter (mm)
3	14	5	1.6
4	16	6	2.0
5	19	8	2.6
6	23	10	3.3
7	27	10	3.3
8	30	12	4.0
9	35	14	4.5
10	38	14	4.5

- Wear protective goggles/facemask especially if infective secretions are suspected.
- The tubing and collection container should be changed every 24 h to minimise further risk of infection (or as per local guidelines).

Patient preparation
- If possible gain consent from the patient. Ensure that adequate explanation in hand is given to the patient. Suctioning is an unpleasant procedure, explanation will minimise distress and enhance co-operation.[12]
- Hyperoxygenation for 3 min prior to suctioning will help to maintain adequate arterial O_2 levels and reduce the risk of hypoxia and cardiac arrhythmia.[1,12,13–15] It should be noted at this point that patients with chronic obstructive pulmonary disease (COPD) should only have a 20% increase in the oxygenation they receive as they may have a dependence on CO_2 levels to maintain their respiratory drive.[16,17]

Equipment preparation
- Check that the suction apparatus is functioning and that the vacuum pressure is set between 13.5–20 kPa/100–150 mmHg (Fig. 1).[11,17] Limiting the negative pressure will help to reduce the risk of mucosal damage, hypoxemia and atelectasis.[1,7,13,17]
- Select a suitably sized sterile catheter, open and attach to the suction apparatus.
- Put a clean disposable glove onto the dominant hand. Avoid touching anything except the catheter with it. This will help to reduce the risk of infection and to ensure the technique is as clean as possible.

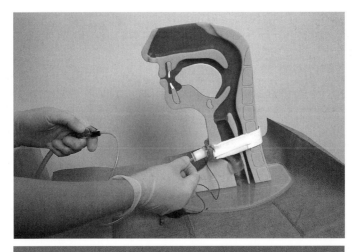

Fig. 3: Insertion of a suction catheter.

Suction technique

- Reassure the patient before proceeding. Ensure that the suction part on the catheter is uncovered before introducing it into the tracheostomy (Fig. 3). The catheter should be introduced quickly and gently to a depth one-third of its length (approximately 15 cm)[3] or until the patient coughs[18,19] or resistance is met indicating the bifurcation of the trachea.[2,20,21] As mucosal trauma can be caused simply by catheter contact during insertion,[22] suction must be off during insertion. Once this point is reached the catheter should be withdrawn approximately 1 cm before suction is applied.[23] Suction should be continuous and last for a maximum of 10–15 s.[19,20] Prolonged suction times may result in hypoxia.[13,14] During this period the catheter should be steadily withdrawn to allow most effective clearance of secretions.[15]
- When the catheter is completely removed from the tracheostomy tube, release suction, wrap around dominant hand, enclose in glove and discard.
- Reapply the patients O_2 supply immediately (within 10 s).[15] This should be maintained until the pre-suctioning oxygen parameters return; this will help to reduce the risk of further hypoxia.[17]
- The suction tubing should then be cleaned by decanting enough clean water into a bowl to flush through the tubing; this will prevent the tubing from becoming blocked and reduce the risk of infection. Excess water should be discarded.
- The suction catheter and glove should be disposed of according to health and safety guidelines.

- If the procedure needs to be repeated, a fresh clean glove and a new sterile catheter will be needed. The process should then be repeated following the above steps as indicated.

The number of suction passes should be limited to three during each episode[13,17] to minimise the potential complications associated with suction. These include hypoxia, cardiac arrhythmias, pneumothorax, ulceration and necrosis of the trachea, pain, excessive coughing, anxiety and infection. (See Table 4 for further information.) The patient should be allowed sufficient time to recover between each suction, particularly if oxygen saturation levels are low, or if the patient coughs several times during the procedure. Suction can be a traumatic experience, reassurance should be given and adequate recovery time allowed to prevent exhaustion and to minimise distress.

Table 4: Potential complications of tracheal suctioning

Complications	Minimising the risks
Hypoxia Suction induces arterial oxygen de-saturation (PaO$_2$ less than 50 mmHg).	• Pre/post-oxygenation with 100% O$_2$.[13,22] • Ensure correct catheter size, i.e. the catheter is half the inner diameter of the tracheostomy tube.[1,6,23] • Suction for no more than 15 s.[2,17,24] • Suction pressure should be 13.5–20 kPa/100–150 mmHg.[17] • The use of CSMU's will allow continual supply of both O$_2$ and ventilatory support.[24,25] • Adequate recovery time between each procedure.
Cardiac arrhythmias Thought to result from a combination of hypoxia and vagal stimulation leading to bradycardia due to introduction of the suction catheter or movement of the tracheal tube.	• Pre-oxygenation with 100% O$_2$.[26,27] • Nebulised atropine can be used to prevent bradycardia and hypotension under medical direction.[13,23,25]
Pneumothorax Reported by Anderson (1976) in neonates secondary to perforation of	• The catheter should be passed carefully and gently. • The catheter should only pass one-third of its length[3] or before meeting with resistance or stimulating a cough reflex, do not force the

Table 4 (continued)	
Complications	**Minimising the risks**
segmental bronchi by the suction catheter. Imperfect suction techniques may increase the incidence in adults.[27,28]	catheters' passage beyond this point as it will increase the risk of pneumothorax[27,28] or damage to the tracheobronchial tree.[13]
Ulceration/necrosis of the trachea The most commonly recognised hazard of tracheal suctioning.	• Only suction when assessed to be necessary. • Minimise the number of times suction is carried out, this should be limited to a maximum of three times each session.[17] • Minimise the effects of negative pressure, both by using the correct size catheter (see Table 3) and setting the suction unit to pressures of 13.5–20 kPa/100–150 mmHg.[17,21] • Once the suction catheter has passed into the tracheostomy tube and stimulated a cough reflex or has met with resistance, it should be withdrawn by 1 cm before suction is applied to prevent tracheal mucosa invagination into the catheter end. • Once suction is applied, the catheter should be kept moving to prevent invagination of the mucosa through the side holes.[15,22] The only recommended suction catheter is a multi-eyed catheter, which has a special tip, which prevents the side holes coming into contact with the tracheal mucosa causing least possible trauma.[10] • If the patient is conscious they should be encouraged to assist with clearance techniques the physiotherapist has suggested, this will help mobilise the secretions towards the end of the tracheostomy tube making clearance easier.
Excessive coughing Can be caused by accidental movement of the tracheostomy tube or suctioning. This can lead to exhaustion and also causes increases in intra-thoracic,	• Ensuring that the tracheostomy is well positioned and fitted and that the tube ties are secure to keep tube movement to a minimum. • Suction only when appropriate. • Ensure that the patient receives adequate analgesia and a sedative if necessary. Morphine or one of its derivatives can provide the answer to both these problems as well as suppression of

Table 4 (continued)	
Complications	**Minimising the risks**
intra-abdominal and intra-cranial pressures. There is also a risk of rib fracture.[13]	the cough reflex. It should be taken into consideration that it also acts as a respiratory depressant.
Anxiety Suctioning can be an uncomfortable, even frightening experience. It may lead to tachycardia and hypertension. The patient may actively resist treatment.	• Adequate explanation and reassurance can reduce stress and assist with patient compliance.
Infection Due to bypass of the upper airway where anti-microbial defence mechanisms are centred.[13]	• Ensure clean technique when suctioning. • Suction catheters are single use only. • Only suction when appropriate. • The use of CSMU's will help reduce the risk of infection transmission. • Dispose of equipment. • Wear eye protection, gloves and apron.

Special considerations

- It is essential that before suction is undertaken by the clinician, they are aware of the type of tracheostomy tube that the patient has in place. If the tracheostomy tube is fenestrated, the clinician must ensure that the unfenestrated inner cannula is in position before proceeding. Suction should not be performed when a fenestrated cannula is present, as this may allow the catheter to pass out of the fenestration, leading to possible damage to the posterior tracheal wall.

Care of the inner cannula

It is recommended that all adult patients with a tracheostomy should have a tube system with an inner cannula, unless contra-indicated. The inner cannula is removed (Fig. 4) and either disposed of, if re-usable, or can be cleaned and replaced. The inner tube should be checked every 4 h to ensure patency.

Warm running water and a tracheostomy cleaning brush should be used for cleaning (Fig. 5). Brushes should be cleaned under use, allowed to air dry, stored in a container and should be replaced daily.

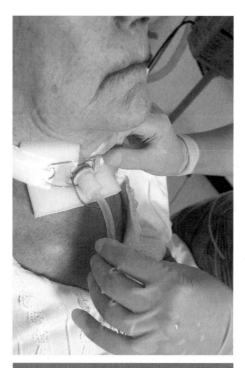

Fig. 4: Removal of the inner tube.

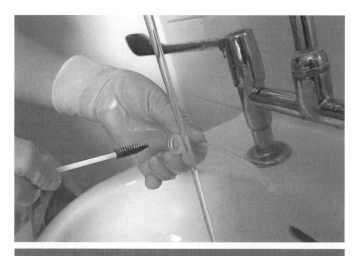

Fig. 5: Cleaning of the inner tube.

Special considerations for care of an inner cannula:

- Changing of the inner cannula can stimulate coughing as a result of pressure being applied to the tube.
- Following suction the inner cannula should be removed and cleaned before being replaced.
- Collection of secretions in the inner cannula may give indication that humidification of the patient is insufficient (see Chapter 8, Humidification).
- Care of the tracheostomy inner cannula is an essential aspect of tracheostomy care by the clinician.

CLOSED SYSTEM MULTIPLE USE SUCTION UNITS (Fig. 6)

This type of suction catheter is predominantly seen in the ITU/critical care environment. Its use is indicated when a patient is highly dependent on ventilatory support to maintain O_2 saturation i.e. those patients receiving IPPV (intermittent positive pressure ventilation) with high levels of PEEP (positive end expiratory pressure). It may also be of benefit when a patient has infected/copious secretions, which may leave those caring for them at risk of cross infection.

The CMSU consists of a catheter contained in a plastic outer sheath, which allows the catheter to be inserted into the patient's tracheostomy on repeated occasion without the need to change it. As the system remains closed to the patient it prevents introduction of external bacteria, exposing the patient only to those, which are common to them. The catheter is attached via an external

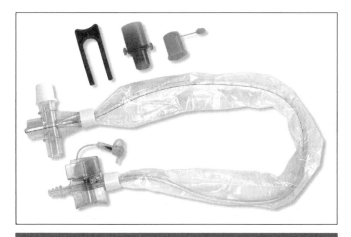

Fig. 6: Closed suction unit (courtesy of Portex).

catheter mount, which is close to the device. The catheters come in two lengths, one suitable for endotracheal tubes and the other being shorter specifically designed for use with tracheostomy tubes. It should be noted that, if an adjustable flanged tracheostomy is present the use of the shorter CMSU might be inappropriate.

The weight of the catheter and mount is liable to cause excessive movement of the tracheostomy tube as the external protrusion or the tracheostomy is greater than that of other types of tracheostomies. The excessive movement could lead to damage of the trachea itself, excessive coughing and discomfort and has been attributed to granulation tissue at the stoma site.

The CMSU sits on a catheter mount and remains closed off to the tracheostomy tube until it is required for use. Before proceeding with suction the HCP should follow the previously discussed steps for safe and clean practice. The patient should be given a full, unambiguous explanation of the procedure, which is about to take place.

Technique for use of a closed system multiple use suction unit

- The suction port of the catheter mount should be opened, and the catheter introduced into the tracheostomy tube (the outer plastic sheath allows repeated re-use of the catheter and provides protection from external pathogens). Bunching of the external sheath may occur on introduction, to prevent this, ensure that the sheath passes behind the hand with each advancement.
- When withdrawing the catheter hold the catheter mount to reduce the risk of disconnection or tube migration, which may cause trauma to the tracheal wall.[18,19]
- The tip of the catheter should be withdrawn 1 cm upon feeling resistance to its advancement, before suction is applied, to reduce the risk of trauma to the tracheal mucosa and carina.[19,20]
- The procedure should be repeated if necessary. Allow adequate recovery time between each suctioning to reduce the risk of hypoxia and tiring the patient.
- Once suctioning is complete the catheter should be withdrawn until the black marking is visible within the chamber of the suction mount. If applicable 'lock off' the port before cleaning the catheter with 5–10 ml of normal saline 0.9%. This can be introduced through the installation port.
- The CSMU should be marked with the date and time at which its use commenced. It should be changed according to manufacturers and local guidelines. This should be every 24 h, unless the nature of the secretions being cleared dictates it sooner.

What to do when a suction catheter cannot be passed?

- In an acute situation when obstruction of the tracheostomy tube by secretions is suspected the following procedures can be undertaken.

  - In the case of a cannulated tracheostomy tube, the inner cannula should be removed and cleaned before being replaced.
  - In the case of a single lumen tracheostomy tube, installation of a small amount of sterile 0.9% saline may be used to initiate a strong cough response, which aids the removal of secretions and subsequent removal by suctioning. Practical experience supports this practice, however, some evidence is contradictory therefore this should not be a routine procedure.

- Passage of a suction catheter can help determine an inner tube patency. It may give early indication of partial occlusion or dislodge a blockage.

Summary

Despite the risks associated with tracheobronchial suctioning it remains an essential aspect of tracheostomy care. The clinicians' awareness of the physiological state of the patient and the factors, which may contribute to the hazards encountered, should ensure a safe approach both to the procedure and the outcome of the patient.[13]

It is crucial that suction is not seen as a benign and routine procedure. Practice must be based on knowledge validated by research since healthcare professionals are accountable for their actions and the quality of care given.[2] A formal process of clinical support, such as clinical supervision, will enable clinicians to develop their knowledge and competence, enabling them to take responsibility for their own practice.

This chapter has attempted to highlight the best practice from the current research available. Many hospitals will have their own established protocols for practice, which the HCP should make him/herself aware of.

Key points

- Tracheal suctioning is a frequent and necessary intervention in the management of a patient with a tracheostomy.
- Suctioning should never be carried out as a routine procedure. Only after assessment has established a need, should the procedure be undertaken.
- Suctioning is not without its hazards. The clinician should be aware of these risks and how to minimise them.

- Suction is a clean technique. Hospital protocols should be acknowledged, along with guidelines for best practice.
- It is the responsibility of the clinician to ensure that their knowledge and training is sufficient to facilitate best and safe practice. A training and education package should be available to meet these needs. This should be constantly reviewed and updated in accordance with research. All practice should be evidence based.

REFERENCES

1. Odell A, Allder A, Bayne R, Everatt C, Scott S, Still B, West S. Endotracheal suction for adult, non-head injured patients: A review of the literature. *Inten & Crit Care Nurs* 1993; 9: 274–278.
2. McEleney M. Endotracheal suction. *Prof Nurs* 1998; 13: 220–227.
3. Hooper M. Nursing care of the patient with a tracheostomy. *Nurs Stand* 1996; 10: 40–44.
4. Ackerman MH. The effect of saline lavage prior to suctioning. *Am J Crit Care* 1993; 2: 326–330.
5. Bostick J, Wendglass ST. Normal saline instillation as part of the suctioning procedure: Effects on PaO_2 and amount of secretions. *Heart Lung* 1987; 16: 532–537.
6. Burglass E. Tracheostomy care: Tracheal suctioning and humidification. *Br J Nurs* 1999; 8: 500–504.
7. Shekelton ME, Neild M. Ineffective airway clearance related to artificial airway. *Nurs Clin N Am* 1987; 22: 167–178.
8. Carroll PF. Safe suctioning PRN. *Regist Nurs* 1994; 57(5): 32–37.
9. Young CS. A review of the adverse effects of airway suction. *Physiotherapy* 1984; 3: 104–105.
10. Landa JF, Kwoka MA. Effects of suctioning on mucociliary transport. *Chest* 1980; 77: 202–208.
11. Sackner MA, Landa JF, Greeneltch N, Robinson MJ. Pathogenesis and prevention of tracheobronchial damage with suction procedures. *Chest* 1973; 64: 3.
12. Regan M. Tracheal mucosal injury – The nurse's role. *Nursing* 1988; 29: 1064–1066.
13. Fiorentini A. Potential hazards of tracheobronchial suctioning. *Inten & Crit Care Nurs* 1992; 8: 217–226.
14. Carroll PF. Lowering the risks of endotracheal suctioning. *Nursing* 1988; 18(5): 46–50.
15. Day T. Tracheal suctioning: When, why and how. *Nurs Times (supplement)* 2000; 96(20): 13–15.
16. Hough A. *Physiotherapy in Respiratory Care*. London: Chapman and Hall, 1996.
17. Glass CA, Grap MJ. Ten tips for safer suctioning. *Adv J Nurs* 1995; 5: 51–53.
18. Fuchs PL. Streamlining your suctioning techniques. Part 2: Endotracheal suctioning. *Nursing* 1984; 14: 46–51.
19. Czarnik RE, Stone KS, Everhart CC, Preusser BA. Differential effects of continuous versus intermittent suction on tracheal tissue. *Heart Lung* 1991; 20(2): 144–151.
20. Fluck RR. Suctioning – Intermittent or continuous? *Resp Care* 1985; 30: 837–838.

21. St. George's Healthcare NHS Trust. *Guidelines for the Care of Patients with Tracheostomy Tubes.* London: St. George's NHS Trust, 2000.

22. Young CS. Recommended guide lines for suction. *Physiotherapy* 1984; 3: 106–107.

23. Meyer-Holloway N. *Nursing the Critically Ill Adult,* 4th edn. California: Addison-Wesley, 1993.

24. Laws-Chapman C. Tracheostomy tube management. *Care Crit Ill* 1998; 14: 120–130.

25. Fuchs PL. Providing tracheostomy care. *Nursing* 1983; 7: 19–23.

26. Naigow D, Dowser MM. The effect of different endotracheal suction procedures on arterial blood gases in a controlled experimental model. *Heart Lung* 1977; 6: 808–816.

27. Rudy EB, Turner BS. Endotracheal suctioning in adults with head injury. *Neuro Asp Crit Care* 1991; 6: 667–674.

28. Anderson K, Chandra K. Pneumothorax secondary to perforation of sequential bronchi by suction catheter. *J Plast Surg* 1976; 11: 687–693.

WOUND CARE

Claire Scase

INTRODUCTION

The aim of managing a tracheostomy wound is to promote healing and prevent complications associated with the surgical stoma or incision. A tracheostomy stoma can be classified as a full thickness wound due to the anatomical level of affected tissue.

This chapter will focus on strategies to promote skin integrity surrounding the tracheostomy stoma and suggested treatments for use in tissue compromise or breakdown. It is important to appreciate the effect the tracheostomy tube has on the stoma and the detrimental effect of continual secretions emanating from the wound directly on to the surface of the skin and the surgical incision.

The following considerations are examined:

- Immediate post-operative care
- Wound assessment
- Skin care
- Dressing products
- Securing the tracheostomy tube
- Hypergranulation
- Decannulation

IMMEDIATE POST-OPERATIVE PERIOD

The following wound care considerations are identified in the initial stages following a tracheostomy:

1. Any incidence of haemorrhage is most likely to occur during the tracheostomy procedure.
2. Post-operatively, the patient may experience oozing from the stoma or blood staining in the tracheal secretions.

3. If oozing persists, the stoma may require surgical packing.
4. In the event of profuse bleeding, surgical haemostasis may be necessary.[1]

Care of a newly formed tracheostomy stoma should include frequent wound cleaning; two or three times a day with saline.[2,3] The neck incision may be sutured on either side of the stoma, which will remain in situ for 5 to 7 days. If the stoma incision has been sutured too tightly, the patient is at risk of surgical emphysema, whereby air will become trapped in the subcutaneous tissues of the thorax.[1,4] To overcome this, the sutures can be removed.[4] To secure the tracheostomy tube, the flange may be sutured directly to the skin. This can be seen particularly with patients with neck swelling to avoid the use of tapes or collars. Additionally, the sutures will provide extra security if difficulties replacing a dislodged tube are anticipated.[4]

If the patient is mechanically ventilated via the tracheostomy tube, the ventilator tubing must be supported to prevent tube displacement or trauma to the stoma site. A recognised cause of tracheal stenosis of the stoma site is excessive traction on the tracheostomy tube from the ventilator tubing.[1] Permanently ventilated patients will benefit from a chest strap with Velcro fastenings, which wraps around and supports the catheter mount.

WOUND ASSESSMENT

Tracheostomy wound assessment will consist of:

1. Ongoing assessment of the stoma and skin during healing stage.
2. Detecting changes/deterioration in surgical incision and peri-stoma tissue.
3. Choosing appropriate dressing type.

At each dressing change, the stoma site should be observed for:

- Bleeding from stoma site or surgical incision
- Increase in stoma size
- Appearance of stoma edges
- Appearance of peri-stoma tissue (e.g. maceration, cellulitis)
- Evidence of surgical incision infection
- Breakdown of surgical incision
- Nature and quantity of stoma exudate
- Offensive odour
- Pain during dressing change
- Allergic reaction to dressing products (e.g. erythema)

If the peri-stoma tissue becomes red, shiny and oedematous, this may indicate signs of cellulitis. The individual may complain of tightness and pain around the area. If cellulitis is diagnosed, a course of antibiotics will be required.

SKIN CARE

'Skin adjacent to tubes, open wounds and taped areas is at risk of chemical and mechanical injury.'[5]

The tracheostomy incorporates a combination of all three of these influences and should be the determining factors in planning and managing the skin care of the tracheostomy patient.

Care of the surgical incision

The stoma site should be assessed at least daily. A healthy stoma will appear red and moist with a healed edge.[6] Measures should be taken to prevent skin breakdown and decrease the risk of infection. The surgical incision and peri-stoma area are vulnerable as they are in constant contact with secretions expelled from the stoma and/or tracheostomy tube, which are potentially infected (Fig. 1). However, the incision should only be cleaned if clinically indicated.[7,8] The surgical incision will require observation for signs of infection. These include:

- Purulent discharge
- Patient experiencing pain
- Odour
- Abscess formation
- Cellulitis and discolouration[7]

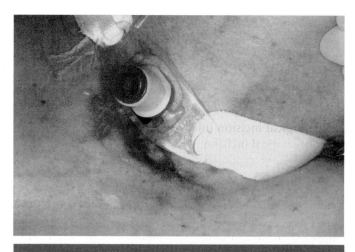

Fig. 1: An infected tracheostomy site.

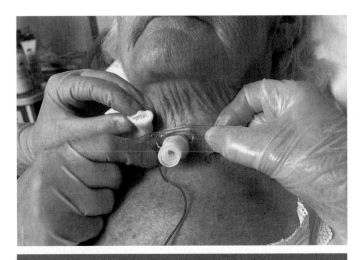

Fig. 2: Cleaning the tracheostomy stoma site.

Cleaning the stoma site

Peri-stoma skin, which is soggy and wet from exudate, may result in maceration or breakdown. However, skin breakdown and incision site infection can be avoided. Regularly removing the secretions from the skin will reduce maceration.[1] There should be no guide to determine how frequently this is performed, but should meet the individual need of the patient.

The skin and stoma is cleaned using aseptic technique[9] with saline and gauze (Fig. 2). However, a report investigating if clean tracheostomy care is more effective than sterile care in preventing infection supports practising clean procedures and questions the need for sterile technique.[10] This is certainly a consideration in the management and care of a tracheostomy at home where patients who self-care are unlikely to carry out aseptic tracheostomy care.

It is important to use gauze instead of cotton wool which has loose fibres which can break off and enter the stoma.[4] Attention should be paid to the skin under the flange (neck plate) as this is at risk of erythema and excoriation. The swivel plate design of some tracheostomy tubes facilitates easy access beneath the flange, e.g. Tracoetwist, Kapitex Healthcare.

DRESSING PRODUCTS

Choosing the dressing

The application of dressings should be carefully considered. It is important to select a dressing, which will *protect* the peri-stoma area while keeping the

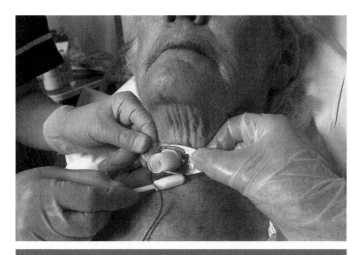

Fig. 3: Application of Cavilon.

stoma edges *moist*. Choose a stoma dressing to accommodate the following properties:

- Slim dressing to prevent movement of tracheostomy tube and potential dislodgement.
- Will not adhere to and cause trauma to stoma edges.
- Absorbs tracheal secretions from skin surface.
- Prevents debris or foreign substance entering stoma opening.
- Will not shed dressing fibres into stoma opening.
- Prevents infection.
- Promotes healing of surgical incision.
- Promotes patient comfort.
- Trauma-free removal.
- Prevents pressure damage from tracheostomy flange.

The macerating effects of stoma and tracheostomy tube secretions can be managed effectively with the use of protective film dressing. *Cavilon*™ (Table 1) can be used to provide a protective film for peri-wound maceration (Fig. 3).

Applying the dressing

A *keyhole dressing* is placed under the flange and around the stoma (Fig. 4). If this proves to be difficult, loosen the collar and while one person holds the tracheostomy tube the second person can slide the dressing into position. The dressing does not need to be taped to the skin as the flange and collar will

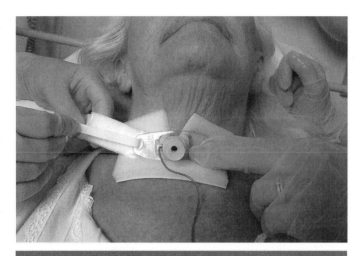

Fig. 4: Application of dressing and Velcro tube holders.

secure its position. If extra protection is required, a transparent film dressing can be applied over the top of the keyhole dressing. It is recommended that modified or self-cut keyhole dressings are avoided to prevent the risk of loose fibres entering the stoma. Instead, it is advisable to use a manufactured pre-formed keyhole dressing. A polyurethane foam dressing will provide an effective healing environment for the granulating wound, e.g. *Lyofoam T.*[8,11] In the event of skin breakdown, a hydrocolloid dressing can be applied (e.g. *Duoderm*™ by Convatec). A range of dressings are available specifically for tracheostomy use. A selection of dressings can be found in Table 1.

It may not be necessary to continue the use of stoma dressings for a long-term or permanent tracheostomy, providing the site has healed and the production of exudate is minimal.[8] In the instance of a clean and dry wound, a dressing is only required for comfort.

Key points of a tracheostomy dressing change are:

1. Remove old dressing and tapes.
2. Clean the stoma and surrounding area with saline and gauze.
3. Dry the peri-stoma area.
4. Apply keyhole dressing around the stoma/under flange of tracheostomy tube.
5. Apply transparent film dressing if required.
6. Inspect dressing frequently.
7. Change dressing when exudate visible.

Table 1: Tracheostomy dressing options

Product name and manufacturer	Properties	Function
Metalline tracheo 8 cm × 9 cm Lohmann Rauscher	Pre-punch hole and slit Non-adherent Fast wicking action	Fibres do not enter stoma Easy and painless dressing changes Absorbs stoma exudate rapidly
Trachi-dress 60 mm × 82 mm 100 mm × 82 mm Kapitex Healthcare Ltd.	Skin contact layer Absorption layer Backing layer Pre-formed dressing Low profile	Non-adherent Absorbs stoma exudate minimising maceration Retains secretions in dressing Fibres do not enter stoma Tube not raised from the neck
Allevyn tracheostomy 9 cm × 9 cm Smith and Nephew	Keyhole aperture Hydrocellular central layer Waterproof outer film Non-fibrous Cushioned	Easy to apply Absorbs stoma exudate Prevents leakage of secretions through front of dressing Prevents fibre shredding Patient comfort
Lyofoam T 6.5 cm × 9 cm SSL International plc.	Pre-formed polyurethane dressing Contact surface layer, hydrophilic layer and outer layer Non-adherent	Fibres do not enter stoma Excess exudate absorbed and then lost by evaporation through the dressing reduces maceration Easy and painless and non-traumatic dressing changes
Cavilon no sting barrier film 1.0 ml (15 cm² coverage) 3M Health Care Ltd.	Foam applicator Quick drying film Non-stinging solvent	Precise application Skin barrier from stoma drainage/secretions and maceration Pain free application

SECURING THE TUBE

If a tracheostomy tube has not been sutured to the skin by the flange, an alternative method of securing the tube is required. Two fastenings are available: *ribbon tapes* or *Velcro collars*. The main drawback with the use of ribbon tapes is the risk of skin ulceration. The alternative Velcro collar is manufactured specifically for tracheostomy use. These are preferable, as they are easy to apply and adjust, are more comfortable for the patient and less abrasive to the skin.[8] They will stretch as the patient coughs or moves, preventing skin damage.

N.B: Remember that an individual who is confused or agitated may pull at the tracheostomy tube. Children may be able to loosen or remove a Velcro collar either accidentally or intentionally. In these incidences a Velcro collar may be an unsuitable fastening to secure a tracheostomy tube.

How to change ribbon tapes

Ribbon tapes are threaded through the slots of the flange, fed around the patient's neck and secured with reef knots.

1. Cut two pieces of cotton tapes each approximately 50 cm in length (dependant on neck size).
2. Divide the tape into thirds and fold the first-third over the remaining two-thirds of the ribbon.
3. Thread the folded edge through one flange hole, forming a loop.
4. Thread the loose tape ends through this loop and pull until tight and secure.
5. Repeat the process for the other side, securing the tapes with reef knots on each side of the neck (knots directly over the spine can cause tissue breakdown).

How to change a Velcro tube holder (Fig. 4)

1. Thread the narrow Velcro tab through the slit in the flange of the tracheostomy tube and fold back to adhere to the main tube holder, repeat on other side.
2. Overlap the shorter length of collar with the longer length of collar and secure with the wider Velcro tab.*
3. Trim any excess length of collar to fit the size of the patient's neck.**

* Some collars are available as one continuous length.
** Available in neonate, paediatric and adult sizes.

Finally, it is important to regularly check how secure the tape or collar feels. The tracheostomy tube should be observed for increased movement or projection from the stoma, indicating that the collar is *too loose*. The tracheostomy tube is then at risk of displacement or dislodgement. In addition, the free moving tube will gradually erode the walls of the stoma and eventually increasing the size of the opening. Stoma site stenosis can also result from loosely secured tubes.[1] However, a collar or tapes which are *too tight* can cause ulceration to the skin, inhibit circulation and cause patient discomfort. A useful indicator to establish the ideal fitting is to be able to insert one to two fingers between the collar and the neck.[8] The use of a film barrier can be used to prevent the shearing effect of the tapes against the neck skin.

Key points for tape/collar changes

- The tapes or collar only require changing when soiled.
- Soiled or wet tapes can cause excoriation of the neck skin.
- It is preferable to ensure two carers are present, as this procedure can make the patient cough and potentially dislodge the unsecured tracheostomy tube.
- One carer can replace the tapes while the second carer holds the tracheostomy in place by the flange.
- Involve the patient/carer who is able to participate in changing the collar by supporting and securing the flange with their hands.

HYPERGRANULATION

Hypergranulation is described as 'exuberance of granulation tissue during the proliferative stage of healing and an absence of epithilisation, thus preventing the maturation stage of wound healing'.[12,13]

Hypergranulation is also referred to as:[14]

- Hyperplasia of granulating tissue.
- Over granulation.
- Proud flesh.
- Hypertrophic granulation.

As with any other wound, hypergranulation can develop around a tracheostomy stoma[15] (Fig. 5). It is suggested[16] that hypergranulation occurs when there is infection, inflammation, oedema or foreign bodies in a wound bed. A tracheostomy stoma can be exposed to any of these factors:

- Excess bacteria in the wound can result in *infection*.[13]
- The tracheostomy tube can cause friction against the stoma edges resulting in *inflammation*.[17]

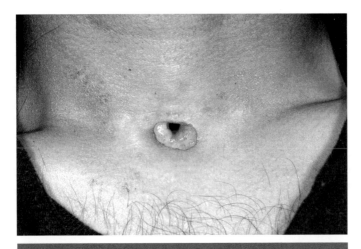

Fig. 5: Hypergranulation of a stoma.

- Loose fibres from an unsuitable stoma dressing can become a *foreign body*.[13]

Hypergranulation of a tracheostomy stoma can cause the following complications:

- Narrowing of the stoma and tract resulting in difficulty/trauma when changing the tracheostomy tube.
- Bleeding with movement of the tube and tube changes.
- Impede the healing of the stoma following decannulation.

Hypergranulation can prevent epithilisation, stop wound healing and extend the inflammatory response.[16] This tissue if left untreated will usually resolve as the granulation tissue contracts.[15]

Management of hypergranulation at the tracheostomy site

- Prevent friction by reducing the movement of the tracheostomy tube with the use of secure tapes or collar.[13,17]
- Topical application of silver nitrate 95% to cauterise hypergranulation (Fig. 6). This form of treatment should be used with caution as:
  - It can leave necrotic tissue in the wound.[13]
  - Leave wound bed with grey discolouration ('Argyria') after repeated applications.[15]
  - May cause discomfort for the patient.
  - Trauma may initiate inflammatory phase of healing.[14,15]

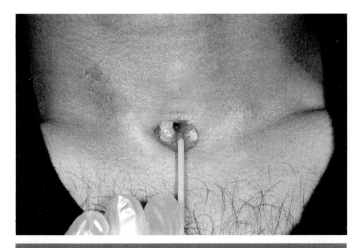

Fig. 6: Application of silver nitrate to hypergranulation tissue.

- It may burn healthy skin surrounding the stoma. The application of petroleum jelly as a protective barrier can help prevent this.

- Polyurethane foam dressing with high moisture vapour transmission rate significantly reduces hypergranulation.[14,15,18] *Lyofoam T™* (Table 1) is a keyhole polyurethane foam dressing designed for tracheostomy use.
- Surgical excision of excessive hypergranulation[16] (particularly relevant if tract has become narrowed or if excessive bleeding of a highly vascular tissue occurs during tube changes).
- Surgical opinion to avoid the development of a significant scar, requiring corrective surgery.[19]

While the tracheostomy tube remains in situ, the hypergranulation is less likely to resolve on its own. The hypergranulation may increase the stoma size and form a scar. This will be significant in managing the closure of the stoma following decannulation. Scar tissue around the stoma edges can cause a delay in the healing process. If the hypergranulation extends internally narrowing the airway, airflow can be compromised. Following decannulation, the individual may have difficulty breathing through their upper airway.

DECANNULATION

Following permanent removal of a tracheostomy tube (decannulation), effective stoma healing will depend on the selection of an appropriate dressing. If the site is left undressed, the patient will continue to be able to breathe, cough and speak through the stoma. Any of these activities will facilitate airflow through the stoma and compromise the healing process.

The following recommendations are required in selecting a dressing to encourage rapid and effective stoma closure:

- The dressing needs to be airtight. This will occlude the stoma opening and prevent any air entering or leaving the stoma.
- The dressing should provide an effective seal to withstand airflow pressure. At the first sign of the dressing becoming dislodged, replace as soon as possible, to prevent air leakage.
- The dressing should adhere effectively to the skin. The use of *Sleek*™ tape may be an effective method of stoma closure, but tends to detach easily when the patient moves.[20]
- The patient should be encouraged to support the dressing and stoma opening with their hand across the dressing whenever they speak or cough. This will help to prevent loosening of the dressing from leaking air through the stoma.
- The dressing should be easy to remove. The adhesive properties of *Sleek*™ can be aggressive to the skin tissue, causing mild erythema.[20] This will be of particular relevance if the peri-stoma tissue is macerated.

Table 2 details dressings which can be used following decannulation.

The stoma will heal from the trachea outwards. An indication of tracheal closure is the cessation of audible or visible air or secretions escaping through the stoma. The stoma will usually be completely healed within two weeks

Table 2: Dressings suitable for decannulation of tracheostomy	
Product and manufacturer	**Properties/function**
Duoderm Convatec Ltd.	Hydrocolloid dressing Suitable for lightly exudating wounds Adhesive Occlusive Provides moist environment for wound healing
Tegaderm 3M Health Care Ltd.	Forms artificial barrier Facilitates oxygen and moisture vapour exchange Impermeable to bacteria/environmental contaminants Provides moist environment for wound healing Impermeable to bacteria Waterproof Adhesive

following decannulation and the site can then be exposed. In the event of only partial closure, an ENT assessment may be required for surgical closure.[19]

Summary of key factors

1. Protect from chemical and mechanical influences on stoma and surrounding tissue.
2. Prevent skin breakdown and infection.
3. Avoid the use of dressing products which can potentially enter the stoma.
4. Treat using aseptic technique in clinical setting.
5. Promote patient comfort.

REFERENCES

1. Tamburri LM. Care of the patient with a tracheostomy. *Orthopaed Nurs* 2000; 19(2): 49–60.
2. Adam S, Osborne S. *Critical Care Nursing: Science and Practice.* Oxford University Press, 1997.
3. Docherty B. Clinical practice review: Trachestomy care. *Prof Nurs* 2001; 16(8): 1272.
4. Serra A. Tracheostomy care. *Nurs Stand* 2000; 14(42): 45–52.
5. Rolstad BS. A comparison of an alcohol-based and siloxane-based peri-wound skin protectant. *J Wound Care* 1994; 3(8): 367–368.
6. Diehl B, Dorsey L, Koller C. Transitioning the client with a tracheostomy from acute care to alternative settings. In Tippett D (ed.). *Tracheostomy and Ventilator Dependency – Management of Breathing, Speaking and Swallowing.* USA: Thieme Medical Publishers Inc., 2000; 237–265.
7. Gould D. Clean surgical wounds: Prevention of infection. *Nurs Stand* 2001; 15(49): 45–52.
8. Docherty B. Tracheostomy management for patients in general ward settings. *Prof Nurs* 2002; 18(2): 100–104.
9. Sigler B. Nursing management of the patient with a tracheostomy. In Tippet D (ed.). *Tracheostomy and Ventilator Dependency – Management of Breathing, Speaking and Swallowing.* USA: Thieme Medical Publishers Inc., 2000; 57–65.
10. Harris R, Hyman R. Clean V sterile tracheostomy care and level of pulmonary infection. *Nurs Res* 1984; 33(2): 80–84.
11. Williams C. Product focus – Lyofoam. *Br J Nurs* 1996; 5(12): 757–759.
12. Young T. Common problems in overgranulation. *Pract Nurs* 1995; 6(11): 14–16.
13. Nelson L. Points of friction. *Nurs Times* 1999; 95(34): 72–75.
14. Harris A, Rolstad BS. Hypergranulation tissue: A non-traumatic method of management. *Ostomy/Wound Management* 1994; 40(5): 20–30.
15. Dunford C. Clinical concepts – Hypergranulation tissue. *J Wound Care* 1999; 8(10): 506–507.
16. Stansfield G. *Wound Management Newsletter – Hypergranulation and its management.* Peterborough; Coloplast Ltd., 2002; 10–11.

17. Hanlon M, Heximer B. Excess granulation tissue around a gastrostomy tube exit site with peritubular skin irritation. *J Wound, Ostomy and Continence Nurs* 1994; 21(2): 76–77.

18. Hampton S. Complex wound care. *Pract Nurs* 1997; 13(14): 205–210.

19. Harkin H, Russell C. Preparing the patient for tracheostomy tube removal. *Nurs Times* 2001; 97(26): 34–36.

20. Vats A, Worley G, Wareing M. Short communication. A novel dressing for tracheostomy decannulation. *J Laryngol Otol* 1999; 113: 999.

SWALLOWING

Pippa Hales

INTRODUCTION

One of the key components of the Speech and Language Therapist's (SLT) role is to identify and manage the factors that may put a patient at risk of aspiration, while also ensuring that the patient can safely meet their nutrition and hydration requirements.

The SLT therefore plays a key role within the tracheostomy team, where the presence of the tracheostomy tube alone can impact significantly on a patient's ability to swallow safely, regardless of any other additional factors that may also be affecting their swallow.

This chapter will identify the mechanisms of a 'normal' swallow, the implication a tracheostomy can have on swallowing, the SLT's assessment and management of the patient with a tracheostomy.

NORMAL HEAD AND NECK ANATOMY (Fig. 1)

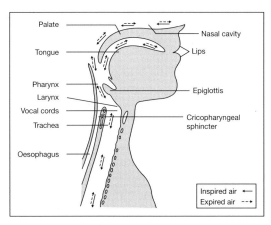

Palate
Tongue
Pharynx
Larynx
Vocal cords
Trachea
Oesophagus
Nasal cavity
Lips
Epiglottis
Cricopharyngeal sphincter

Inspired air ←
Expired air --→

Fig. 1: The anatomy of the head and neck demonstrating the direction of airflow.

CRANIAL NERVE INVOLVEMENT FOR SWALLOWING (Table 1)

Table 1: The cranial nerves involved in swallowing	
Cranial nerve	**Summary of function**
I Olfactory	Smell.
II Optic	Vision.
V Trigeminal	Mastication, sensation to the face, movement of the soft palate, anterior and upward movement of the larynx.
VII Facial	Movement of facial muscles, movement of the larynx up and back, taste, salivary glands.
IX Glossopharyngeal	Lateral dilation of the pharynx, taste to posterior third of the tongue, elevation of the pharynx and larynx, parotid salivary gland, sensation to upper pharynx.
X Vagus	Pharyngeal constriction, sensation to the epiglottis, taste, swallowing, elevation of palate, phonation.
XII Hypoglossal	Movement of tongue, phonation.

Collated from Love and Webb.[1]

THE NORMAL SWALLOW

The primary function of the swallow is to transfer material from the mouth to the stomach via the pharynx and the oesophagus in order to maintain adequate nutrition and hydration.

This process can be broken down into four clear stages:

I. Oral preparatory stage
II. Oral stage
III. Pharyngeal stage
IV. Oesophageal stage

I. The oral preparatory stage (Fig. 2a)

The oral preparatory stage begins as the material approaches the mouth. Sensory feedback is provided on its appearance, smell and texture, which in turn prepares the oral cavity to receive the bolus. For example, saliva is produced to lubricate the oral cavity and to keep the bolus moist.

When the material enters the oral cavity:

- The lips are used to help draw the material into the oral cavity.
- The lips form a seal to prevent food/fluid falling out of the oral cavity.
- The tongue and mandible move in a rotary pattern to masticate the material, if required, to form a cohesive bolus.
- If the consistency requires minimal preparation the tongue maintains the original cohesion of the bolus by forming a seal around the lateral alveolus and controlling it between the hard palate and the midline of the tongue.
- The tone in the lips and cheeks is used to prevent the bolus falling into the sulci between the lips and cheeks and the teeth.
- The soft palate and the back of the tongue make contact to seal the oral cavity and prevent the bolus from prematurely entering the pharynx. This results in nasal breathing.
- For a bolus that requires a considerable amount of mastication it is within normal limits for the lingual-palatal seal to be absent, allowing some of the bolus to prematurely fall into the pharynx to the level of the valleculae.
- Sensory receptors supply feedback on the taste, temperature, texture, volume, shape and position of the bolus.

II. The oral stage (Fig. 2b)

- The tongue tip is elevated and held against the alveolar ridge.
- The blade of the tongue moves in a series of wave-like motions, elevating against the hard palate in order to propel the bolus backwards.
- The bolus is transferred in the midline as the rolling pressure of the tongue against the hard palate squeezes it posteriorly towards the faucial arches.
- The oral cavity remains sealed posteriorly with the back of tongue making contact with the soft palate.
- Nasal breathing is necessary as a result of the lingual-palatal seal.

III. The pharyngeal stage (Fig. 2c)

The pharyngeal swallow is triggered as the head of the bolus travels between the faucial arches and where the tongue base crosses the lower edge of the mandible.[2] The specific point of the trigger is considered to vary with age, with the point of trigger being closer to the faucial arches in the young and closer to where the mandible and the tongue base cross in the older population.[3]

When the swallow triggers:

- The soft palate elevates to seal off the nasal cavity.
- The base of tongue retracts posteriorly to make contact with the pharyngeal wall to move the bolus into the pharynx.

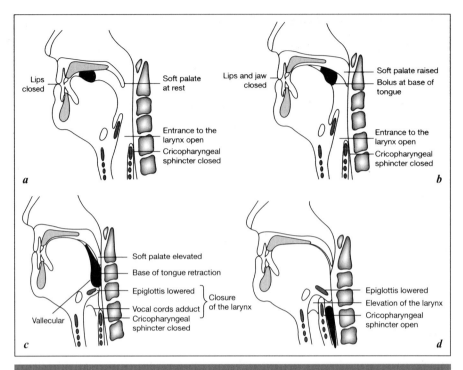

Fig. 2: Line drawings depicting (***a***) the oral preparatory stage, (***b***) the oral stage, (***c***) the pharyngeal stage and (***d***) the oesophageal stage of the normal swallow.

- The larynx and hyoid move superiorly and anteriorly resulting in:

  - the epiglottis closing down over the airway entrance to prevent material penetrating the airway.
  - the vocal cords adducting.
  - the laryngeal entrance constricting.
  - the cricopharyngeal sphincter opening to allow the bolus to pass through into the oesophagus.
  - there is a progressive peristaltic contraction of the pharyngeal constrictor muscles that moves the bolus through the pharynx.

IV. The oesophageal stage (Fig. 2d)

This stage begins as the bolus passes through the cricopharyngeal sphincter, into the oesophagus at which point the peristaltic wave moves the bolus along the length of the oesophagus to the stomach.

THE LEVELS OF AIRWAY PROTECTION

The following terms are used to describe material entering the airway:

1. *Penetration* – material entering the laryngeal vestibule, but not passing below the level of the vocal cords.
2. *Aspiration* – material passing below the level of the vocal cords.

In order to prevent material entering the airway, the following protection mechanisms are in place:

- The epiglottis closes over the top of the airway entrance as the larynx elevates.
- The vocal cords adduct as a result of laryngeal elevation.
- The breath is held.
- The laryngeal entrance constricts.
- The cough reflex is triggered in the presence of any penetrated or aspirated material.

THE RELATIONSHIP BETWEEN RESPIRATION AND SWALLOWING

Due to the presence of the lingual-palatal contact sealing the oral cavity during the oral stages of the swallow, breathing is nasal, but as the swallow is triggered, breathing stops completely to prevent the bolus being inhaled into the airway.

Studies have shown that this apnoeic period occurs most frequently during the expiratory phase of the respiratory cycle after which the vocal cords abduct and the expiratory phase continues.[4,5] This is believed to further aid airway protection by clearing any residue in the larynx post-swallow.[4,6]

The swallow is clearly a very complex process and therefore any anomaly occurring outside the parameters of the normal swallow can have a significant impact on a person's swallow function and ultimately the safety of their swallow.

THE IMPACT OF THE TRACHEOSTOMY TUBE ON SWALLOW FUNCTION

It is well documented that the presence of the tracheostomy tube alone can have a significant impact on a patient's swallow function:

This can be divided into two categories:

- Mechanical impact
- Physiological impact

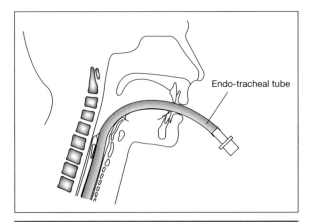

Fig. 3: A drawing of the head and neck to demonstrate the positioning of an endo-tracheal tube.

The mechanical impact

Changes affecting laryngeal function post-endo-tracheal intubation

Endo-tracheal intubation is used to provide and maintain a stable airway by passing a tube through the mouth, into the pharynx and then into the trachea by way of the larynx (Fig. 3). A cuff is then inflated to ensure there is a closed circuit for ventilation and/or to prevent aspiration of secretions. The patient can potentially remain intubated for several weeks before a trial extubation takes place and a tracheostomy will be considered if the patient is unable to self ventilate or protect their own airway post-extubation.

Prolonged intubation can result in changes to the laryngeal mucosa which can ultimately manifest in vocal cord and supraglottic oedema, desensitising the larynx and pharynx and blunting its response to material entering the airway, resulting in aspiration.[7–9]

The intrinsic and extrinsic laryngeal and pharyngeal musculature can also atrophy when their natural movement is restricted for a prolonged period of time while the endo-tracheal tube holds the glottis open.[10]

Restriction of laryngeal elevation

As stated in the section describing 'the normal swallow' laryngeal elevation is fundamental to the swallow mechanism, and is necessary to protect the airway, however, the following aspects of a tracheostomy may impede swallow function and safety by restricting the elevation of the larynx:

- Surgical technique – a horizontal incision is more likely to restrict vertical movement than a vertical incision.[11]
- Tube size – an oversized tube will leave minimal space between its outer circumference and the tracheal wall resulting in inhibited movement that may subsequently anchor the larynx.
- Weight of the equipment – the weight of the tracheostomy tube as well as any additional equipment such as a speaking valve or humidification system could be enough to restrict the elevation of the larynx.
- Cuff inflation – an inflated cuff and more significantly an over inflated cuff may tether the larynx restricting its vertical movement.

Obstruction of the oesophagus

An over inflated cuff can impinge on the tracheal-oesophageal wall to the extent that it can obstruct the passage of the bolus as it passes through the oesophagus (Figs 4, 5). It must therefore be deflated for oral intake and inflated using either a cuff pressure manometer and/or the minimal leak technique.

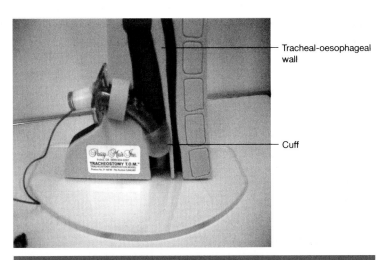

Tracheal-oesophageal wall

Cuff

Fig. 4: A model of the head and neck demonstrating how accurate inflation of the cuff does not lead to the obstruction of the oesophagus.

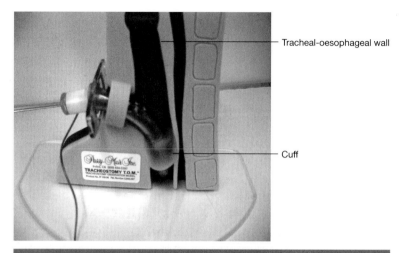

Tracheal-oesophageal wall

Cuff

Fig. 5: A model of the head and neck demonstrating how over inflation of the cuff can impinge on the tracheal-oesophageal wall.

Physiological impact

Loss or reduction of airflow into the upper airway

The laws of physics stipulate that airflow will always take the path of least resistance. In the unaltered anatomy air passes through the upper airway, through the nose and mouth and back again. However, when a tracheostomy tube is in situ, the anatomy is altered in such a way that the path of least resistance is now through the tube, therefore redirecting all or the majority of the airflow away from the larynx (Fig. 6).

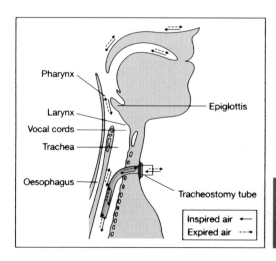

Pharynx

Larynx

Vocal cords

Trachea

Oesophagus

Epiglottis

Tracheostomy tube

Inspired air ←
Expired air --→

Fig. 6: A drawing to demonstrate airflow being redirected along the path of least resistance.

This can result in the following:

- Absent or weak cough – little or no air can pass above the level of the tube to reach the larynx in order to clear any material that may have collected there.
- Absent smell and taste – these senses are dependent on air flow through the oral and nasal cavities to stimulate the chemoreceptor cells in the nasal mucosa and the taste buds.[11] The absence or reduction of airflow through the upper airway will therefore significantly affect an individual's sense of taste and smell and potentially result in a loss of appetite.

Altered airway pressures

- Subglottic air pressure is created by air pressure building up below adducted vocal cords. This pressure can then be utilised, e.g. to cough to clear residue. In the presence of an open-ended tracheostomy tube the subglottic air pressure is disrupted due to the additional air passage through the tube reducing the patient's ability to build up sufficient pressure. This can therefore affect the safety of the swallow as the patient's ability to cough to clear residue can be reduced.
- Pharyngeal air pressure – the base of tongue is used to create pressure to aid the passage of the bolus through the pharynx and into the oesophagus. With an open tracheostomy tube this pressure is reduced and can result in increased pharyngeal residue post-swallow.

Loss or reduction of airflow through the larynx

- Reduction in the glottic closure reflex – the glottic closure reflex is triggered when material penetrates the laryngeal entrance. In response the vocal cords reflexively adduct to prevent the material falling below the level of the vocal cords, thus preventing aspiration. Subglottic pressure then increases and the material is coughed clear of the larynx. Studies have shown that the presence of the tracheostomy tube can affect the speed of this response, making aspiration of material a potential hazard.[12,13]

THE IMPACT OF MECHANICAL VENTILATION ON SWALLOWING

The mechanical impact

Reduced laryngeal elevation

The weight of the equipment attached to the tracheostomy tube required for ventilation can restrict laryngeal elevation, consequently affecting swallow function and swallow safety.

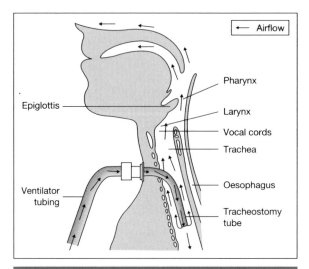

Fig. 7: A drawing to demonstrate how air delivered by the ventilator can leak up into the upper airway to potentially disrupt the swallow.

The physiological impact

Disrupted apnoeic period

As described in the sections 'the normal swallow' and 'the relationship between respiration and swallowing' the swallow commonly occurs during the expiratory phase of the respiratory cycle. During the inspiratory phase of ventilation air enters through the tracheostomy tube and into the lungs, however if the cuff is deflated some of this air will also leak into the upper airway (Fig. 7). Swallowing at this point can result in the air leak blowing the bolus back into the oral or nasal cavity, disrupting the swallow. The ventilated patient therefore has to learn to co-ordinate their swallow with the different phases of the ventilator. Air pushed through the upper airway can then be used to clear any residue remaining post-swallow.

THE SWALLOWING ASSESSMENT (Refer to appendix for 'Outline of the SLTs assessment of a non-ventilated patient with a tracheostomy tube')

The assessment of a tracheostomy patient's swallow involves the SLT examining the following areas:

- Oro-motor function
- Tolerance of secretions
- Tolerance of oral intake

The oro-motor assessment

The oro-motor assessment provides a good indication of function of the oral stages of the swallow and will highlight any potential areas of break down in these stages.

In this assessment the SLT assesses:

- Rate, range and strength of movement of the lips, cheeks, tongue, jaw and palate.
- Dentition, e.g. presence or absence of teeth or dentures.
- Saliva control in the oral stage.
- Oral hygiene – poor oral hygiene is a predictor of aspiration pneumonia.[14]
- The presence of primitive reflexes.

N.B: The presence or absence of the gag reflex is not indicative of swallow function.[15,16]

Assessing tolerance of secretions – cuff deflation trials

The majority of patients with a tracheostomy tube will need to undergo cuff deflation trials, in which case the patient's ability to tolerate their own secretions will be assessed.

Cuff deflation

Cuff deflation should only be carried out with medical consent to do so. The cuff can then be deflated by a designated member of the tracheostomy team and the patient suctioned as required. If the patient is ventilated a designated member of the tracheostomy team, trained in the use of mechanical ventilators, will be required to make the necessary modifications to the ventilator settings. The patient's physiological and clinical response to cuff deflation will be monitored for indications of intolerance, e.g. increased work of breathing, fatigue, decreasing O_2 saturation levels and/or a change in skin pallor. The cuff will be reinflated if signs of intolerance are observed.

Assessment of upper airway patency

Upper airway patency is assessed to ascertain whether a patient is able to pass sufficient air into the upper airway to be able to clear any unwanted material.

By lightly occluding the end of the tracheostomy tube with a gloved finger (do not do this if the patient is ventilated) or with a one way speaking valve, the patient is asked to voice or breath out onto the therapist's arm. Expiratory airflow, if present, can then be felt. If minimal or no airflow is felt adjustments will be made to maximise airflow into the upper airway (refer to Chapter 12, Communication).

Gross assessment of laryngeal function

- The SLT will assess vocal cord function by asking the patient to voice while breathing out, e.g. count to 3 or say 'aahhh'.
- The patient will be asked to cough or clear their throat. The SLT will listen for vocal cord adduction and will observe the effectiveness of the voluntary cough.
- The SLT will also ask the patient to produce a variety of different sounds to assess the range of laryngeal movement.

A positive outcome from this assessment can ultimately lead to the use of a speaking valve or digital occlusion in conjunction with the swallowing assessment.

Tracheostomy tube occlusion during cuff deflation trials and oral intake assessments

Studies shows that occlusion of the tracheostomy tube with a gloved finger or a one-way speaking valve restores subglottic pressure, normalises pharyngeal pressures and resensitises the glottic reflex, therefore normalising laryngeal and swallow function.[17,18] However, other studies have shown that tracheal occlusion does not improve the safety of the swallow in all cases, suggesting that the beneficial effects of tracheal occlusion are variable.[19,20]

Tube occlusion must therefore be used cautiously with regards to swallowing as, although it has many physiological benefits, it is also an additional variable for the patient to tolerate and will not necessarily have a positive impact on the safety of their swallow. Thus if a patient is unable to tolerate tube occlusion for a sufficient period of time the SLT will assess whether they can undergo the oral intake assessment without it.

Assessment of swallow function

- The SLT will observe the frequency of spontaneous saliva swallows.
- The SLT will ask the patient to swallow the saliva in their mouth while assessing laryngeal movement with regards to swallow function and airway protection (Fig. 8).
- Approximately 0.1 ml of blue food dye can be dropped onto the patient's tongue in order to dye the secretions to potentially help track them if the secretions are aspirated (see section on 'The blue dye test').
- If the assessment shows that the patient is at risk of aspirating their secretions the cuff will be reinflated and the patient will be reassessed at a later stage.
- If the patient tolerates cuff deflation at the initial trial the tracheostomy team will set up a programme for further cuff deflation trials with the aim of increasing the length of time tolerated and to ultimately achieve continuous cuff deflation.

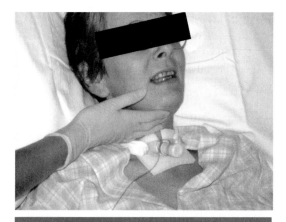

Fig. 8: A picture to demonstrate assessment of the swallow at bedside.

Assessing tolerance of oral intake

Indications for assessment of tolerance of oral intake
- The patient can tolerate cuff deflation.
- The patient can safely manage their secretions.
- The tracheostomy team deem the patient medically and cognitively able to tolerate the assessment.

Contraindications for assessment of tolerance of oral intake
- If the patient cannot tolerate cuff deflation.
- If the patient is unable to tolerate their secretions.
- If the tracheostomy team deem the patient medically or cognitively unable to tolerate the assessment.
- If the patient is unable to maintain a safe position for oral intake.

The oral intake assessment follows the same procedures as the saliva assessment and, other than being able to use blue dye, as an additional assessment tool, the assessment remains the same as it does for the non-tracheostomised patient.

The SLT will be looking for:

- Any areas of break down in the stages of the swallow resulting in swallowing difficulties (dysphagia).
- Altered physiology of the swallow resulting in dysphagia and risk of aspiration.
- Evidence of aspiration.
- Techniques to safely manage the dysphagia.

- The patient's ability to safely tolerate a range of different consistencies.
- Indications for the need for further assessment techniques, e.g. Video-fluoroscopy.

THE BLUE DYE TEST

Routine care of the tracheostomy patient involves suctioning tracheal secretions via the tracheostomy tube in order to maintain a clear airway and it is this tracheal opening that can potentially provide the therapist with additional information regarding the safety of the patient's swallow.

The theory behind the blue dye test is:

- If a tracheostomised patient were to aspirate it would be very difficult to tell the aspirated material apart from the existing tracheal secretions, hence the material is dyed an atypical colour (i.e. blue) so that the aspirated material can be distinguished from any other secretions.

Saliva assessment

In order to distinguish aspirated secretions from the secretions already present in the trachea, the saliva needs to be dyed blue. This involves introducing approximately 0.1 ml of blue food dye into the oral cavity to stain the secretions. This should not be significant enough to stimulate saliva production, but should be enough to adequately stain the secretions within the oral cavity.

The patient's tracheal secretions can then be monitored over time for any traces of blue. If blue tracheal secretions are observed it can be assumed that the blue dyed oral secretions have been aspirated.

Oral intake assessment

The same principle applies to the oral intake assessment as it does to the saliva assessment. Blue food dye can be added to the consistency being trialled and the tracheal secretions can then be monitored for evidence of blue, aspirated material.

Signs to look for

A slight tinge of blue in:

- The secretions suctioned through the tube.
- Secretions coughed through the tube.
- Secretions leaking around the tracheal stoma.
- Evidence of blue on the stoma dressing.
- Blue staining of the inner cannula.

The colour of the blue dye will be less distinct as it becomes further diluted by additional secretions. An effective way to look for blue dyed secretions in the suction catheter is to hold the catheter against something white, e.g. the bed sheet.

Monitoring the secretions

The tracheal secretions should be monitored for any signs of blue for approximately 24 h after the assessment using a tracking sheet (see Appendix). This time period allows for any residual blue that may have been residing above the level of the tube to show up in the tracheal secretions.

If blue dyed tracheal secretions are found

If blue tracheal secretions are found it is known as a 'positive' result. This means that the trialled substance, e.g. saliva, food or fluid, has been aspirated.

If evidence of blue dye is found in the tracheal secretions the cuff should be reinflated and the SLT should be contacted who will then modify the management and assessment of the patient accordingly.

If blue dyed tracheal secretions are not found

If no evidence of blue has been found in the tracheal secretions it is known as a 'negative' result. In theory this means that the patient has not aspirated any of the blue material below the level of the vocal cords, but this could potentially be a 'false-negative' result (see the section on 'The value of the blue dye test').

Trialling different consistencies

If two or more consistencies were trialled at one time and the patient's tracheal secretions were later found to be blue, it would be difficult to distinguish which consistency they aspirated. It is for this reason that approximately 24 h are left between each test to allow for the blue to potentially show up before testing the next consistency.

The value of the blue dye test

Most people who have worked with patients with tracheostomies have heard of the 'blue dye test' and it is often treated as the test that will provide all the necessary information about a tracheostomised patient's swallow. This is not the case.

- When the blue dye test can be relied on – only if blue dye is found in the tracheal secretions can you assume that the patient has aspirated the blue stained substance. However it will not tell you why, when or how they aspirated.
- When the blue dye test cannot be relied on – studies have shown that if the result is negative (i.e. no blue dye is found) aspiration cannot be ruled out, i.e. it may be a false-negative.[21] It is possible that the aspirated material has gone undetected, e.g. the material is still pooled above the level of the tube, diluted with secretions beyond detection or has simply been missed.

The blue dye test is a useful assessment tool, but it is one that must only be used and interpreted in conjunction with other swallowing assessment techniques.

COMPLEMENTARY SWALLOW ASSESSMENTS

In addition to the traditional bedside assessments and the blue dye test there are a number of assessment tools and techniques that the SLT can use to gather information on the tracheostomised patient's swallow function. None of these tools should be used in isolation.

Cervical auscultation

Cervical auscultation involves listening for pharyngeal and laryngeal sounds using a stethoscope by placing it on the side of the neck approximately in line with the lateral surface of the larynx. The most useful elements of this tool are:

- To determine if the person has any upper airway sounds prior to the swallowing trial.
- To determine at which point in the respiratory cycle they swallow.
- To determine if there is a change in upper airway sounds post-swallow.
- It can be used to detect a swallow on a person whose larynx is difficult to palpate, e.g. due to excessive amounts of soft tissue around the area of the neck.

Videofluoroscopy

This is a radiographic assessment that enables the SLT and the radiologist to observe the anatomy and physiology of the swallow in motion. Penetration and aspiration of the bolus can be observed and the cause identified and potentially modified. The moving image is also recorded to enable the therapist to analyse the assessment in greater detail.

It must be remembered that although videofluoroscopy provides detailed information about a patient's swallow function it is only a 'snap shot' in time during a relatively demanding procedure that, due to exposure to radiation has limitations on how frequently it can be repeated.

Fiberoptic endoscopic evaluation of swallowing (FEES)

This is an invasive assessment tool that involves passing a flexible nasendoscope via the nose and down into the pharynx and larynx to view the pharyngeal stage of the swallow. This allows the SLT to view the anatomy and function of the palate, pharynx and larynx and assess the swallow in a more functional environment, observing for pooling and residue and assessing effectiveness of therapeutic techniques. FEES, however, cannot be used to view mid-swallow as the pharyngeal constriction and the bolus passing the nasendoscope blocks its view.

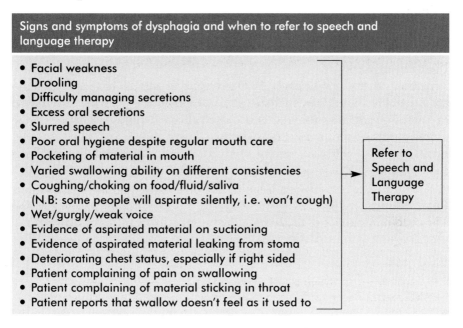

Signs and symptoms of dysphagia and when to refer to speech and language therapy

- Facial weakness
- Drooling
- Difficulty managing secretions
- Excess oral secretions
- Slurred speech
- Poor oral hygiene despite regular mouth care
- Pocketing of material in mouth
- Varied swallowing ability on different consistencies
- Coughing/choking on food/fluid/saliva
  (N.B: some people will aspirate silently, i.e. won't cough)
- Wet/gurgly/weak voice
- Evidence of aspirated material on suctioning
- Evidence of aspirated material leaking from stoma
- Deteriorating chest status, especially if right sided
- Patient complaining of pain on swallowing
- Patient complaining of material sticking in throat
- Patient reports that swallow doesn't feel as it used to

→ Refer to Speech and Language Therapy

MANAGEMENT OF DYSPHAGIA

After the SLT has assessed the patient's swallow function, recommendations regarding management will be made. This will take into consideration the results of the swallow assessment and the team's holistic assessment of the patient.

The SLT may recommend a range of therapeutic interventions depending on the individual and the presentation of the dysphagia.

Indirect therapy
Indirect therapy does not involve directly introducing a bolus, but works on the aspects of the swallow that have been identified as being outside the parameters of the 'normal' swallow. These generally include exercises to increase rate, range and strength of movement as well as those that aim to normalise sensation and develop the patient's ability to self-monitor.

Tube manipulation
Manipulation of the tracheostomy tube is used in an attempt to normalise the patient's swallow and therefore increase swallow safety. This will be dependant on the individual and what they are able to tolerate.

For example the SLT might recommend down sizing the tracheostomy tube, light occlusion of the tracheostomy tube with a gloved finger when the patient swallows or attachment of the speaking valve when eating/drinking.

N.B: The cuff must be deflated for all oral intake.

Diet changes
According to the presentation of the dysphagia the SLT may recommend modified food/fluid consistencies in order that the patient can receive oral nutrition/medication/hydration safely. This requires liaison with the dietitian regarding available food consistencies, nutritional value, supplements etc. This can also involve modifications to the presentation of the food/fluid.

Positioning
The optimum, safe position for swallowing is upright with the chin slightly dropped down towards the chest. This is not possible for some patients and the SLT will make recommendations as to the safest position for each individual patient.

The SLT will also recommend postural techniques and manoeuvres that can be used to increase the patients swallow safety. This will be dependent on the individual patient and their dysphagia.

Non-oral feeding
If the SLT recommends that the patient should be nil by mouth or that they can only commence on oral trails the patient may require an alternative form of feeding in order to maintain their nutrition and hydration needs. The SLT will refer to the dietitian in this instance. The SLT will also be involved in the decision for placement of longer-term methods of non-oral feeding, depending on the prognosis of the patient's swallow function.

QUALITY OF LIFE

In the circumstance where quality of life is considered the patient's primary issue, the tracheostomy team will weigh up the positive impact that oral intake will have on quality of life against the negative and potentially life threatening impact of aspirating any oral intake.

Summary

The identification and management of factors that put a patient at risk of aspiration is one of the key roles of the SLT working with patients with tracheostomies. In order for them to do this effectively, however, it is essential that they work closely with the rest of the tracheostomy team, utilising their specialist knowledge and skills to achieve the optimum outcome for the patient.

REFERENCES

1. Love R, Webb W. *Neurology for the Speech and Language Pathologist*, 3rd edn. Newton, MA: Butterworth and Heinmann, 1996.
2. Logemann J. *Evaluation and Treatment of Swallowing Disorders*. Austin, TX: Pro.ed, 1998.
3. Robbins J, Hamilton JW, Lof GL, Kempster GB. Oropharyngeal swallowing in normal adults of different ages. *Gastroenterology* 1992; 103: 823–829.
4. Martin BJW, Logemann JA, Shaker R, Dodds WJ. Co-ordination between respiration and swallowing: Respiratory phase relationships and temporal integration. *J Appl Physiol* 1994; 76(2): 714–723.
5. Preiksaitis HG, Mayrand S, Robins K, Diamant NE. Co-ordination of respiration and swallowing: Effect of bolus volume in normal adults. *Am J Physiol* 1992; 263: R624–R630.
6. Selley WG, Flack FC, Ellis RE, Brooks WA. Respiratory patterns associated with swallowing: Part 2. Neurologically impaired dysphagic patients. *Age Ageing* 1989; 18: 173–176.
7. Lundy DS, Casiano RR, Shatz D, Reisberg M, Xue JW. Laryngeal injuries after short versus long term intubation. *J voice* 1998 (Sep); 12(3): 360–365.
8. Ellis P, Bennet J. Laryngeal trauma and prolonged endo-tracheal intubation. *J Laryngol* 1997; 91: 69.
9. De Larminat V, Montravers P, Dureuil B, Desmonts J. Alteration in the swallow reflex after extubation in intensive care patients. *Crit Care Med* 1995; 23: 486–490.
10. Goldsmith T. Evaluation and treatment of swallowing disorders following endotracheal intubation and tracheostomy. *Int Anaesthesiol Clin* 2000 (Summer); 38(3): 219–242.
11. Dikeman K, Kazandjian M. *Communication and Swallowing Management of Tracheostomized and Ventilator Dependent Adults*. CA: Singular Publishing, 1995.
12. Shaker R, Milbrath M, Ren J, Campbell B, Toohill R, Hogan W. Deglutive aspiration in patients with tracheostomy: Effect of tracheostomy on the duration of vocal cord closure. *Gastroenterology* 1995; 108(5): 1357–1360.
13. Saski C, Suzuki M, Horiuchi M, Kirshner J. The effects of tracheostomy on the laryngeal closure reflex. *Laryngoscope* 1997; 8: 1429–1433.
14. Langmore SE, Terpenning MS, Schork A, Chen Y, Murray JT, Lopatin D, Loesche WJ. Predictors of aspiration pneumonia: How important is dysphagia? *Dysphagia* 1998 (Spring); 13(2): 69–81.
15. Leder SB. Gag reflex and dysphagia. *Head Neck* 1996; 18: 138–141.
16. Leder SB. Videofluoroscopic evaluation of aspiration with visual examination of the gag reflex and velar movement. *Dysphagia* 1997; 12: 21–23.
17. Stachler RJ, Hamlet SL, Choi J, Fleming S. Scintigraphic quantification of aspiration reduction with the Passy Muir valve. *Laryngoscope* 1996 (Feb); 106(2): Part 1.

18. Eibling DE, Gross RD. Subglottic air pressure: A key component of swallowing efficiency. *Ann Otol Rhinol Laryngol* 1996 (Apr); 105(4): 253–258.
19. Leder SB, Tarro JM, Burrell MI. Effect of occlusion of a tracheostomy tube on aspiration. *Dysphagia* 1996; 11: 254–258.
20. Leder SB. Effect of a one way tracheostomy speaking valve on the incidence of aspiration in previously aspirating patients with a tracheostomy. *Dysphagia* 1999; 14: 73–77.
21. Thompson-Henry S, Braddock B. The modified Evan's blue dye test procedure fails to detect aspiration in the tracheostomised patient: Five case reports. *Dysphagia* 1995; 10: 172–174.

APPENDIX: BLUE DYE TRACKING SHEET

Speech and language therapy department			

Patient's Name:	Trial Given:		Date: Time:
Ward:	Named Nurse:		

Consistency Trialled: 1) saliva   2) water   3) yoghurt   4) _____

Instructions: _____

_____

_____

Suctioned		Evidence of blue dye present around the stoma site, tube or in suction catheter	
Date	Time	YES	NO

OUTLINE OF THE SPEECH AND LANGUAGE THERAPISTS ASSESSMENT OF A NON-VENTILATED PATIENT WITH A TRACHEOSTOMY TUBE

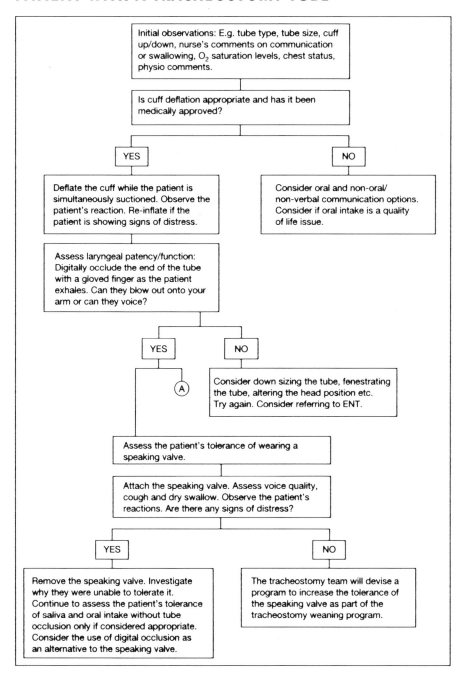

Initial observations: E.g. tube type, tube size, cuff up/down, nurse's comments on communication or swallowing, O_2 saturation levels, chest status, physio comments.

Is cuff deflation appropriate and has it been medically approved?

YES

Deflate the cuff while the patient is simultaneously suctioned. Observe the patient's reaction. Re-inflate if the patient is showing signs of distress.

NO

Consider oral and non-oral/ non-verbal communication options. Consider if oral intake is a quality of life issue.

Assess laryngeal patency/function: Digitally occlude the end of the tube with a gloved finger as the patient exhales. Can they blow out onto your arm or can they voice?

YES

(A)

NO

Consider down sizing the tube, fenestrating the tube, altering the head position etc. Try again. Consider referring to ENT.

Assess the patient's tolerance of wearing a speaking valve.

Attach the speaking valve. Assess voice quality, cough and dry swallow. Observe the patient's reactions. Are there any signs of distress?

YES

Remove the speaking valve. Investigate why they were unable to tolerate it. Continue to assess the patient's tolerance of saliva and oral intake without tube occlusion only if considered appropriate. Consider the use of digital occlusion as an alternative to the speaking valve.

NO

The tracheostomy team will devise a program to increase the tolerance of the speaking valve as part of the tracheostomy weaning program.

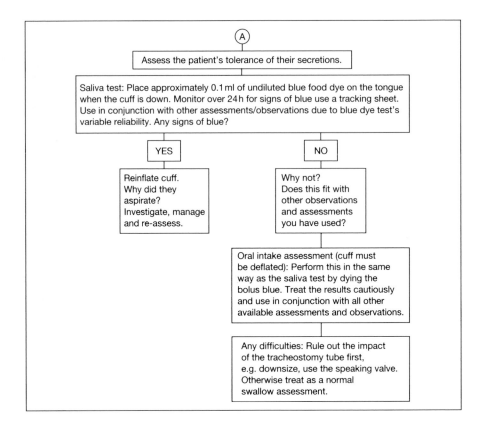

(A)

Assess the patient's tolerance of their secretions.

Saliva test: Place approximately 0.1 ml of undiluted blue food dye on the tongue when the cuff is down. Monitor over 24 h for signs of blue use a tracking sheet. Use in conjunction with other assessments/observations due to blue dye test's variable reliability. Any signs of blue?

YES

NO

Reinflate cuff.
Why did they
aspirate?
Investigate, manage
and re-assess.

Why not?
Does this fit with
other observations
and assessments
you have used?

Oral intake assessment (cuff must
be deflated): Perform this in the same
way as the saliva test by dying the
bolus blue. Treat the results cautiously
and use in conjunction with all other
available assessments and observations.

Any difficulties: Rule out the impact
of the tracheostomy tube first,
e.g. downsize, use the speaking valve.
Otherwise treat as a normal
swallow assessment.

COMMUNICATION

Pippa Hales

INTRODUCTION

One of the Speech and Language Therapist's (SLT) key roles is to maximise a patient's ability to communicate consistently and effectively with the people around them. The patient is as much a part of the multi-disciplinary team as the professionals involved in their care and it is therefore essential that the patient's ability to communicate their needs, opinions and feelings is identified and facilitated.

The SLT, therefore, has a pivotal role within the tracheostomy team, as the presence of the tracheostomy tube alone can impact on the patient's ability to communicate.

This chapter will identify the 'normal' mechanisms of voice and speech production, the impact of the tracheostomy tube on communication and the SLT's assessment and management of a patient with a tracheostomy tube.

NORMAL HEAD AND NECK ANATOMY (Fig. 1)

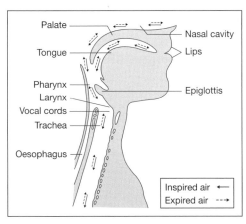

Palate
Nasal cavity
Tongue
Lips
Pharynx
Larynx
Epiglottis
Vocal cords
Trachea
Oesophagus

Inspired air ⟵
Expired air ⤍

Fig. 1: The anatomy of the head and neck demonstrating the path of airflow.

CRANIAL NERVE INVOLVEMENT FOR COMMUNICATION (Table 1)

Table 1: The cranial nerves involved in communication	
Cranial nerve	**Summary of function**
II Optic	Vision.
III Oculomotor	Innervation of muscles to move the eye lid, eyeball and pupil.
IV Trochlear	Innervation of the superior oblique muscle of the eye.
V Trigeminal	Mastication, sensation to the face, movement of the soft palate, anterior and upward movement of the larynx.
VII Facial	Movement of facial muscles, movement of the larynx up and back, taste, salivary glands.
VIII Vestibulocochlear	Hearing and equilibrium.
IX Glossopharyngeal	Lateral dilation of the pharynx, taste to posterior third of the tongue, elevation of the pharynx and larynx, parotid salivary gland, sensation to upper pharynx.
X Vagus	Pharyngeal constriction, sensation to the epiglottis, taste, swallowing, elevation of palate, phonation.
XI Accessory	Head movement, shrugging of shoulders.
XII Hypoglossal	Movement of tongue, phonation.

Collated from Love and Webb.[1]

NORMAL VOICE AND SPEECH PRODUCTION

The production of voice requires three main components:

The Generator – The lungs and air stream
The Vibrator – The vocal cords
The Resonator – The pharynx and the nasal and oral cavities

Speech sounds are then formed by:

The Articulators – The palate, tongue, cheeks, teeth, lips

The generator – the lungs and air stream

Respiration is fundamental to the production of voice, as it can only be achieved as air passes through the larynx. As the air flows through the larynx it sets the adducted vocal cords into motion, causing them to vibrate and consequently create voice.

The vibrator – the vocal cords

The vocal cords are found within the cartilaginous structure of the larynx and are made of two-folds of highly elastic tissue covered in a mucous membrane.

The vocal cords have two main functions:

- *Airway protection:* The vocal cords are essential in expelling unwanted material from the airway. This is achieved by the vocal cords reflexively adducting, causing pressure to build up below them, until they are explosively blown apart to expel the unwanted material.
- *Voicing:* Prior to voicing the vocal cords are abducted to enable the inhalation of air. As the expiratory phase of the respiratory cycle begins the vocal cords adduct, causing pressure to build up below them. They are then rapidly forced apart and into vibration, setting sound waves into motion, creating voice.

The resonators – the pharynx, nasal cavity, oral cavity

The sound then resonates throughout the pharynx and oral and nasal cavities causing the sound waves to become progressively more complex.[2]

Articulators – the palate, tongue, cheeks, teeth, lips

Speech sounds are ultimately formed by the voiced and unvoiced air stream being shaped by the articulators, i.e. the palate, tongue, cheeks, teeth, lips.

As the generator of the voice runs out, the vocal cords abduct allowing for inhalation of air and the cycle of voice production to continue (Table 2).

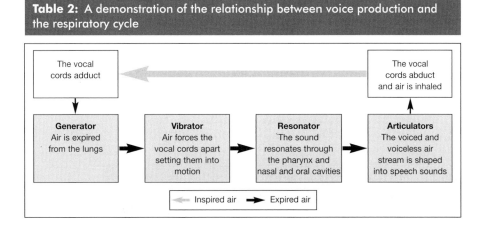

Table 2: A demonstration of the relationship between voice production and the respiratory cycle

THE IMPACT OF THE TRACHEOSTOMY TUBE ON COMMUNICATION

The presence of the tracheostomy tube within the trachea can have a significant impact on a patient's ability to communicate.

This can be divided into two categories:

- Mechanical impact
- Physiological impact

The mechanical impact

Laryngeal tissue changes as a result of endo-tracheal intubation

Endo-tracheal intubation is used to provide and maintain a stable airway by passing a tube through the mouth, into the pharynx and then into the trachea by way of the larynx (Fig. 2). A cuff is then inflated to ensure there is a closed circuit for ventilation and/or to prevent aspiration of secretions. The patient can potentially remain intubated for a matter of weeks before a trial extubation takes place and a tracheostomy will then be considered if the patient is unable to self-ventilate or protect their airway post extubation.

Studies have revealed that endo-tracheal intubation can damage the vocal cords causing granuloma, nodules, oedema or polyps that can ultimately

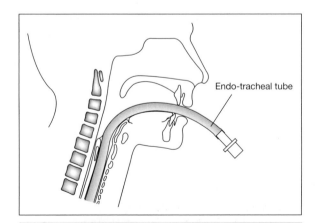

Endo-tracheal tube

Fig. 2: A drawing of the head and neck to demonstrate the positioning of an endo-tracheal tube through the larynx.

result in incomplete laryngeal closure, impacting on voice quality and airway protection.[3,4,5] Similarly, endo-tracheal intubation using an oversized tube and/or an over inflated cuff can result in temporary or long-term vocal cord paralysis as a consequence of the recurrent laryngeal nerve being compressed between the inflated endo-tracheal tube/cuff and the thyroid cartilage.[6,7]

Tracheal injury

Long-term tracheostomies (in place for 6 months or more)[3] requiring cuff inflation can result in damage to the wall of the trachea such as tracheal stenosis and tracheal malacia.[3,5,8] These can ultimately result in reduced airway patency, therefore reducing the airflow into the upper airway, required to produce voice. This type of tracheal injury can remain after decannulation and may require surgical intervention.

Reduced laryngeal elevation

The vertical movement of the larynx during speech alters the length of the vocal cords resulting in pitch variation.[2] The presence of the tracheostomy tube alone is believed to significantly restrict laryngeal elevation and consequently restrict pitch change.

Laryngeal elevation is considered to be restricted as a result of:

- *Surgical technique* – a horizontal incision is more likely to restrict vertical movement of the larynx than a vertical incision.[9]
- *Tube size* – an oversized tube will leave minimal space between its outer circumference and the tracheal wall resulting in inhibited movement that may subsequently anchor the larynx.
- *Weight of the equipment* – the weight of the tracheostomy tube as well as any additional equipment such as a speaking valve or humidification system could be enough to restrict the elevation of the larynx.
- *Cuff inflation* – an inflated cuff and, more significantly, an over inflated cuff, may tether the larynx, restricting its vertical movement (see section on 'Cuffed talking tubes' in Chapter 6, Tracheostomy Tubes).

The physiological impact

Loss or reduction of voice production

The laws of physics stipulate that airflow will always take the path of least resistance. In the unaltered anatomy air passes through the upper airway, through the nose and mouth and back again (Fig. 1). However, when a tracheostomy tube is in situ, the anatomy is altered in such way that the path of

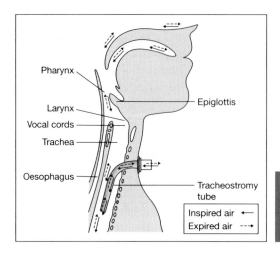

Pharynx

Larynx

Vocal cords

Trachea

Oesophagus

Epiglottis

Tracheostromy tube

Inspired air ←
Expired air ⇢

Fig. 3: A drawing to demonstrate airflow being redirected along the path of least resistance.

least resistance is now through the tube, therefore redirecting all or the majority of the airflow away from the larynx (Fig. 3). This alteration to the respiratory system can ultimately impact on communication in the following ways.

Aphonia – This is the inability to produce voice and will happen as a result of a tracheostomy tube with an inflated cuff being in situ. An inflated cuff will prevent all of the expired air from passing through the larynx by redirecting it from the lungs, through the tracheostomy tube. In doing so the patient becomes aphonic (Fig. 4).

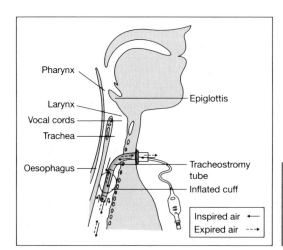

Pharynx

Larynx

Vocal cords

Trachea

Oesophagus

Epiglottis

Tracheostromy tube

Inflated cuff

Inspired air ←
Expired air ⇢

Fig. 4: A drawing to demonstrate the redirection of air away from the larynx in the presence of an inflated cuff.

Dysphonia – Dysphonia is an alteration in a person's voice quality and in this instance it is the result of insufficient airflow passing above the level of the tube. This can result from there being insufficient space between the outer circumference of the tube and the tracheal wall, such as in the presence of an oversized tube or as a result of a narrowed trachea caused by damage to the tracheal wall.

Reduced subglottic air pressure

Subglottic air pressure is the build up of pressure created by adduction of the vocal cords in conjunction with expiration. This is required for normal speech production and coughing. The presence of the tracheostomy tube, however, introduces an outlet below the level of the vocal cords for the air to escape, thus reducing subglottic pressure.

THE IMPACT OF MECHANICAL VENTILATION ON COMMUNICATION

The mechanical impact

Reduced laryngeal elevation

The weight of the equipment attached to the tracheostomy tube required for ventilation may restrict laryngeal elevation and consequently affect voice quality by restricting the mechanism involved in altering pitch.

The physiological impact

Loss of voice

In the majority of cases, a fully inflated cuff is required for ventilation to ensure that the air delivered by the ventilator does not escape and alter the ventilatory pressures. Air cannot, therefore, reach the upper airway in order to create voice, making the patient aphonic.

Co-ordinating ventilation and phonation

A patient requiring mechanical ventilation can achieve voice by the use of cuff deflation in conjunction with appropriate ventilator modifications, allowing airflow to reach the upper airway to create voice.

Voicing occurs during the expiratory phase of the respiratory cycle (Table 2). Ventilated patients, however, often find that their expiratory flow is not strong enough to initiate voicing and therefore have to learn to co-ordinate voicing with the inspiratory phase of the ventilators' cycle. This is known as *leak speech*.

Leak speech – During the inspiratory phase of ventilation the air passes from the ventilator, through the tracheostomy tube and into the lungs. When the

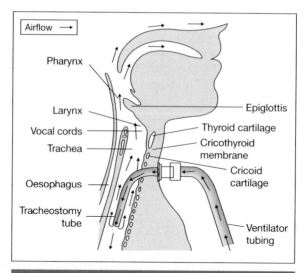

Fig. 5: A drawing to demonstrate how air delivered by the ventilator can also be used to create leak speech.

cuff is deflated some of this air will also leak upwards, past the tube, into the upper airway and can consequently be used to create voice (Fig. 5). However, the resulting change in the relationship between respiration and voice can ultimately cause dysphonia.

ASSESSING THE COMMUNICATIVE ABILITIES OF THE PATIENT WITH A TRACHEOSTOMY

The initial communication assessment of a tracheostomised patient will often take place in an intensive/critical care setting. In this environment the process of assessment differs from that of most other settings, due to the patient's critical and fluctuating medical status. Assessment therefore, needs to be functional and time efficient, as well as adaptable to all levels and aspects of each individual's changing communicative abilities.

Assessment needs to answer the following questions:

- What are the patient's communicative needs?
- What is the patient's current pattern of alertness?
- Are they already communicating?
- If so, how and is it effective?
- Do they have a method of attracting someone's attention?
- Do they have a consistent yes/no response?

- What is their level of cognition? E.g: Is it sufficient to use a communication aid?
- What are the patient's physical/motor abilities? E.g: Oro-motor movement, eye movement, limb movement, has their dominant hand been affected?
- What are the patient's current linguistic abilities? E.g: Are their receptive or expressive language skills within normal limits?
- Who are the patient's main communication partners?

The answers to these questions will help build up a picture of the patient's communicative needs, abilities and potential. This information will then be used to assess which mode or combination of modes would be the most suitable and efficient communication option.

COMMUNICATION OPTIONS

The ultimate goal, with regards to communication, is to restore the patient's ability to communicate verbally, consistently and effectively. This goal is seldom achieved immediately and alternative communication options may therefore need to be considered in order to substitute or support verbal communication in the interim.

The communication options available to the tracheostomy patient are:

- *Verbal communication* – uses natural voice production.
- *Oral communication* – requires sufficient oro-motor skills, without the use of natural voice production.
- *Non-oral/non-verbal communication* – does not require natural voice or oro-motor movements.

Combinations of all of these options are likely to be used in the majority of tracheostomised patients throughout the weaning process.

VERBAL COMMUNICATION OPTIONS

Indications for use

- Medical agreement for cuff deflation.
- Cuff deflation tolerated (see Chapter 11, Swallowing).
- Patent upper airway.
- Air can pass above the level of the tube into upper airway, i.e. around the sides of tube or through a fenestration.
- Able to maintain satisfactory baseline respiratory status with digital occlusion/attachment of the one way speaking valve.
- Ability to produce voice on tube occlusion.
- Sufficient oro-motor function to produce intelligible speech.
- Ability to use language effectively to communicate.

Contraindications for use

- Medical consent for cuff deflation refused.
- Unable to tolerate cuff deflation.
- Patient unable to produce voice.
- Upper airway obstruction.
- Unstable medical/respiratory status.
- Insufficient oro-motor function to produce intelligible speech.
- Severe language or cognitive impairment that affects the patient's ability to use language to communicate effectively.

Assessment of upper airway patency and voice production

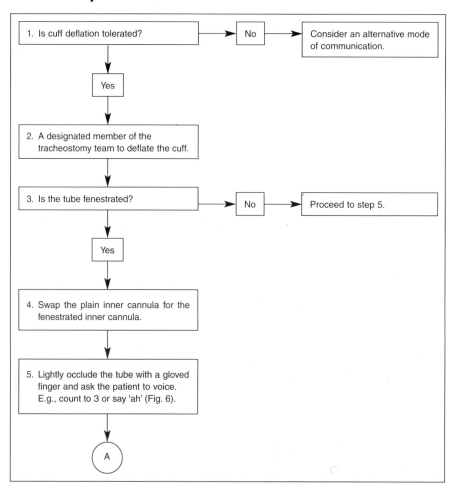

1. Is cuff deflation tolerated? → No → Consider an alternative mode of communication.

Yes

2. A designated member of the tracheostomy team to deflate the cuff.

3. Is the tube fenestrated? → No → Proceed to step 5.

Yes

4. Swap the plain inner cannula for the fenestrated inner cannula.

5. Lightly occlude the tube with a gloved finger and ask the patient to voice. E.g., count to 3 or say 'ah' (Fig. 6).

A

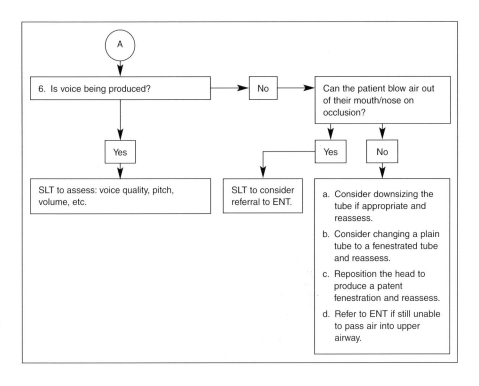

6. Is voice being produced? → No → Can the patient blow air out of their mouth/nose on occlusion?

Yes → SLT to assess: voice quality, pitch, volume, etc.

Yes → SLT to consider referral to ENT.

No →
a. Consider downsizing the tube if appropriate and reassess.
b. Consider changing a plain tube to a fenestrated tube and reassess.
c. Reposition the head to produce a patent fenestration and reassess.
d. Refer to ENT if still unable to pass air into upper airway.

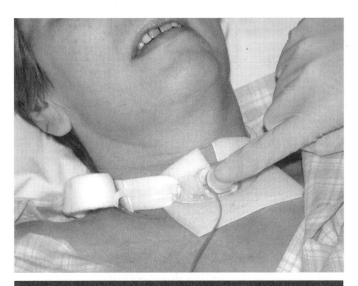

Fig. 6: A picture to demonstrate the use of digital occlusion to assess patency of the upper airway and voice quality.

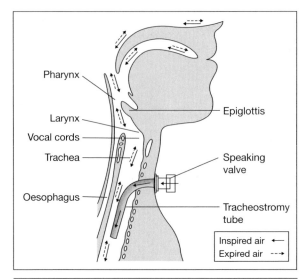

Pharynx

Larynx

Vocal cords

Trachea

Oesophagus

Epiglottis

Speaking valve

Tracheostromy tube

Inspired air ←
Expired air ---→

Fig. 7: A drawing to demonstrate air passing around the sides of the tracheostomy tube to reach the upper airway when a one way speaking valve is attached.

Maximising airflow into the upper airway

When the cuff is deflated and the end of the tracheostomy tube is occluded by a gloved finger or a one way speaking valve, air from the lungs is directed up, past the cuff and through the larynx to potentially create voice.

The presence of the tracheostomy tube alters the anatomy of the trachea so that where air could once pass freely, it is now impeded by the tube and forced to pass around it (Fig. 7).

To increase the column of air able to reach the upper airway two things can be done.

1. Downsize the tube

If the tracheostomy tube is oversized, therefore taking up a large proportion of space within the trachea and restricting airflow into the upper airway, an option would be to downsize the tube to one with a smaller outer circumference. This will increase the space between the tube and the tracheal wall, allowing more air to pass up into the upper airway.

However, downsizing the tube can significantly impact on work of breathing. By downsizing the outer circumference of the tube the inner circumference of the tube is often also reduced, increasing the resistance to airflow. This option must therefore be discussed with the relevant members of the tracheostomy team to best meet the patient's individual needs.

2. Fenestrate the tube

If the patient is not considered a candidate for downsizing the tube then a fenestrated tube can be considered.

A fenestrated tube consists of an outer cannula with a fenestration (one large or several small holes on the outer curvature of the tube), one fenestrated inner cannula and one plain inner cannula. When the fenestrated inner cannula is inserted it allows air to pass through the tube, out of the fenestration and into the upper airway thereby increasing the column of air passing through the larynx (Fig. 8).

A fenestrated tube will only be effective if the fenestration is patent. In some patients the position of the fenestration is such that it interacts with the wall of the trachea, thereby blocking the fenestration and causing trauma to the tracheal wall. In this instance the position of the patient's head can be readjusted in an attempt to unblock the fenestration. If this fails, an alternative tube type will need to be considered.

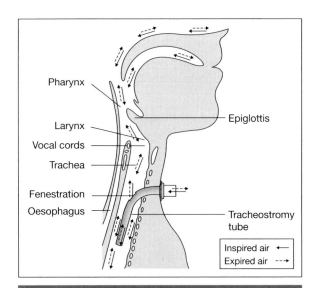

Fig. 8: A drawing to demonstrate air passing through the fenestration and into the upper airway.

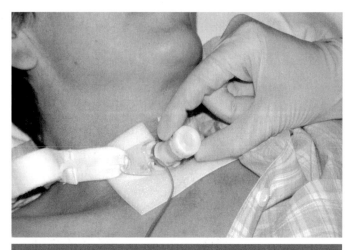

Fig. 9: A picture demonstrating the attachment of the one way speaking valve onto the hub of the tracheostomy tube.

The one way speaking valve

The one way speaking valve attaches to the hub of the tracheostomy tube, altering the path of expired air and providing the potential to produce voice (Fig. 9).

The one way speaking valve works in the following way:

- Air is inspired through the tracheostomy tube.
- On exhalation the valve shuts and the expired airflow is redirected past the tube and/or through the fenestration, into the upper airway allowing voice production (Fig. 10).

N.B: The cuff must be deflated prior to fitting the speaking valve. If the cuff remains inflated the valve will allow the person to breathe in but will prevent them breathing out (Fig. 11).

The benefits of using a one way speaking valve are as follows:

- Provides the facility to produce voice.
- Eliminates the use of digital occlusion.
- Normalises the pathway of expired air.
- Restores subglottic pressure.

Use of the one way speaking valve with non-ventilated patients

1. Obtain medical agreement for cuff deflation.
2. Inform the patient of the procedure and the sensations they can expect.

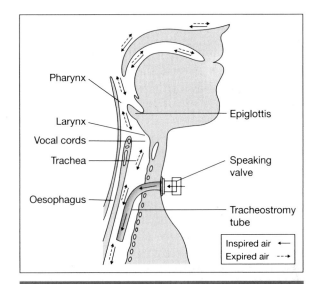

Fig. 10: A drawing to demonstrate how the one way speaking valve alters the respiratory pattern.

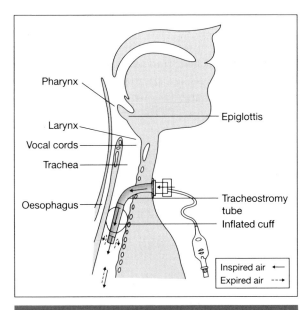

Fig. 11: A drawing to demonstrate why the cuff should not be inflated when the speaking valve is attached.

225

3. The cuff must be fully deflated by a designated member of the tracheostomy team and the patient suctioned if indicated.
4. Change the plain inner cannula to a fenestrated inner cannula if applicable.
5. Assess upper airway patency using digital occlusion.
6. The SLT will assess gross vocal cord function using digital occlusion.
7. Attach the speaking valve to the hub of the tracheostomy tube if the upper airway is deemed patent.
8. Verbally reinforce the change in the respiratory pattern, i.e. breathing in through the tracheostomy tube and out through the nose and mouth.
9. Encourage the patient to produce voice, i.e. counting to 3, saying 'ah'.
10. The SLT will assess voice quality.
11. Monitor the patient's physiological and clinical response to the use of the speaking valve for indications of intolerance, e.g. increased work of breathing, fatigue, decreasing O_2 saturation levels, a change in skin pallor.
12. Remove the speaking valve if/when these occur.
13. The Tracheostomy Team will determine a programme for weaning and increasing the tolerance of the speaking valve according to the patient's response to its use.

Use of one way speaking valve with ventilated patients

Ventilated patients can also benefit from using a speaking valve by using the #007 Passy Muir speaking valve.

1. Obtain medical agreement for cuff deflation.
2. A designated member of the Tracheostomy Team will fully deflate the cuff and will suction the patient if indicated.
3. A designated member of the Tracheostomy Team trained in the use of mechanical ventilators will make the necessary modifications to the ventilator settings.
4. Disconnect the ventilator tubing from the hub of the tracheostomy tube.
5. Place the #007 Passy Muir speaking valve onto the hub of the tracheostomy tube or as close to the tube as possible using the necessary attachments.
6. Re-attach the ventilator tubing to the speaking valve.
7. Monitor the patient's physiological and clinical response and adjust the ventilator settings accordingly.
8. Encourage the patient to produce voice, i.e. counting to 3, saying 'ah'.
9. The SLT will assess voice quality.
10. The Tracheostomy Team will determine a programme for weaning and increasing the tolerance of the speaking valve according to the patient's response to its use.
11. Remove the speaking valve when considered appropriate, e.g. if the patient is seen not to be tolerating the valve.

12. Re-attach the ventilator tubing to the hub of the tracheostomy tube.
13. Restore the cuff status and ventilator settings to their previous status/ levels.

ORAL COMMUNICATION OPTIONS
Indications for use

- Sufficient oro-motor function to produce intelligible speech as assessed by the SLT.
- Ability to use language effectively to communicate.
- Aphonia, e.g. the patient is unable to produce voice due to vocal cord dysfunction.

Contraindications for use

- Insufficient oro-motor function to produce intelligible speech.
- Severe language or cognitive impairment that may affect the patient's ability to use language to communicate effectively.

Mouthing

Mouthing can be effective and is an innate form of oral communication.

The benefits of mouthing
- It is immediately accessible.
- It is innate.
- Improvements to clarity of mouthing can be made quickly, e.g. by repositioning or adding dentures.

The limitations of mouthing
- Not all of the patient's communication partners will be able to 'lip read' consistently and effectively.
- Altered dentition, e.g. removed dentures, can alter the structure of the mouth making mouthing less intelligible.
- Inadequate positioning can make mouthing difficult to see to read. It can also reduce intelligibility.
- Not all speech sounds are visible to lip read.

Ways of making mouthing more effective and successful
- Ensure you are clearly able to see the patient's mouth.
- Replace dentures if appropriate.

- Encourage the patient to use shorter phrases.
- Encourage the patient to look for acknowledgement from the listener that they have understood.

Electro larynges

An electro larynx gives those patients who are aphonic but can mouth sufficiently, the ability to create speech sounds.

The electro larynx vibrates the air in the airway (in place of the vocal cords), creating sound, which can then be shaped into speech sounds by the articulators.

There are two types of electro larynx:

- Neck/cheek.
- Oral.

A neck/cheek-type electro larynx is placed on the side of the patient's neck in the approximate region of the larynx or on the cheek, according to what the patient finds most successful. It is then switched on while the patient mouths. This aid requires good arm and hand function to be used effectively. Alternatively a communication partner can be trained to operate it. Maximum intelligibility is often achieved when the patient reduces their rate of speech and concentrates on clear articulation of each speech sound.

An oral-type electro larynx works on the same principle as the neck/cheek-type but the vibrations are sent along a thin tube that is placed into the oral cavity to vibrate the air within it. This type requires less manual dexterity. Some versions can also be operated with remote switches making it accessible to patients with restricted upper limb movement.

NON-VERBAL/NON-ORAL COMMUNICATION OPTIONS

There will be periods of time for most tracheostomised patients when they will be unable to rely 100% on oral or verbal communication. It is, therefore, essential that an alternative method of communication is made accessible in order to ensure that communication continues.

Indications for use

- Insufficient oro-motor function.
- Inability to successfully use oral or verbal communication options 100% of the time.

Contraindication for use

- Severe language or cognitive impairment that may affect the patient's ability/desire to use language to communicate effectively.

Handwriting

Handwriting will be a natural and familiar mode of communication to the majority of tracheostomised patients and is readily accessible, i.e. requires only a pen and paper. It is therefore the first alternative mode to be considered.

This option requires the patient to be literate, with adequate vision, fine motor movement, the ability to use the non-dominant hand if the dominant hand has been affected, and can be positioned adequately.

If the patient is to rely on handwriting as their main mode of communication the team needs to evaluate whether it is legible in all circumstances and whether they need additional equipment to assist in positioning the pen, the paper and the patient. Confidentiality also needs to be considered as the written word will leave a tangible record unless the message can be easily erased, e.g. by using a wipe clean board.

Drawing

Drawing can be used to supplement written and spoken language when other modes fail, e.g. if a patient is dysphasic and has word finding difficulties they may be able to draw a picture of the message they are trying to convey.

This will require the same physical abilities and evaluation as handwriting will and cannot be relied upon as the sole mode of communication.

Gesture

Gesture can be used to support other modes of communication in the same capacity as drawing can and requires sufficient upper limb movement.

Gesture needs to be used more specifically by people with language impairments than it does when it accompanies natural, unimpaired speech, e.g. in normal speech we use gesture to emphasise stress and mark out the intonation and rhythm of our speech whereas a language impaired person may need to use gesture to act out specific words or point to items in their immediate environment. Ultimately this could be developed into a form of sign language if this was considered the preferred mode of communication.

Direct selection

If a patient has any form of voluntary motor movement this can be utilised to enable them to create a message by selecting a letter, word, phrase picture, photo etc. and is ideal for those who are unable to rely on handwriting.

- *Communication board* – This low tech board can display, letters, words, pictures etc. which can be selected by pointing with digits, limbs, pointers etc (Fig. 12).
- *Electronic keyboard* – This can be operated by switches, digits, pointers etc. to convey a message (Fig. 13).

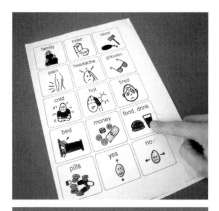

Fig. 12: A low tech communication chart.

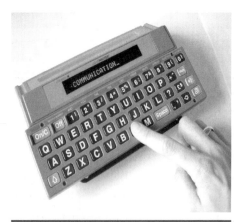

Fig. 13: An electronic communication aid.

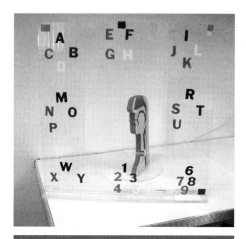

Fig. 14: An E-tran frame using encoding.

- *E-tran* – This is a transparent frame with letters, words etc. positioned on it in groups. The message is conveyed by the message sender selecting the desired component of the message using eye pointing, while the communication partner deciphers the message by standing in front of them, tracking their eye gaze. This allows those with the most minimal movement to communicate effectively (Fig. 14).

Scanning

This form is dependent on the person having a reliable way to signal for the scanning to stop, such as closing the eyes, nodding or operating a switch. A sequence of items such as letters or pictures are pointed to or passed in front of the message sender until they signal for the scanning to stop as the desired item is shown. This process continues until the message is completed. Some electronic communication aids have the benefit of a scanning mode that can be operated by way of a switch.

Encoding

This method can be incorporated into both direct selection and scanning methods. It involves using a simple code to deliver a more complex message.

For example, a message board may display ten, numbered, set phrases depicting a person's basic needs. The person then needs to select a number in order to communicate a set message. They could do this by blinking or tapping their finger the specified number of times to make the selection. Colour coding can also be used in order to develop the code further (Fig. 14). E.g. 'red 1' means 'what time is it?' where as 'yellow 1' means 'I need to be suctioned'.

It is advisable to record each selected component, e.g. by writing it down to ensure that the message is successfully pieced together without part of it being forgotten.

TRAINING COMMUNICATION PARTNERS

Communication, in its simplest form, is a two way process, consisting of a message sender and a message receiver. Thus, to send or receive a message successfully, the mode of communication must be known and understood by both parties.

It is the SLT's responsibility to train all relevant communication partners, supporting them in their learning.

To accomplish this, the patient's key communication partners, e.g. the patient's family, friends, and members of the medical team, need to be identified and trained in the specific mode and instructions need to be placed in the patient's immediate environment to target any partners who have not been trained directly. These interactions need to be observed and monitored so that any communication breakdowns can be identified and rectified immediately with the intention of maintaining its consistency and effectiveness.

WHEN TO REFER TO SPEECH AND LANGUAGE THERAPY?

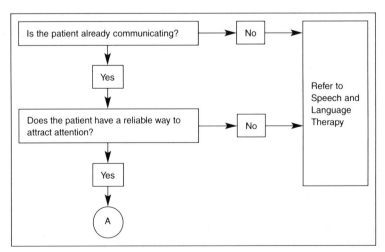

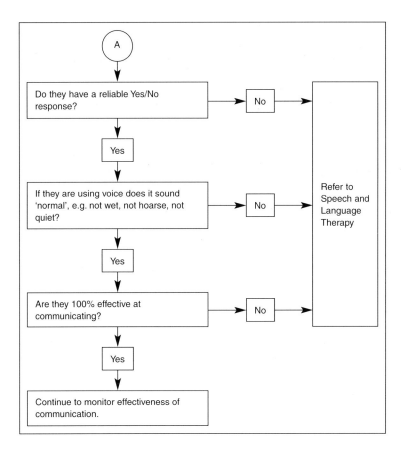

Summary

A key part of the SLT's role with patients with tracheostomies is to optimise the patient's ability to communicate successfully. Ultimately, the patient is the pivotal member of the Tracheostomy Team and their capacity to communicate with the people around them is paramount to their care, psyche and general well-being. It is therefore essential that their communication needs and abilities are identified and maximised at the very outset of their care.

REFERENCES

1. Love R, Webb W. *Neurology for the Speech and Language Pathologist*, 3rd edn. Newton, MA: Butterworth and Heinmann, 1996.
2. Greene M, Mathieson L. *The Voice and its Disorders*, 5th edn. London: Whurr, 1997.
3. Logemann J. *Evaluation and Treatment of Swallowing Disorders*. Austin, TX: Pro. ed, 1998.

4. Colice GL. Resolution of laryngeal injury following translaryngeal intubation. *Am Rev Respir Dis* 1992; 145: 361–364.
5. Kazandjian M, Dikeman K. Communication options for tracheostomy and ventilator dependent patients. In: Myers E, Johnson J, Murry T (eds). *Tracheotomy: Airway Management, Communication and Swallowing*. San Diego, CA: Singular Publishing, 1998; 97–118.
6. Ellis P, Bennet J. Laryngeal trauma and prolonged endo-tracheal intubation. *J Laryngol* 1977; 91: 69.
7. Cav J. True vocal cord paralysis following intubation. *Laryngoscope* 1985; 95: 1352.
8. Devita MA, Spiere-Rundback L. Swallowing disorders in patients with prolonged orotracheal intubation or tracheostomy tubes. *Crit care med* 1990; 18: 1328–1330.
9. Dikeman K, Kazandjian M. *Communication and Swallowing Management of Tracheostomized and Ventilator Dependent Adults*. San Diego, CA: Singular Publishing, 1995.

TRACHEOSTOMY TUBE CHANGES

Claudia Russell

Changing a tracheostomy tube carries significant risk. Complications associated with tube changes usually occur when there is inadequate preparation of patient and facilities. If the tube exchange fails and there is an excessive delay to intubate, it can be fatal.[1]

This chapter will discuss the indications for tube changes including both elective and emergency situations. Preparation and practice guidelines to assist with the management of the tube change will also be included.

Along with the straightforward tube change procedure, the chapter identifies risk factors for difficult tube changes and will make suggestions for appropriate precautions and management techniques.

The practitioner preparing for changing a tracheostomy tube should have a good understanding of the anatomy and physiology of the upper airway. Support from a clinical manager and from the relevant professional body is required in order to confirm whether it is appropriate and within the individual's scope of practice to change a tracheostomy tube without direct supervision. Ongoing supervision and support with clinical practice will allow the individual to improve their practice and be able to appropriately evaluate any problems that may arise.

Some consideration should be given to clearly identify the benefits to the patient by taking on this skill and also the feasibility of maintaining the skill within their own clinical practice.

INDICATIONS FOR A TUBE CHANGE

Changing a tracheostomy tube is not without risk or anxiety for the patient. It is therefore only advocated when there is a clinical need. Tube changes can be divided into the elective and emergency indications (see Table 1).

Table 1: Indications for changing a tracheostomy tube

Elective:
- Facilitate weaning/speech production
- Maximum recommended time in situ as set by EEC Directives[2]
- To increase patient comfort
- To allow non-routine cleaning and dressing of a tracheostomy wound
- To allow treatment of granulation tissue at stoma site and/or fenestration

Emergency:
- Blocked tube
- Misplaced or displaced tube
- Cuff failure
- Faulty tube
- Resuscitation

THE PROCEDURE

Each tube change requires the same preparation and careful consideration of potential risks. Every tube change should be carried out with at least two suitably trained staff. This will enable one person to hold the tube securely while the tapes and dressings are being removed and changed. Where a child or adult is likely to struggle or become agitated, a third person may be needed to offer further assistance.

An individual's preference and confidence needs to be considered, along with the clinical situation, when deciding whether the person to insert the tube will also remove the old one. It is recommended that the practitioner who is to insert the tube should also remove the previous tube. This allows the practitioner to assess the position and angle of the tract and alerts them of any ledge or resistance that they may encounter. Whichever method is chosen, clear responsibilities should be identified between the team and the patient before the procedure is started.

PREPARATION

Preparation for a tube change should include the patient, the staff and carers. In addition to this, the equipment that may be required should be at hand, in case complications occur (see Table 2). Complications can occur at any tube change, the same precautions need to be in place before every tube change irrespective of the individual's experience and the number of previous tube changes.

Table 2: Complications of tube changes

- Trauma and bleeding
- Aspiration
- Coughing
- Hypoxia
- Misplacement of tube
- Failure to re-insert tube
- Respiratory arrest
- Anxiety
- Discomfort

Team preparation

Communication with the patient, colleagues and carers prior to the procedure, needs to include a description of what is to happen, the rationale for the positioning and precautions used. The likely side-effects of the procedure should be explained prior to the procedure to alleviate anxiety during the procedure. The most common side-effects of a tube change are coughing and local discomfort, which for most will resolve spontaneously. A well-informed patient will promote compliance during the procedure and also reduce any anxiety for future tube changes. Communication between the team, including the patient, is paramount for a safe and successful procedure.

The elective tube change should be planned for a time of day to suit the necessary staff involved and also the staff who may be needed in the event of any complications. If the patient is ventilator dependent, an anaesthetist should be aware of the planned procedure, in the event that the patient requires intubation.

The choice of tube size and style should have been considered, prior to the procedure, by the relevant members of the multi-disciplinary team to ensure the most appropriate tube is inserted to promote safe management and care. The patient's quality of life will be addressed by considering comfort, potential for speech and/or swallowing and any potential weaning or decannulation trials with the chosen tube.

Patient preparation

Clinical assessment
Prior to the tube change, thorough assessment and preparation of the patient will promote a safe and timely procedure. The patient should be clinically stable and should be able to tolerate the short period of cuff deflation and absent ventilatory support. A review of the mode of ventilation and oxygen

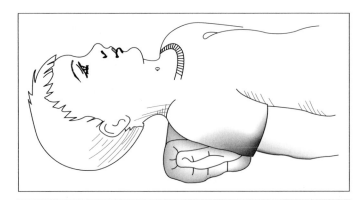

Fig. 1: Child positioned for a tube change (courtesy of Mallinckrodt).

administration is required and an increase in both may be necessary pre- and post-procedure to reduce significant hypoxia.[3] If the patient is at risk from vomiting and/or aspirating any gastric contents, then the patient should have been kept nil by mouth (NBM) for at least 3–4 h and aspirate the nasogastric tube if present.[4] If the situation has not allowed for a period of NBM and the patient is at risk of aspiration, then it is suggested to apply cricoid pressure to further protect the airway.[3]

Patient positioning

The ideal position to change a tube is with the patient in the supine position with the neck in hyperextension. This will place the trachea closer to the skin and re-align the tracheal and skin openings as when the procedure was performed.[1] A sandbag or rolled towel underneath the patient's shoulders will allow neck hyperextension as shown in Figures 1 and 2.

Before positioning the patient it is important to ascertain whether it is contra-indicated, e.g. unstable spine, cervical osteoarthritis. For some patients it may be advisable to sit them upright for the procedure to promote the comfortable clearance of secretions.[1]

Psychological preparation

A tube change can be a worrying time for a patient and their carers. An adequate explanation and preparation for the patient are essential in helping to alleviate these concerns. Appropriate information will allow informed verbal consent and promote co-operation with the procedure. If the patient is anxious it may be useful to use a local anaesthetic to the throat, e.g. xylocaine spray.[1]

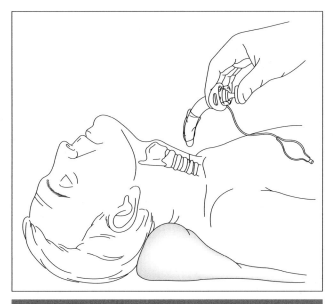

Fig. 2: Adult positioned for a tube change (courtesy of Shiley, Mallinckrodt).

Equipment preparation

Due to the speed at which both elective and emergency procedure needs to be carried out the patient must have with them, or by their bedside, the appropriate emergency equipment (see Table 3).

TRACHEOSTOMY TUBE CHECKS

- The inner tube and introducer (where available) must be inserted into the outer tube to check fit and ease of removal, prior to insertion.
- The patency, uniformity and shape of the inflated cuff must be assessed and confirmed prior to insertion to ensure safe use as a cuffed tube. The appropriate test volume for each tube is indicated within the manufacturers product leaflet.
- All air must be removed prior to insertion to ensure the cuff does not inhibit tube insertion.
- Tube size (when changing type and/or manufacturer it is important to cross reference the outer diameter of each tube as this will determine the tube size inserted (see Chapter 6, Tracheostomy Tubes)).
- Check for cracks tears and decreased flexibility especially if using a re-usable tube.[5]

The tube change procedure is detailed in Table 4.

Table 3: Equipment list

Item	Rationale
Tracheal dilators	May be used to support the tracheal opening
Same size tube	To be inserted (if cuffed then check uniformity and patency of cuff with test volume as recommended in the product leaflet)
Smaller size tube	For use if unable to insert 'same size' tube
Stitch cutters	To remove skin and tracheal sutures (where appropriate)
10 ml syringe	To inflate and deflate cuff (where appropriate)
Cuff pressure manometer	To measure cuff pressure (where appropriate)
Blunt ended scissors	To allow safe cutting of tracheostomy tapes
Sandbag or rolled up towel	To be placed underneath shoulders to extend the neck (unless contra-indicated)
Gloves, apron and eyeshield	To prevent cross infection
Tracheostomy ties/tapes	To secure the tube
Suction equipment	To clear oropharyngeal, tracheal or chest secretions
Water soluble lubricating gel	To ease tube insertion
Normal saline	To clean peri-stomal skin
Pre-cut tracheostomy dressing and barrier solution	To provide an absorbent wound dressing, protect skin and to aide comfort
Additional equipment	
Guidewire or bougie	To ensure correct placement of a tube in an early or difficult tube change
Re-breath bag	For resuscitation post tube change
Stethoscope	To assist with chest auscultation and correct cuff inflation
Intubation equipment	In case of unsuccessful tube insertion

Table 4: The tube change procedure

Action	Rationale
Put on gloves, apron and eye protection	To adhere to infection control guidelines
Remove clothing that obstructs the neck	To allow good visualisation and access to the tracheostome
Prepare tube with introducer in place on a prepared sterile surface	To allow ready access to a prepared tube and dressing pack

Table 4 (continued)

Action	Rationale
Apply a small amount of water soluble lubricating gel along the length of the shaft, deflated cuff and introducer tip (Optional: attach tapes/straps)	To minimise trauma to tracheal mucosa during insertion of the tube, excessive amounts will cause aspiration and coughing
Lie the patient flat with neck extended and pillow underneath the shoulders (unless contra-indicated)	To ensure correct positioning for insertion of the tube
Cut/untie the tapes/straps and remove the soiled tube while asking the patient to breathe out	Conscious expiration relaxes the patient and reduces the risk of coughing[3]
Observe stoma site	To identify signs of infection, wound breakdown and/or granulation tissue
Insert new tube in an 'up and over' action	Introducing the tube in this way is less traumatic as this directs the tube along the contour of the tracheostomy tract
Remove the introducer	The patient cannot breathe with the introducer in situ
Assess for correct positioning: • Chest rising? • Expired breath observed/heard/felt • Equal and bilateral air entry	To assess patency of new tube and correct placement
If correct position confirmed then proceed to next steps. If not refer to attached flowchart.	
Re-inflate cuff to within 15–25 cmH$_2$O, check with pressure manometer	To assist with positive pressure ventilation and protect from aspiration
Place the inner tube in position	The inner tube maintains patency of the tube
Suction mouth and tracheostomy as required	To clear secretions following tube change and cuff deflation
Re-attach required ventilation equipment	To recommence ventilation support
Clean around the stoma and gently dry	To prevent wound infection and promote comfort and skin integrity
Replace dressing if appropriate	To protect the patients skin from secretions and improve comfort
Secure the tube with tracheostomy tape or velcro ties	To prevent dislodgement of the tube

CUFF INFLATION

The following techniques are recommended when inflating the cuff to provide an adequate seal to allow positive pressure ventilation and/or protection from aspiration. Both techniques require an experienced practitioner to auscultate, with a stethoscope, the trachea above the level of the tracheostomy tube. The practitioner listens carefully to monitor the moment airflow ceases and starts as each 0.5 ml of air is instilled. The cuff is then inflated until either: *minimal leak technique* (MLT) inserts the smallest volume of air that allows a small leak on inspiration, or *minimal occlusive volume* (MOV) inserts the smallest amount of air that prevents air leak on inspiration.[6]

The cuff pressure is then checked using a cuff pressure manometer to ensure the pressure of the cuff on the tracheal mucosa does not exceed 25 cmH$_2$O (18 mmHg). Tracheal capillary obstruction occurs at 37 mmHg, leading to tissue necrosis, stenosis and/or fistula formation.

POST TUBE CHANGE

Return oxygen delivery to the previous level, as clinically indicated, and where indicated arrange for a chest X-ray to allow visual confirmation of the position of the tube (in particular the distance of the tube tip from the carina).[6] Clear away all equipment with special note to sharps, such as stitch cutters.

Document appropriately in the patient's care plan the following information:

- Reason for tube change
- Type, manufacturer and size of tube inserted
- Ease of insertion
- Cuff pressure after inflation
- If any sedation was required, the dose and type
- SaO$_2$ and vital signs during and after the procedure
- Condition of the stoma site
- Amount and colour of any secretions
- Date of next planned change/assessment

EARLY TUBE CHANGES

A newly formed tracheostomy will close more quickly than the more established tracheostomy tract.[7] Indeed in the first 48 h it is recognised that a tube change can be difficult or even impossible.[8] If a change is necessary within the first 48 h then it is recommended that a good light source, good patient positioning and a bougie or guidewire be used.[8] Complications of premature tube changes can lead to the creation of a false passage, developing subcutaneous air collection, pneumothorax and an inability to control the airway and to ventilate the patient.[9]

There are two methods of forming a tracheostomy, a surgical opening and a percutaneous dilatational approach. The latter can prove to be a more challenging early tube change due to the stoma site shrinking down as the tube supporting the stoma is removed. This may potentially make it harder to re-insert the tube and also increasing the risk of tube misplacement.[10]

For both techniques it should be ascertained, by reading the operation note, details of the position and size of the thyroid isthmus and whether it was divided or retracted during surgery, which may allow it to fall down and obscure the tracheal opening once the tube is removed.[1] The clinician should also have made note of any tracheal deviation, presence of scar tissue and/or tumour presence which may affect the success of subsequent tube changes.

WHO SHOULD CARRY OUT THE FIRST TUBE CHANGE?

The first tube change, dependent on the patient's clinical needs and condition, may take place between 5–7 days post-formation. This first tube change should ideally be carried out by the clinician/individual who performed the tracheostomy. This clinician will establish that the stoma has healed sufficiently and to assess whether other trained personnel can safely carry out subsequent tube changes without direct supervision.[9] Experienced ear, nose and throat (ENT), surgical or critical care nurses or physiotherapists may also carry out tube changes with the surgeon/anaesthetist in agreement and close at hand.

Following the first successful change the tube can be changed by a suitably trained nurse with the carer involved at the agreed and required level to suit the patient, the team and themselves. Whoever is to carry out the procedure should have access to ongoing specialist training, advice and support.

FREQUENCY OF TUBE CHANGES

Subsequent tube changes will depend on the patient's condition, clinical needs and the suitability of the current tube to accommodate these needs. The majority of adult patients with a tracheostomy, especially on the general ward, are recommended to have a tube with an inner cannula.[11] This system facilitates the maintenance of the patent airway due to the ability to remove and clean/replace the inner cannula. It is recommended that these tubes be changed every 28–30 days, depending on the manufacturers guidelines.[2] Tubes without an inner cannula need to be changed more frequently to ensure a patent airway. It is recommended that single lumen tubes are changed every 7 to 10 days.[4]

PAEDIATRIC CONSIDERATIONS

For the paediatric age group (0–15 years) a smaller airway can pose a greater risk (see Chapter 17, Paediatric Tracheostomy). To help prevent difficulty in inserting the tube within the crucial first week while the tract is forming, a 'stay' suture is placed at either side of the vertical incision. They are then clearly labelled and secured to the chest. These 'stay' sutures (Fig. 3) can be used to open up the incision by applying gentle tension laterally making the tube insertion easier. Once this first tube change has been successfully performed these sutures are removed.

Due to the narrower inner diameter of the paediatric tracheostomy tube (2.5–5.0 mm) the tube has a higher risk of partial or complete occlusion from the build up of secretions. In the event of a build up of secretions which cannot be cleared by suctioning an urgent tube change may be indicated. To reduce the likelihood of this occurring effective humidification and suction are required along with regular tube changes every seven days.[12]

In order to choose an appropriate tube for each child, some may need the length to be adjusted/trimmed to ensure adequate ventilation without causing damage to the carina. In instances where tubes are trimmed to fit, it is important that the length is noted and the bedside 'emergency' tube is also trimmed to this length ready for use.[5]

With elective tube changes it is recommended to allow a one and a half hour period of NBM prior to a tube change due to the risk of increased

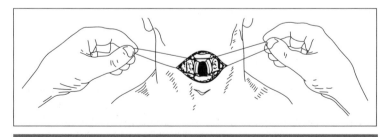

Fig. 3: Stay sutures.

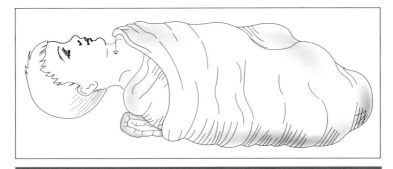

Fig. 4: Child swaddled for a tube change.

coughing which may induce vomiting and aspiration.[13] Some children may go into spasm after the tube has been removed, usually waiting a second will allow the child to relax and allow the tube to be inserted smoothly.[5] The young child may require gentle but firm holding or swaddling to allow the parents or practitioners to carry out the tube change, see Figures 1 and 4.

The early involvement of a play therapist can reduce anxiety in children related to this regular and necessary procedure. Whether or not the parents or carers are present for the first tube change will depend on the clinical issues and the needs of the child and parents/carers.

When the child continues to require a tracheostomy on discharge, the parents/carers should be trained in all aspects of tracheostomy care including tube changes. Training should include appropriate theoretical knowledge with adequate practical skills and should start as soon as they are comfortable and it is clinically appropriate. All parents and significant carers should have observed a tube change prior to carrying out one themselves. Each main carer is required to have carried out 2–3 supervised tube changes prior to discharge. These tube changes can be carried out as frequently as the child and carers are comfortable with, and in line with any planned discharge date. The caregiver must also be trained to identify problems and how to manage tracheostomy tube complications including tube misplacement, a blocked tube, difficulty to re-pass the tube and also resuscitation techniques.

Training should be extended to all those who will have sole responsibility of the child and may include, grandparents, childminders, teachers, teaching assistants and neighbours. The benefit in providing an ongoing training programme commenced at an early stage means that safe discharge into the community is less likely to be hindered by delays.[9]

TROUBLESHOOTING

Thorough preparation of the patient, equipment and carers will usually be sufficient for the straight forward tube change. However where difficulties are predicted and/or occur (Table 5), additional strategies can be required to ensure the successful re-insertion of a tube.

Table 5: Risk factors for a difficult tube change
• Obstructed upper airway, e.g. tumour growth, infection, oedema, bilateral vocal cord palsy
• Large pre-tracheal space, e.g. obese patients, enlarged thyroid
• Thyroid isthmus not divided, may slip down over tracheal opening
• Paediatric or neo-natal age group
• Lack of patient compliance, e.g. patient is hypoxic, in pain, scared or confused
• Deviated/narrow trachea
• Insertion of a larger tube
• Patient unable to extend neck or tilt jaw, e.g. patient with an unstable spine
• New tracheostomy (performed less than 5 days ago)
• Evidence of scarring, calcification or granulation tissue at stoma site
• Lack of training and/or preparation for the procedure
• Emergency scenario

MISPLACED TUBES

The tracheostomy tube in certain incidences may become displaced or misplaced (in a false tract). Tube misplacement during a tube change may occur when the caudal turn is carried out prematurely creating a false tract into the medistinum.[1] A tube may become misplaced if the tube is not of an adequate length to allow ventilation upon patient re-positioning or coughing. Table 6 identifies risk factors of a misplaced tube and Table 7 lists signs of a misplaced tube.

Table 6: Risk factors for a misplaced tube
• Short, thick necks
• Coughing
• Patient movement
• Low stoma placement
• Loose tracheal tapes
• Traction on the tube by ventilator and/or humidification attachments
• Positive pressure ventilation on non-compliant lungs[7]

Table 7: Signs of a misplaced tube

- Voice with cuffed tube, when previously no voice
- Increased tube extending from the stoma
- Decreasing saturation's
- Patient's pallor
- Absent or reduced expired air from tracheostomy
- Suction catheter unable to pass down below end of tube
- Respiratory distress
- Stridor
- Agitation

Strategies used to prevent tube misplacement of the new tracheostomy include suturing the tube in situ, securing the tube with ties which allow the insertion of only 1–2 finger between the tapes and skin and adequate support of all attachments applied to the distal end of the tube, e.g. ventilator tubing, humidification circuits. Tube misplacement is a rare and potentially fatal complication of new tracheostomies which will necessitate urgent management to re-establish the tracheostomy or an alternative airway. Even a short period of hypoxia may lead to brain damage or cardiac arrest.[6]

BOUGIES AND GUIDEWIRES

The benefit of using a bougie/guidewire is to allow a secure passageway for the new tube in the instance where difficulty in passing the new tube is predicted. This can make the procedure more uncomfortable and lengthy for the patient so it should only be used when necessary and by a competent practitioner. The use and selection of either a bougie or guidewire will depend on the practitioner's clinical judgement, suitability of tube system and the inner diameter of the tube.

The bougie should first be checked to ensure it will allow the smooth movement of the tube over it. The bougie will need to be moulded to mirror the natural curvature of the tube (Figs 5, 6).

Guidewires are a more flexible method of ensuring the correct passage of the tube and for certain tube systems they can be combined with the introducer which allows a more comfortable tube insertion for the patient (Portex Blueline Ultra) (Fig. 7).

When using a bougie or guidewire, care must be taken not to remove the device on withdrawal of the tube to ensure that the bougie/guidewire stays in the correct position within the tracheal opening.

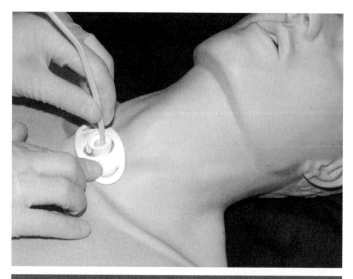

Fig. 5: Bougie inserted into tube lumen.

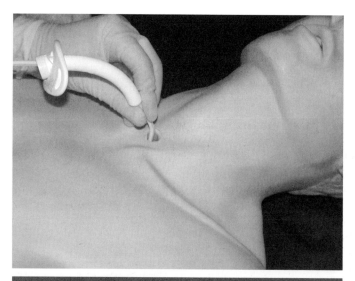

Fig. 6: Tube removal over bougie.

TRACHEAL DILATORS

Tracheal dilators should be found at the bedside of every patient with a tracheostomy. They may be required in an early, complicated or initially unsuccessful tube change. They are inserted closed, into the visualised stoma, with care taken

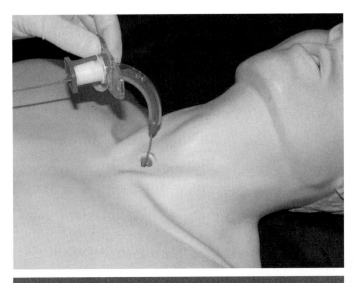

Fig. 7: Insertion of tube with obturator using a guidewire.

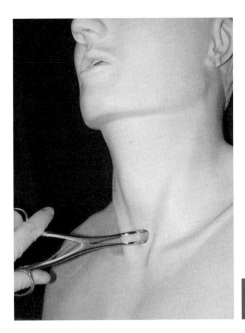

Fig. 8: Tracheal dilators supporting the stoma opening.

not to rest the dilators on the posterior tracheal wall. They are then opened at either 3 o'clock or 9 o'clock position by squeezing the dilator arms together until slight pressure is exerted upon the tracheal opening. The dilators will support the tracheal cartilage rings open and prevent rapid stoma closure (Fig. 8).

Dilators are available in adult and paediatric sizes, although the size of an infant stoma may not permit the insertion and opening of the dilators to allow a tube to be passed through.

STRATEGIES TO HELP WITH A DIFFICULT TUBE CHANGE

Difficulties may arise with any tube change, however with a sound knowledge of alternative techniques these difficulties should be able to be safely managed. In the event of either the tube entering a false tract or the tube not entering the stoma at all it is vital that assistance is requested immediately. While help is being obtained further attempts should be made to re-gain the patent tracheostomy once more.

Tips to assist the management of a difficult tube change
- Re-positioning the patient (fully extending the neck and/or lying flat).
- Tracheal dilators can be used to hold open the stoma while attempts to re-insert the tube continue.
- Using your fingers, gently spread the skin either side of the stoma.
- Attempt tube insertion as the patient inhales.
- If partly inserted, remove the tubes introducer, to allow the patient to breath while attempts continue, and then fully insert the whole tube.[14]
- Following three or more unsuccessful attempts with the same sized tube, attempt inserting the smaller sized tracheostomy tube already prepared at the bedside.
- If a tube can be inserted but air entry cannot be confirmed on several attempts, then the tube should be removed to prevent obstruction of the airway by the tube in the pre-tracheal space and re-inserted into the correct position, a longer length tube may be required in this instance.
- If no suitable tube is at the patient's bedside then while awaiting the required tube of further assistance the use of a suction catheter, plain inner tube, small uncuffed endotracheal tube or a Yankeur sucker may be used to prevent complete lose of the stoma opening and enable O_2 delivery.
- If no tube can be inserted then insert a suction catheter, trim and secure and administer O_2 as required.[7]
- If oxygen therapy and or resuscitation are required while awaiting tracheostomy re-insertion, cover the stoma and provide ambu bag and facemask ventilation or mouth to mouth ventilation.[15]
- If your patient has no patent upper airway due to vocal cord palsy, upper airway oedema or tumour, then deliver required O_2 via stoma supported by tracheal dilators.
- If an alternative airway is needed then urgently seek the assistance of your on-call anaesthetist or ENT Surgeon to re-establish an airway.

See flowchart in Appendix 1 to assist with a misplaced or displaced tube.

Summary

Changing a tracheostomy tube is a routine procedure that is necessary to promote patient safety and comfort. However there are, like many other health care procedures, associated risks which should be made aware to all practitioners and carers wishing to undertake this skill. However when carried out by competent practitioners with appropriate training and ongoing support the risks associated with changing the tube are minimised.

To become a competent practitioner in changing a tracheostomy tube you should have a sound understanding of the related anatomy and physiology, the pathological changes of each patient and a sound knowledge of the products available to best suit each individual patient's needs.

The procedure should be taught by an experienced surgeon, anaesthetist or nurse and time should be spent observing a variety of procedures and then themselves be observed carrying out tube changes under direct supervision until both feel confident with the practitioner's competence.

Complications can occur at any tube change and therefore it is necessary for all practitioners to carry out the same preparation before each procedure.

Key points

- Changing a tracheostomy tube is a skill that requires appropriate training, assessment and ongoing support.
- There are risk factors to a difficult tube change which should be acknowledged prior to the procedure.
- Each tracheostomy patient should have an equipment box with them at all times, with equipment for an emergency tube change.
- Preparation for a tube change will minimise complications and allow a quick and efficient response to problems.
- Practitioners changing tubes should know how to manage an unsuccessful tube insertion and how to access further assistance.
- Parents and patients routinely change their child's and their own tubes along with a wide range of care needs with the support of hospital and/or community based health care teams.

REFERENCES

1. Mirza S, Cameron DS. The tracheostomy tube change: A review of techniques. *Hospital Medicine* 2001; 62(3): 158–163.
2. EEC Directive – Class IIA, Rule 7. *Council Directive Concerning Medical Devices*, 93/42 EEC.

3. Addenbrooke's NHS Trust. *Tracheostomy Care: Information Pack and Nursing Protocols.* Addenbrooke's Cambridge University Teaching Hospital Trust, 1996.
4. St. Georges Healthcare NHS Trust. *Guidelines for the Care of Patients with Tracheostomy Tubes.* St.Georges Healthcare NHS Trust, 2000; 47–51.
5. Bissell CM. *Pediatric Tracheostomy Home Care Guide.* Grafton: Twin Enterprises, 2000.
6. Myers E, Johnson J, Murry T. *Tracheotomy.* San Diego: Singular Publishing Group, 1998.
7. Seay SJ, Gay SL, Strauss M. Tracheostomy emergencies: Correcting accidental decannulation or displaced tracheostomy tube. *Am J Nurs* 2002; 102(3): 59–63.
8. Eisenhauer B. Actionstat dislodged tracheostomy tube. *Nursing* 1996 (Jun); 25.
9. Fagan JJ, Johnson SE, Myers EN. *Post-Operative Care in Tracheotomy*, 3rd edn. Alexandria, VA: American Academy of Otolaryngology-Head and Neck Surgery Foundation Inc., 1997; 42–45.
10. Deutsch ES. Early tracheostomy tube change in children. *Arch Otolarygol Head Nec Surg* 1998; 124: 1237–1238.
11. Heafield S, Rogers M, Karnik A. Tracheostomy management in ordinary wards. *Hospital Medicine* 1999; 60(4): 261–262.
12. Myers EN, Johnson J, Murry T. *Tracheotomy: Airway Management, Communication and Swallowing.* San Diego: Singular Publishing Group, 1998.
13. Mallinckrodt Medical. *A Parents Guide to Pediatric Tracheostomy Home Care Guide.* Mallinckrodt Medical, 1999.
14. Adamo-Tumminelli P. *A Guide to Pediatric Tracheotomy Care*, 2nd edn. Springfield, IL: Charles C Thomas, 1993.
15. Tippett DC (ed.). *Tracheostomy and Ventilator Dependency: Management of Breathing, Speaking and Swallowing.* New York: Thieme, 2000.

APPENDIX 1: FLOWCHART TO ASSIST TUBE DISPLACEMENT

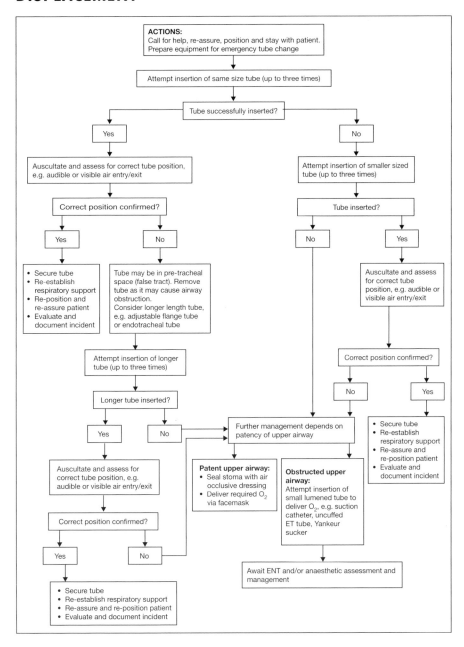

14

DECANNULATION

Hilary Harkin

Decannulation is the deliberate and permanent removal of the tracheostomy tube. It should only be considered when the indication for the insertion of the tracheostomy has resolved.

This chapter will support the multi-disciplinary approach to weaning from a tracheostomy with the aid of a systemised approach, which, opposed to a random approach is associated with fewer weaning attempts and less post removal complications.[1] The chapter will include patient selection criteria, patient assessment, multi-disciplinary involvement, how to carry out the process, recommendations for documentation and associated complications.

Tracheostomy tubes are inserted into patients from varying specialities (Table 1) and for many different clinical conditions involving inflammatory, physiological and anatomical processes.

Table 1: Indications for tracheostomy	
Specialty affected	**Indications for tracheostomy**
Surgical	Prolonged and assisted ventilation; tracheostomy reduces the risks associated with long-term intubation and enables vocalisation and suction.
ENT	Relief of upper airway obstruction, congenital malformation, inflammation and malignancy.
Medical	Aspiration pneumonia. Respiratory insufficiency caused by pulmonary, cardiovascular or muscular disease.
Neurological	Pharyngeal or laryngeal paralysis as a result of neurological deficits. Head injuries.
Paediatrics	Congenital malformation, tracheal stenosis, epiglotitis, long-term ventilation.

Due to the physiological changes caused by the presence of a tracheostomy and the associated morbidity and mortality it is important to commence weaning as soon as the patient's condition indicates.

Some of the changes that a tracheostomy can cause include:

- reduction of the motility of the epithelium which reduces the ability to waft secretions up into the pharynx.
- reduced intratracheal pressure reducing the ability to cough and expectorate.
- affected cough reflex due to the shortened trachea.

MULTI-DISCIPLINARY ASSESSMENT AND MANAGEMENT

Members of the team managing the weaning and decannulation process may include the Ward Nurse, Tracheostomy Nurse Specialist, Respiratory Physician, Ear, Nose and Throat (ENT) Surgeon, Speech and Language Therapist (SLT) and Physiotherapist. Weaning can commence once it has been established that there is no clinical indication that would prevent successful removal of the tube.

The assessment can be instigated by any appropriate member of the team, following team consultation and agreement that the patient's clinical status supports the commencement of weaning.

The SLT is crucial to the success of the procedure if the patient has had swallowing or speech difficulties. With suspected laryngo-tracheal and/or vocal cord pathology it is appropriate to carry out nasendoscopy examination of the upper airway, vocal cord movement and the tracheal mucosa.

The involvement of the dietician in the patient undergoing weaning will help monitor the patient's nutritional status and ensure that the patient is well hydrated with a sufficient fluid intake. This will help to reduce thickened secretions assisting the patient with expectoration.[2] With the tracheostomy occluded, secretions will bypass the tube. Thick secretions entering into the pharynx can be difficult to clear and can increase anxiety and a feeling of choking.

PATIENT SELECTION CRITERIA

In order for the patient to understand and co-operate with the forthcoming process the patient should be alert and orientated.

Some patients will develop a psychological dependence on their tracheostomy and often a clear explanation will help to alleviate any anxiety.

The patient should be able to cough sputum around the tube and into their mouth. This demonstrates a sufficient respiratory expiration and expectoration to tolerate tube removal. To indicate the ability of the patient to reuse their upper airway for ventilation the patient should be able to tolerate a speaking valve or digital occlusion. This uses the tracheostomy for inspiration only and, on expiration the tube becomes occluded. This occlusion can be by a gloved finger or the one-way valve within the speaking valve. Expiration then has to occur around the tracheostomy and up and out through the nose and mouth. The patient should be able to tolerate digital occlusion of the tube or the use of a speaking valve for a minimum of 10 min with no signs of respiratory distress, decrease in oxygen saturations or stridor.

Indications to proceed with weaning:

- Reason for the tracheostomy resolved.
- Patient alert, responsive and consenting.
- Patient tolerating cuff deflation for a minimum of 12 h.
- Patient managing to protect their airway and have a clear chest.
- Patient maintaining oxygen saturations.
- Patient tolerating the use of a speaking valve and/or digital occlusion.
- Patient able to expectorate around the tube into their mouth.
- Tracheostomy tube type and size is appropriate.

The patient assessment needs to include a swallow test, which is explained below. An example of a blue dye assessment sheet has been included (see Chapter 11, Swallowing).

SWALLOW ASSESSMENT

A swallow assessment including the 'blue dye' test aides the team in identifying a patient who is aspirating saliva and/or diet. The safe swallow and/or management of their own secretions is usually required prior to commencing the weaning process. Prior to the swallowing assessment the patient should be alert and have tolerated the cuff of the tracheostomy tube deflated for at least 12 h.

Evidence of saliva on suctioning or expectoration from the tube would indicate that the patient is aspirating. Tracheal secretions are thin and liquid and can be mistaken for saliva. To assess that the secretions are not salivary in origin, a blue food colouring can be mixed with the patient's drinks or instilled into the mouth. Evidence of the colouring being suctioned or expectorated will support the referral to the speech and language therapy department. The patient should be nil by mouth until considered safe to swallow.

The blue dye test is not fool-proof in detecting aspiration in all tracheostomy patients. In some patients aspiration was only detected using either videofluoroscopy or fibreoptic endoscopic evaluation of swallowing (FEES).[3] With this in mind the blue dye test results should be reviewed in conjunction with other signs of aspiration. These will include a wet voice, watery secretions and/or signs of aspiration on chest examination. Regardless of the outcome of the blue dye test if there is any doubt regarding the patient's ability to protect their airway a referral to speech and language therapy should be made. If the patient manages to protect their airway, the multi-disciplinary team may proceed with weaning when removal of the tube is in the best interest of the patient.

It should be noted that in a small group of patients with tracheostomies the presence of the tube in the larynx can itself, disrupt the swallow leading to aspiration.[4] In these cases it is only when the tracheostomy has been removed that the patient can regain a safe swallow. Indeed, it has been reported that for some patients a tracheostomy will cause more aspiration than they prevent.[3]

Each healthcare provider will have individual policies on referral to speech therapy departments and may have blue dye assessment sheets for ward staff.

TYPE AND SIZE OF TUBE FOR WEANING

It is recommended that patients nursed outside the critical care environment have a tracheostomy tube with an inner cannula (unless contraindicated). The inner tube can be removed and either cleaned or replaced to minimise the risk of blockage with secretions, thus reducing the likelihood of tube obstruction.

It is necessary to establish that the tracheostomy tube size and type is suitable for weaning. The ideal tube to use for the weaning process is one that allows adequate airflow around the tube while the tube is occluded. An uncuffed fenestrated tube will offer the least resistance. This allows air to pass from the lungs through the fenestration and around the tube into the upper airway. A large plain-cuffed tube will offer the greatest resistance to airflow and will increase respiratory effort on tube occlusion and so may hinder weaning.

It is recommended that the tube size used for successful weaning with an average sized adult is no larger than 32 French gauge/Shiley 6/Portex 7.5 mm and for a large adult no larger than 34 French gauge/Shiley 6/Portex 8 mm.

Individual assessment is paramount, two patients the same size, age and sex may require different tube styles and/or sizes whilst still obtaining successful tube occlusion.

A daily chest examination should be carried out in order to identify any signs of chest deterioration.

The patient should be able to maintain SaO_2 above 90%. A chest X-ray may be necessary to further assess respiratory status. It is recommended that patients with neuromuscular disease should have the ability to generate peak cough flows of at least 160 l/min irrespective of their ability to breathe.[6]

PATIENT PREPARATION AND INVOLVEMENT

The assessment process and procedure should be explained to the patient and verbal consent obtained. The patients' anxieties should be discussed and identified and a full explanation of the weaning process should be given to the patient and his/her family. The patient may be taught how to cap off the tube and how to document their own progress.

Insertion of the tracheostomy can adversely affect the patient's independence. They may feel as if they have lost control of their breathing, voice and/or swallowing. This can lead to dependence on the tube itself and the healthcare team. Teaching the patient to assist with weaning is promoting their independence in preparation for discharge. The family should also be included in this aspect of care as it can fulfil their need to demonstrate care and reassure the patient. The skin around the tracheostomy tube will need to be cleaned regularly with a clean technique and teaching the patient this aspect of care will assist with their acceptance of the tube and post-decannulation, the scar.

The confidence the patient has in the structured, shared approach to the weaning will encourage their co-operation.

PRACTICAL ISSUES

Having explained the procedure to the patient in order to reduce anxiety and gain compliance the patient should also be informed that it may be a slow process taking at least three days and that over exertion may be counter productive. For this reason the process is best started in the morning after the patient has carried out their hygiene needs. It is advisable to start the process at the beginning of the week in order to access advice and support if needed during weaning and post-decannulation. It may prove more difficult to obtain a specialist assessment over a weekend and there are often fewer staff available on the ward.

The patient should be nursed close to the nurse's station with an adequate number of staff to allow close monitoring. The weaning procedure needs to be documented (see Appendix 1).

This chart allows all members of the team to observe and monitor the patient's progress and observe whether interventions need to be put into place to assist the patient and to assess for difficulty. In a comparative study of systemised vs. random tracheostomy weaning it was found that there were fewer weaning attempts and less post removal complications in the systemised procedure.[1]

THE WEANING PROCESS

Following team agreement the weaning process can commence. Ideally, at the beginning of the week and in the morning time when the patient is rested. All stages in the procedure should be documented in the weaning chart (included as Appendix 1).

The patient should be comfortably positioned and as upright as possible. If they require supplementary oxygen or saline nebulisers then these should be continued via nasal speculum or an oral mask.

The term cap will be used to describe the spigot/plug placed over the tracheostomy. This will occlude the tube ensuring that all airflow is via the upper airway (Fig. 1). A speaking valve on the end of the tube will divert expired air to the upper airway allowing the patient time to adjust to breathing through the mouth and nose while inspiration is continued via the tracheostomy.

1. Ensure the cuff, if present, is deflated.
2. Insert fenestrated inner tube if appropriate.
3. Whilst reassuring the patient, place an occlusion cap over the end of the tracheostomy tube (Fig. 1). Observe for signs of respiratory distress and stay with the patient for at least the first 10 min. The patient's oxygen saturation and vital signs should be recorded after 15 min. Expect a mild increase in heart rate and blood pressure and it is normal to feel some anxiety.
4. If tolerated and the patient is in agreement, continue to occlude tube for 12 h, allowing the patient to breathe via the tracheostomy and rest over the first night.
5. Day 2 should start as day 1 but with the aim of maintaining the occlusion cap in situ for 24 h. If the patient is tolerating the spigot for shorter periods of time, continue at a slower pace, gradually increasing the period of time the tube is occluded. If there is no improvement in the toleration of the spigot after three days, look at the section on troubleshooting and if necessary refer to the ENT team.
6. If by day 3 the patient has tolerated the tracheostomy tube occluded (without experiencing respiratory distress) for a period of 24 h, then a collaborative assessment should be made in order to predict the patient's ability to cope with the removal of the tube.

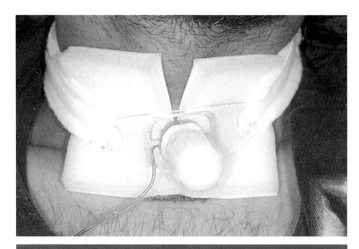

Fig. 1: Tracheostomy tube 'capped off'.

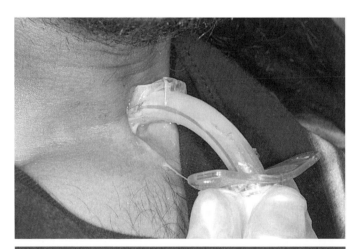

Fig. 2: Removal of tracheostomy tube.

7. With team agreement the tube should be removed in a firm yet gentle action (Fig. 2). The trachea should then be examined with a pen torch or other appropriate light source. In the unlikely event of a tracheoesophageal fistula the tract will be seen through the stoma and the colour of the tracheal mucosa can be observed for granulation tissue (Fig. 3), crusting or stenosis. If any abnormality is found a referral to the ENT team will be required.

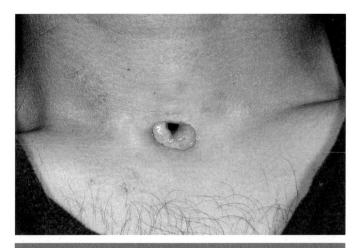

Fig. 3: Granulation tissue at tracheostomy site.

If suction is required via the tracheostomy it is encouraged to continue tube occlusion after performing suction, as tolerated by the patient. It may be necessary to administer regular saline nebulisers via an oral mask in order to loosen secretions and facilitate expectoration. If the patient becomes anxious and starts to hyperventilate, apply oxygen therapy through an oral mask and offer plenty of reassurance rather than instinctively remove the spigot. Secretions can become trapped within the larynx and the patient may panic. At the early stage of weaning the patient may benefit from using a Yankeur sucker at the back of the throat to assist in removal of these secretions.

The benefit of occasional capping over three days prior to 24 h occlusion is not indicated by current research. It is, however, recommended that the weaning procedure is performed at the pace of the patient's ability to maintain occlusion.[7] If after 24 h of tube occlusion there are no clinical signs indicating a continued need for the tracheostomy, the tube can be removed. The tube should be removed in the morning during the week to ensure that a specialist assessment can be readily sought in the unlikely event that the patient needs tube re-insertion.

Difficulty with weaning/troubleshooting

Respiratory insufficiency

- If the patient has respiratory distress or decreased oxygen saturations and is not tolerating the spigot – the weaning procedure may have been commenced earlier than the patient's condition indicates. Ensure the reason for the tracheostomy has resolved and the patient's condition is stable.

The patient may not have the respiratory capacity to manage without the tracheostomy and a referral to ENT will be necessary for continued patient support and management of the permanent tracheostomy. If there is any doubt about the patient's tracheal condition a referral can be made to ENT for an assessment and assistance with further management.

Airway obstruction

- If the patient tolerates the speaking valve with a good voice but not tube occlusion due to respiratory distress or stridor, an ENT assessment will be required to assess for vocal cord damage. There is a greater risk of damage to the vocal cords post-thyroid, parathyroid, or cardio-thoracic surgery due to damage of the recurrent laryngeal nerve intra-operatively.
- If the patient has a poor voice and difficulty with tolerating either the speaking valve or tube occlusion – an ENT assessment will be required to assess for mucosal or vocal cord damage as a result of a traumatic intubation or extended endotracheal intubation.

In a study of the weaning process, 75 patients were monitored, 12 of the patients who could not tolerate capping had significant tracheal obstruction to airflow and required ENT input.[8]

Retention of secretions

- If the patient continues to require suctioning, the physiotherapist may feel that the patient's chest needs to improve before weaning. A mini-tracheostomy (a 16 French gauge single lumen tube) may be indicated as it permits suctioning of retained secretions.

Evidence of blood in secretions

- If the patient has small amounts of bleeding from the stoma site or there are traces of blood in the secretions on suctioning or coughing – a chest X-ray will be required to exclude a thoracic cause. Nasendoscopy will also be indicated to assess for mucosal damage which may have occurred as a result of trauma from suctioning, granulation tissue occurring at the site of the fenestrations and/or the stoma site.

Patient anxiety

- If time has been spent with the patient in the initial stage of the weaning process the patient will be more confident in their ability to cope without the tracheostomy. Nasendoscopy by the ENT surgeon, SLT or specialist nurse to rule out tracheal or laryngeal abnormality can help to allay the patients' fears.

It should be noted that for certain patients decannulation is not possible. In these instances the patients require ongoing support and training and are usually followed up by a specialist respiratory or ENT department.

Following removal of the tracheostomy tube

For 48 h following tube removal, it is recommended that the tracheostomy equipment, including tracheal dilators should be kept by the bedside, in case the patient requires reinsertion.[5]

The patient should be closely monitored for up to 48 h after removing the tube to ensure tolerance for decannulation.[9]

The wound should be dressed twice daily with an occlusive dressing. This is required to promote closure and prevent airflow through the healing tract after the tube has been removed. This tract is referred to as the fistula. Sleek is no longer advocated, as it can cause blistering of the skin and does not promote healing. An alternative dressing, e.g., Duoderm, will promote epithelial-isation and wound healing while allowing for moisture permeability but not inspiration. Air can usually be heard escaping or secretions may bubble up through the tract until it closes. Encourage the patient to apply gentle pressure to the dressing especially when coughing and talking to help prevent loosening of the dressing. Remove the dressing when the wound is clean and dry with no escaping air. The length of time the tracheostomy has been formed will affect the length of time the tract and skin will take to heal. If a fistula remains after two weeks refer to ENT for an assessment for surgical closure.

If there is an overgrowth of healing tissue around the wound refer to the ENT team for treatment of the granulation tissue (see Figure 3). If the wound is not treated there is an increased likelihood of the patient developing an unsightly scar that may require treatment by the plastic surgeon. Figure 4 is

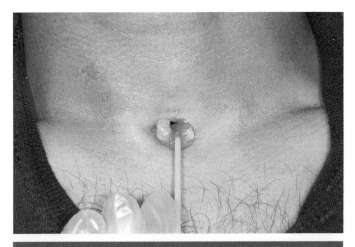

Fig. 4: Silver nitrate cautery applied to granulation tissue.

demonstrating silver nitrate cautery to granulation tissue at the stomal site after the tube has been removed.

It is essential to ensure that the patient has had time to adjust to the removal of the tube and the presence of a scar.[10] Once the wound has been exposed to air and there is no crusting or scab formation the patient can systematically massage the area using small circular movements. Although there is no substantial research massage is said to break up collagen fibres, soften, flatten and fade scars.[11] It may also help to reduce the likelihood of tethering. A small amount of cream to assist the massage can be used. At the first sign of a hypertrophic scar (scar raised above level of skin, excessive itching, redness and increased discomfort) silicone gel can be applied over the wound.

On discharge patients should be given contact numbers in case of problems and an outpatient appointment within six weeks. Further information can be found on the tissue viability websites listed at the end of the chapter. Reassurance should be given regarding healing and scar shrinkage over time.

Summary

The ability to decannulate the patient will be affected by various factors:

1. Selection of patients for the weaning procedure.
2. Reason why the tracheostomy was formed.
3. Type and size of the tracheostomy tube.
4. Support from the SLT, physiotherapist, dietician, tracheostomy specialist nurse, physician and ENT surgeon.
5. A systematic, standardised approach to the weaning procedure by all members of the multi-disciplinary team.
6. Accurate and appropriate documentation of the procedure.
7. Patient and family involvement.

REFERENCES

1. Doerksen K, Ladyshewsky A, Stansfield K. A comparative study of systemized vs. random tracheostomy weaning. *Axone* 1994; 16(1): 5–13.
2. Dikeman KJ, Kazandjian MF. *Communication and Swallowing Management of Tracheostomized and Ventilator-Dependent Adults.* London: Singular Publishing Group Inc., 1995.
3. Thompson-Henry S, Braddock B. The modified evans blue dye test fails to detect aspiration in the tracheostomized patient: Five case reports. *Dysphagia* 1995; 10: 172–174.

4. Nash M. Swallowing problems in the tracheostomized patient. Aspiration and swallowing disorders. *Otolaryng Clin N Am* 1998; 21(4): 701–709.

5. Serra A. Tracheostomy care. *Nurs Stand* 2000; 14(42): 45–52.

6. Bach JR, Saporito LR. Criteria for extubation and tracheotomy tube removal for patients with ventilatory failure. *Chest* 1996; 110: 1566–1571.

7. Harkin H, Russell C. Guidelines for removal of a tracheostomy tube. *Nurs Times* 2001; 97(26): 34–36.

8. Rumbak M, Graves A, Scott M, Sporn G. Tracheostomy tube occlusion protocol predicts significant tracheal obstruction to airflow in patients requiring prolonged mechanical ventilation. *Crit Care Med* 1997; 25(3): 413–417.

9. Heffner JE. The technique of weaning from tracheostomy. Criteria for weaning; practical measures to prevent failure. *J Crit Ill* 1995; 10(10): 729–733.

10. Price B. Living with altered body image: The cancer experience. *Br J Nurs* 1992; 1(13): 641–645.

11. Edwards J. Scar management: What are the available options? *Nurs Pract* 2003 (Jan/Feb); 69–70.

USEFUL WEBSITES

Changing faces	www.changingfaces.co.uk
Scar information service	www.scarinfo.org
British association of skin camouflage	www.skin-camouflage.net

APPENDIX 1: TRACHEOSTOMY WEANING CHART

Patient: . . . .   Hospital no: . . . .

Tube size and type . . . .

Pre-wean criteria

Liase with appropriate members of the multi-disciplinary team . . . . ☐

Maintaining saturations above 90% . . . . ☐

Strong, spontaneous cough . . . . ☐

Passed swallow assessment . . . . ☐

Cuff deflated at least 12 hours . . . . ☐

Should have **fenestrated** tube with **fenestrated** inner tube in situ . . . . ☐

Clear chest . . . . ☐

Weaning process

Apply occlusion cap to inner tube and observe and document progress.

DAY 1 Keep cap on for up to 12 hours depending on how tolerated. (Administer humidified oxygen or saline nebulisers orally/nasally if needed).
Uncap overnight.

DAY 2 Cap 0800 and plan to keep in situ for 24 hours if tolerated by patient. Review chest with physiotherapist.

DAY 3 If cap tolerated for 24 hours, with team and patient approval, remove the tube.

- If suctioning is required aim to replace the cap immediately after suctioning to re-start the weaning process. Consider replacing the tracheostomy with a mini-tracheostomy for access to bronchial toilet.
- Please record duration that tracheostomy is capped to chart progress.

Time/date	Example	_/_/_	_/_/_	_/_/_	_/_/_
Overnight					
08–09.00					
09–10.00					
10–11.00					
11–12.00					
12–13.00					
13–14.00					
14–15.00					
15–16.00					
16–17.00					
17–18.00					
19–20.00					
20–21.00					
21–22.00					
22–23.00					
23–24.00					

Causes of distress:	**Codes:**	C	*Capped*
Suction is required		U	*Uncapped*
Cuff is inflated		SV	*Speaking valve*
Respiratory insufficiency		S	*Suction*
Unready for weaning			
ENT referral required	Yes/no		
Appointment arranged	Yes/no		

Claudia Russell
Tracheostomy Practitioner
Addenbrooke's Hospital
Bleep 152–459

Chart devised by Claudia Russell and Hilary Harkin.

TRACHEOSTOMY AND HEAD & NECK CANCER

Tova Prior and Simon Russell

INTRODUCTION

The management of head and neck malignancy is one of the most challenging areas of oncology. If the patient has a tracheostomy this must be considered in every aspect of patient management, further adding to the complexity of an already difficult treatment.

There are three main modalities used in the management of head and neck cancer, surgery, radiotherapy and chemotherapy. Surgery and radiotherapy are commonly combined in a complimentary manner, and more recently there has been a trend to use all three modalities. Following diagnosis treatment is planned, with either radical or palliative intent. Radical treatment is treatment with the aim of curing disease. It may therefore be acceptable to treat with techniques with considerable toxicity. Palliative treatment is aimed at improving symptoms. Treatment where possible should be quick and simple, with minimal side effects. This is not always the case in head and neck cancer when uncontrolled disease can be extremely distressing and short courses of radiotherapy offer little benefit. In this situation, radical radiotherapy can be given with palliative intent.

PRINCIPLES OF RADIOTHERAPY

Radiotherapy is a treatment using ionising radiation. Ionising radiation kills cancer cells by damaging DNA. Cells respond to this damage by attempting repair, if they are unable to do this they die. The DNA damage is alike in both cancer and normal cells, but in general, cancer cells are less able to repair the damage and so there is a greater chance of killing a cancer cell than a normal cell. Radiation dose is measured in terms of absorbed energy (Joules) per unit mass (kg) and is measured in Gray (J/kg).

There are two main ways of giving radiotherapy, external beam radiotherapy (teletherapy) and interstitial radiotherapy (brachytherapy). By far the most commonly used is external beam radiotherapy (EBRT). EBRT uses a radiation beam directed by a machine to the patient who is usually lying on a couch a short distance away. In general the radiation is high energy electromagnetic radiation, produced by accelerating electrons across a voltage gradient and aiming them at a target of tungsten. The energy of the X-ray is measured in volts and is used to classify therapy into superficial, orthovoltage and megavoltage. Simply, the higher the voltage the more penetrating the radiation beam is. The majority of radiation used to treat head and neck cancer is megavoltage produced by a linear accelerator.

The commonly used particulate radiation is electrons, produced by a linear accelerator. Electrons are sometimes preferable to photons because of the marked difference in dose distribution they have. They deposit their energy in a fairly uniform manner with a specific depth of penetration depending on the energy. Electrons have a rapid dose fall off which means they are good for treating superficial tumours where it is desirable to spare underlying tissue. Electrons are particularly useful when treating disease overlying the spinal cord.

Radiotherapy is usually given in daily treatments called fractions. This is because the amount of radiation that can be given in a single dose is limited by the tolerance of the surrounding normal tissues. If the total dose is divided into daily fractions the maximum dose to the normal tissues increases and cure becomes more likely. Precise fractionation schedules vary from centre to centre with overall results remaining similar. Currently alternative schedules are being investigated with the aim of improving tumour control and decreasing the side effects. Treating the patient more than once a day is called hyperfractionation and decreasing the overall treatment time is called acceleration. Combining the two in continuous hyperfractionated accelerated radiotherapy (CHART) has shown promise in head and neck cancer.[1]

The aim of radiotherapy is to give as high a dose as possible to the tumour at the same time minimising the dose to the surrounding normal tissues in order to avoid complication. This is a particular challenge in head and neck radiotherapy for a number of reasons. First because of regional anatomy, it is often the case that tumour lies in close proximity to normal structures that are critically radiosensitive. Secondly squamous carcinoma of the head and neck is not terribly radiosensitive, that is high doses are required for cure, which is often in excess of the critical tolerance of the surrounding structures. For example cancer of the maxillary antrum can be millimetres from the eye and optic chiasm. A dose of 66 Gy may cure the cancer but complications to the lens become frequent at 8 Gy and retina and optic chiasm at 50 Gy.

This also demonstrates the choices that must be made regarding complications. A high risk of a less serious complication, e.g. cataract of the lens may be acceptable if one is attempting cure, but a low risk of a serious complication, e.g. loss of vision following radiotherapy to the optic chiasm may be quite unacceptable.

PRINCIPLES OF CHEMOTHERAPY

There are more than 40 chemotherapy drugs in common use today, they work by different mechanisms, their activity varies depending on the tumour type and they have different toxicity profiles. Table 1 shows the types of chemotherapy commonly used in the treatment of head and neck cancer.

The administration of chemotherapy is a highly specialised area of medicine. It should only be given in a setting where there is necessary support staff, which would include an oncologist, a specialist pharmacist, and a specialist chemotherapy nurse. Prior to the administration of chemotherapy a full assessment of the patient must be made. The patient must be fit enough to withstand the potential side effects of treatment. The commonest chemotherapeutic drug used in the UK is Cisplatin.

Squamous carcinoma of the head and neck is not very chemo-sensitive, chemotherapy is therefore rarely curative but is used as an adjuvant to surgery or radiotherapy,[2] concurrently with radiotherapy or palliatively. There is significant interest in the use of concurrent chemoradiation,[3] this is

Table 1: The chemotherapy drugs commonly used in the treatment of head and neck cancer

Drug	Mechanism of action	Route of administration	Major side effects
Cisplatin	Forms DNA cross-links	I.V. Infusion	Emesis, Ototoxicity, Nephrotoxicity
5-Fluorouracil	Inhibits thymidylate synthase	I.V. Bolus I.V. Infusion	Stomatitis, Diarrhoea, Skin rashes
Methotrexate	Dihydrofolate Reductase inhibitor	Oral, I.V. Bolus Intrathecal	Myelosuppression, Mucositis
Bleomycin	DNA strand breaks	I.V. Infusion	Lung fibrosis, Fever
Vincristine	Microtubule poison	I.V. Bolus	Neuropathy
Doxorubicin	DNA intercalation, Topoisomerase II inhibition	I.V. Bolus	Myelosuppression, Alopecia, Cardiotoxicity

the treatment with chemotherapy during a fractionated course of radiotherapy. Chemoradiation is thought to work by a number of different means. By inhibiting the repair of the radiation induced DNA damage, by the synchronisation of cancer cells into more radiosensitive phases of the cell cycle, by recruiting non-proliferating cells into the cell cycle and therefore making them more radiosensitive, by reducing the fraction of hypoxic cells in a tumour there may be an improved response to radiotherapy and finally by debulking the tumour, that is if one treatment modality decreases the cell population the second is likely to be more effective as there are fewer cells to kill to achieve a cure.

THE TREATMENT PROCESS

Once the diagnosis of cancer has been made, a treatment plan will be formulated in a multidisciplinary setting. The patient's situation is usually discussed in a forum where all specialist healthcare professionals can add their expertise to the plan. The team usually consists of:

- Specialist head and neck surgeon
- Clinical oncologist (radiotherapist)
- Histopathologist
- Radiologist
- Clinical nurse specialist
- Speech and language therapist
- Dietician
- Macmillan nurse
± Plastic surgeon, prosthetics technician, special dentist

The patient, of course, plays the most important role in the team. From the moment a cancer is suspected, the patient is actively encouraged to become part of the team. Treatment recommendations are just that, recommendations. What is ideal for the cancer may not be ideal for the patient; therefore all treatment plans are tailor made for that individual right at the start of the patient pathway.

The team will consider the treatment modalities appropriate to the patient. In general, the management of the primary tumour is considered separately from the management of the regional neck nodes. Either can be treated with primary surgical excision, or with primary radiotherapy. The most common approach in the UK is to combine primary surgical treatment with postoperative radiotherapy for patients who are at risk of local recurrence of their cancer.

Preparation for treatment

Once the decision to treat with radiotherapy has been made, the patient will meet with the radiotherapist to discuss further the indications for this treatment modality, the treatment planning process, the acute and long-term side effects of radiotherapy and the expected outcome of treatment. Once the patient has considered this and consented to treatment, a number of pre-treatment investigations and checks are carried out.

Airway assessment

Prior to radiotherapy the patient's airway must be assessed. In order to receive radiotherapy they must be able to lie flat comfortably and be able to maintain their airway so that they can be safely left alone in the treatment room safely.

Once radiotherapy has commenced, tumours have a tendency to swell as a result of induced oedema. If the tumour is partially occluding the airway, a judgement must be made as to whether airway compromise may occur as a result of the treatment. It is not uncommon for a patient to have a tracheostomy procedure prior to radiotherapy to prevent acute airway compromise. In this situation, the patient's life is not only at risk, but the effectiveness of the radiotherapy is greatly reduced if there are interruptions to the course of prescribed radiotherapy to allow for treatment of such an event.

The tumours that most commonly cause airway compromise are large, advanced, midline tumours for example transglottic or supraglottic laryngeal tumours, extensive tumours of the base of tongue or hypopharynx.

Should airway compromise occur acutely, the mainstay of management prior to obtaining the advice and support of ENT colleagues is corticosteroid medication. This may reduce oedema and may avoid any other intervention. Antibiotics may also be considered.

There are no hard and fast rules when assessing a patient in this way. Patients who have clinical symptoms and signs of airway occlusion should be assessed further without delay. If the airway is found to be occluded to any significant degree, the patient should be commenced on steroids and discussed with the ENT surgeons. It may be in this situation that primary radiotherapy is no longer appropriate and surgical resection would be safer, either as a debulking procedure or as a definitive resection. Alternatively, a tracheostomy may be appropriate in order to maintain the airway during treatment, leaving the primary tumour in situ. This is avoided if at all possible due to the fear that this may encourage tumour spread and seeding.[4] Radiotherapy fields then have to take this into account to ensure that this area is treated adequately. Subglottic extension of tumour confers the highest risk of this.[5]

Nutritional assessment

The advice of a dietician should be sought and a baseline nutritional assessment done prior to a course of radiotherapy. Radiotherapy may cause a very sore mouth and throat, depending on the area treated and therefore swallowing may become difficult during treatment. Therefore, if the radiotherapy technique is going to irradiate a large volume of either the oral cavity or oropharynx, or both, to a significant dose then prophylactic placement of a percutaneous entero-gastrostomy (PEG) tube is recommended in order to support their nutritional needs at the height of the radiotherapy reaction.[6]

Additionally there are patients who have required nutritional support during and after a major surgical procedure and those who are unable to swallow due to problems of aspiration (either because their tumour has destroyed the protection of the airway on swallowing or the resection of their tumour has left their airway vulnerable) and who are already 'PEG dependent'. The dietician plays a central role in monitoring these patients during their course of post-operative radiotherapy.[7,8]

Dental assessment

A dental opinion is sought prior to radiotherapy. One of the potential long-term side effects of radiotherapy to both sides of the head and neck is a dry mouth secondary to destruction of the salivary glands, which are sensitive to radiation. Without the protective effects of saliva, teeth are more prone to dental caries. If a tooth is subsequently extracted from a bone that has been irradiated, it does not heal well due to the altered blood supply in the region and osteoradionecrosis may develop.

Prevention of these complications is very important. Although it is sometimes possible to spare the salivary glands from damage, it is possible to minimise the risks. Advice and support from an oral hygienist is given and extraction of teeth that may be in bad condition prior to treatment may be carried out. Should extraction be required following radiotherapy, it should be done by a specialist dentist/oral surgeon who is familiar with the potential problems.[9]

THE RADIOTHERAPY PLANNING PROCESS
The mould room

In order to increase accuracy of delivery of the radiotherapy beam, ensuring that the target is consistently hit and the critical structures missed, the patient must be immobilised in the treatment position and thus treated in exactly the same reproducible position each day. A movement of just 5 mm may mean that a critical structure receives too much dose or that the tumour does not receive an adequate dose.

The treatment position is decided according to the tumour site and the beam arrangements that are going to be used. It usually requires the patient to lie supine with arms by their side and their head placed on a custom made head-rest. The patient may be immobilised using a variety of methods, but the commonest system in the UK is to fashion a thermoplastic mask or 'shell' for the patient to wear each treatment.

The patient first attends the mould room in the radiotherapy department. This is where a specialist technician or radiographer will make equipment needed for radiotherapy delivery such as shells and lead used for shielding.

Here, an impression is made of the patient's face, neck and shoulders using plaster of Paris bandages. A space is left around the nose and mouth and any tracheostomy or stoma site so they may breathe comfortably. Once the ban-dages have dried, they are removed in one piece, *forming a mould into the mould plaster is poured which dries and forms a replica model* of the patient's face and neck. The replica of the patient's shape then has a thermoplastic sheet stretched over it, which moulds to its shape and forms a see-through plastic mask which the patient wears at every treatment. It is fixed onto the treatment couch so that the patient's head is in exactly the same position for each treatment.

It is important that a shell is not made too soon after dental extractions or major surgery as the facial contour may change dramatically in the post-operative period with oedema and bruising. Ideally it should be made when all such swelling has subsided so that the shell is snug and comfortable. If the shell is made too soon, subsequent resolution of post-operative oedema may leave the shell with gaps between the patient and shell and thus allow movement.

Simulation

Once the patient has had their shell made with them lying in the treatment position they are brought back to the planning department so that their treat-ment may be planned. This is done with the aid of a simulator, which enables the radiographers and clinicians to simulate what a treatment machine can do without irradiating the patient to the same extent.

Modern planning may use a CT simulator. Here, the patient has a CT scan performed of the region while wearing the mask. Once the CT images have been obtained and reference marks applied to the shell. The radiotherapist, planning radiographers and physicists then use these images to draw up a treatment plan for the patient. In general the radiotherapist defines which area needs to be treated to what dose and the radiographers and physicists use the treatment planning computers to calculate what beam arrangements are required and the dose to the critical structures.

The patient then returns to the department and a 'plan check' is performed. X-rays and measurements are taken to confirm that the treatment proposed is accurate and reproducible. This planning process may take up to two weeks.

Radiotherapy planning

Once the treatment plan is ready, the patient then returns for their first treatment. This appointment is usually longer than subsequent appointments as all positions, doses and beam arrangements are rechecked before treatment. The patient is put into their position, wearing the mask and when all checks have been completed, receives the first treatment. The radiographers leave the room, leaving the patient alone, so they are not exposed to radiation. There are cameras in the room so that the patient is visually monitored and the radiographers can communicate with the patient using an intercom system.

Several beams are treated each session, for example two lateral beams and an anterior beam, each beam taking several minutes to administer. For each beam the head of the linear accelerator has to be moved to the correct position and aligned accordingly and any lead shielding be placed in the correct position between the patient and the beam on a special tray attached to the gantry.

During the first treatment, check beam radiographs are taken by placing an X-ray film under the patient. These radiographs are then checked against the original plan so that the treatment position is checked and verified for accuracy. When the patient has had their first treatment and the check films have been verified the treatment process becomes quicker. An appointment slot of 10–15 min is allowed for such patients once the course is underway.

Treatment schedules

Treatment conventionally is given daily, Monday to Friday for a total of 5–7 weeks, which involves 25–35 fractions of treatment. The dose, and therefore the treatment course length depends on the patient's disease and previous treatment. This gives the patient a total dose of 50–70 Gy for a radical treatment. Currently researchers are devising alternative radiotherapy schedules, the aims of which are to reduce acute and late side effects and increase efficacy of the radiation.

On treatment monitoring

Head and neck oncology patients experience a wide range of problems from their treatment and must be supported before, during and after their radiotherapy by the multidisciplinary team. The patients are seen on treatment every day by the therapy radiographers and at least once a week by the on treatment clinic team. This includes the radiotherapist, radiotherapy nurses, the dietician and the speech therapist. At these clinics each patient is reviewed. Their treatment plan and acute reaction is assessed and patients are given any medications or advice required to control their symptoms. They are usually monitored in this clinic until the acute reaction has settled which may be up to 12 weeks after the beginning of treatment.[10]

Acute side effects of radiotherapy

Patients may expect a variety of acute effects. Initially, fatigue may be their only complaint during the first two weeks. However, during the remainder of the course side effects gradually accumulate, reaching their peak during the final week of treatment and the week or two following completion. These side effects gradually resolve in the subsequent six weeks following completion of treatment.

Airway management

There are three types of patients who have a tracheotomy when undergoing radiotherapy.

1. Patients where a tracheostomy has been fashioned as an emergency to protect the airway and the primary tumour is left in situ.
2. Patients who have had a laryngectomy and are receiving routine post-operative radiotherapy, these patients obviously have a permanent tracheostome.
3. Patients who have had a procedure leaving the airway vulnerable, e.g. a total glossectomy and require a tracheostomy to protect the airway.

Those patients who have a laryngectomy usually have a stoma unencumbered by appliances. A stoma bib may be worn to humidify inspired air. A stoma button may be in situ in the early post-operative period to support the newly formed stoma. Those patients without a permanent stoma usually have a tracheostomy tube in situ and this must be considered in the planning and treatment process. If the patient has a tracheostomy tube, treatment is given with a plastic tube in situ rather than a silver tube. A silver tube will interfere with the radiotherapy beam and cause an increased dose to be given to the under-lying stoma and surrounding skin due to the production of secondary elec-tron scatter. If the patient has a foam or other dressing around the tube, then the radiotherapist should be consulted as to whether this should be removed prior to treatment as this too can increase the dose to the underlying skin and cause a more severe acute reaction. Great caution must be exercised to ensure that the tube is still secure as in inexperienced hands the tube may be left vul-nerable to accidental removal. Patients do not tend to have extra problems with their treatment if these precautions are taken.

Careful consideration needs to be given to the dose to the stoma. Dressings and tracheostomy tubes may modify this. Tissue equivalent material known as bolus may be placed deliberately around the edge of the stoma with the intention of increasing the dose here. The stoma is at high risk of tumour recurrence if the tumour extended into the subglottic region and possibly if the tube was inserted without definitive surgery. If the disease is generally advanced with heavy nodal spread to the neck or there is a large primary tumour there is also a greater risk of stomal recurrence. As this situation is notoriously difficult to treat, prevention is very important. In order to deliver a high dose to the posterior mucosa of the stoma, tissue equivalent bolus is placed around the stoma, or a plastic tracheostomy tube may be inserted during treatment. Both methods are used and have their different advantages and disadvantages.

Skin toxicity

During a course of radiotherapy the skin goes through a well-recognised sequence of changes prior to healing. Initially the skin appears unaffected but from the end of second week the skin becomes progressively more erythem-atous. Subsequently it may desquamate and in a significant minority moist desquamation occurs with a loss of the superficial skin layers and production of exudate. During this time patients are advised to keep the skin moist and supple with the application of aqueous cream initially, but as the reaction pro-gresses dressings may be required. A week or two after radiotherapy has been completed the skin begins to heal leaving a tanned appearance. Over time the tanned appearance subsides and resembles normal skin again. Tube changes should where possible be avoided during the last two weeks of radiotherapy and for two weeks after radiotherapy when the radiation reaction is at its peak.

Mucositis

Perhaps the most disabling side effect of radiotherapy is the effect on the delicate oropharyngeal mucosa lining the oral cavity and oropharynx.

Initially, as with the skin reaction, there is little in the way of symptoms. After the second week the mucositis begins to increase in severity, commencing with erythema and soreness and building up to a confluent mucositis with ulceration and oedema and contact bleeding at its worst. Again, side effects are dependent on the dose and site of treatment. Pain is controlled using both local and systemic methods. Local treatments include such things as aspirin gargles and lignocaine mouthwashes. Systemic treatments are given according to the WHO analgesic ladder working up from simple non-opiate analgesia to opiates.[11]

If the oral cavity is treated then speech and swallowing may be affected. If the neck is treated then the pharyngolaryngeal mucosa is affected causing difficulty with swallowing due to pain, soreness or oedema. As a result most patients require a change of diet to a soft or liquid diet in order to maintain their nutrition during treatment. Use of a PEG tube is required to support patients at this time.

LATE EFFECTS OF RADIOTHERAPY

Once a radical course of radiotherapy has been given, the acute side effects usually settle within three months of completion. However, as a consequence of the damage to the normal cells within the treated field there are late effects seen within the normal tissue. Late effects are defined as those radiation side effects occurring six or more months after commencing radiotherapy. It is thought that damage to the slowly proliferating cells of the supporting stroma is the main mechanism of the changes seen, and these changes may occur gradually over years. As a result, patients who are irradiated at a young age for a potentially curable tumour are most at risk of the effects.

The likelihood of late effects depends on several factors:

- The dose per fraction of radiotherapy
- The total dose given
- The volume of tissue treated
- The addition of chemotherapy to radiotherapy
- The overall treatment time
- The condition of the normal tissues prior to treatment

Skin and subcutaneous tissues

Changes to the skin may be seen as depigmentation, thinning, fibrosis and telangiectasia. Damage to such skin is slow to heal and therefore trauma to irradiated skin should be avoided. Sun exposure of irradiated skin should be kept to a minimum.

If the neck has been irradiated then the subcutaneous tissues may become gradually more fibrosed and less pliable. There may be some lymphoedema as a result, manifesting itself as a swelling beneath the chin. The hair growth in the high dose volume will be permanently affected.

Other complications

Other complications include osteoradionecrosis, cartilage necrosis, temporomandibular joint problems, eye problems, hypothyroidism and rarely spinal cord radiation myelitis.

RETREATMENT

Retreatment with radiotherapy after a radical dose has been given is rarely possible. Although some normal tissues in the treated region show a degree of recovery over time in their tolerance level, it is rarely enough to allow retreatment to a significant dose without a high risk of radiotherapy induced long-term complications.

DISEASE COMPLICATIONS

Head and neck cancer tends to be a loco-regional disease, which metastasises via haematogenous spread to the lungs and less commonly to the bones. Therefore, loco-regional disease control is the primary aim of treatment. Unfortunately, some patients may present with advanced disease or their disease persists through, or recurs after, primary treatment.

Locally advanced head and neck tumours, either at presentation or at recurrence can cause unpleasant, distressing symptoms, which may be difficult to palliate. These tumours may be large and necrotic, leading to compression of surrounding normal tissues and disruption of organ integrity and functional ability. Symptoms will depend on the site and size of the tumour.

The patients' performance status is an important factor in how the patient tolerates advanced disease. Often, a combination of factors contributes to poor nutritional status in the patient, rendering them less able to physically cope with advanced disease.

The treatment of advanced disease is a challenge. Firstly a full assessment of the patient to establish the diagnosis and stage of the disease is made. Once this is established, then the treatment aim must be considered.

If the patient is considered to have a potentially curable cancer then radical treatment options are considered. However, if the chance of cure is small, then management is aimed at achieving an often difficult balance of potential treatment benefit and the side effects of giving such treatment. Treatment involving radical surgery with functional loss is not often performed if the chance of cure is low. As a result, many such patients in this position are treated with radiotherapy or chemoradiation with the aim of long-term palliation. Some patients will not be fit for any such treatment and their symptoms are managed with the involvement of the palliative care services without surgery or radiation.

All patients should have the opportunity to be referred to Macmillan specialist nurses early on in their cancer journey.

Uncontrolled neck disease may be extremely unpleasant for patients. Large lymph node masses or primary tumours may erode cutaneous skin, leaving a necrotic wound. These wounds are often malodorous and painful. At presentation, such wounds are not usually curable. Surgery is rarely carried out due to the advanced nature of the disease and difficulty of tumour clearance once extranodal structures are involved. A course of palliative radiotherapy may shrink the disease and allow a reduction in the need for dressings and analgesia.

If a course of radiotherapy is not possible a number of measures may be taken. Adequate analgesia is mandatory, especially when the wound is being dressed. Support in the community by district and Macmillan nurses reduces the number of hospital attendances for wound management. Antibiotics, systemically or topically, may reduce unpleasant odours emanating from the wound. Dressings may reduce odour, protect the patients clothing and protect the wound from additional trauma, as well as reducing the chance of infection.

Advanced neck disease may infiltrate extranodal structures, including the carotid artery. Erosion of the arterial wall may be more likely following combined treatment with surgery and radiotherapy as the normal tissue planes are disturbed allowing infiltration without natural barriers to tumour spread.

A fungating neck tumour may cause warning or 'herald' bleeds prior to a major catastrophic bleed. If this occurs then prophylactic anxiolytic medication may be considered, such as diazepam. If a large bleed occurs then direct pressure to the wound should be applied and anxiolytic medication prescribed, such as midazolam. The patient should obviously not be left unattended until the flow has stopped.

Usually fatal a carotid 'blow-out' is the term applied to sudden massive haemorrhage from the carotid artery.[12] Exsanguination and death usually occurs within minutes. Staff should stay with the patient and attempt to calm the patient and any attending relatives. The administration of any medication to the patient is usually not possible in the time available, but midazolam and diamorphine are sometimes administered to alleviate pain and distress. Clearly, such an event is very distressing and therefore if the clinicians feel that such an event is likely, those involved in the care of the patient should be warned to allow a degree of practical and psychological preparation.

Metastatic disease

Treatment options will be different in a patient who has distant metastases as palliation of their local symptoms will be the priority, rather than considering radical treatment options with the aim of cure. Surgery rarely plays a role here, but may be useful in palliating airway symptoms. More commonly, palliative radiotherapy is helpful at reducing symptoms for the patient without the side effects of a radical course of treatment. Palliative chemotherapy is rarely given. This is because many patients are not fit enough to receive it safely and the potential benefit is very small at the expense of significant side effects.

It is important to involve the palliative care services as soon as possible in the care of such patients and their families. Macmillan nurses play a vital role in the support of patients both in hospital and in the community. Palliative care physicians and the hospice network provide valuable services in the care of patients with need of symptom control and support.

Conclusion

The patient journey from referral through diagnosis, treatment planning, treatment, rehabilitation and follow-up requires all the members of the multidisciplinary team to be involved. This includes oncologists, therapy radiographers, surgeons, radiologists, pathologists, physicists and nurses. Many other health care professionals may also be called on to help with the physical, psychological and emotional reactions the patient may experience. The management of the patient with head and neck cancer can be challenging and even more so if the patient requires a tracheostomy.

REFERENCES

1. Dische S, Saunders M, Barrett A, et al. A randomised multicentre trial of CHART versus conventional radiotherapy in head and neck cancer. *Radiother Oncol* 1997; 44: 123–136.
2. The Department of Veterans Affairs Laryngeal Cancer Study Group. Induction chemotherapy plus radiation compared with surgery plus radiation in patients with advanced laryngeal cancer. *N Eng J Med* 1991; 324(24): 1685–1690.

3. Henke M. Controlled trials of synchronous chemotherapy with radiotherapy in head and neck cancer: Overview of radiation morbidity. *Clin Oncol* 1997; 9: 308–312.

4. Fagan JJ. Tracheostomy and peristomal recurrence. *Clin Otolaryngol* 1996; 21(4): 328–330.

5. Amatsu M, Makino K, Kinishi M. Stomal recurrence – Etiologic factors and prevention. *Med Pregl* 1994; 47(5–6): 197–199.

6. Piquet MA, Ozsahin M, Larpin I, Zouhair A, Coti P, Monney M, Monnier P, Mirimanoff RO, Roulet M. Early nutritional intervention in oropharyngeal cancer patients undergoing radiotherapy. *Support Care Cancer* 2002; 10(6): 502–504.

7. Fietkau R. Principles of feeding cancer patients via enteral or parenteral nutrition during radiotherapy. *Strahlenther Onkol* 1998; 174(Suppl 3): 47–51.

8. Lees J. Nasogastric and percutaneous endoscopic gastrostomy feeding in head and neck cancer patients receiving radiotherapy treatment at a regional oncology unit: A two year study. *Eur J Cancer Care (Engl)* 1997; 6(1): 45–49.

9. Carl W, Ikner C. Dental extractions after radiation therapy in the head and neck area and hard tissue replacement (HTR) therapy: A preliminary study. *J Prosthet Dent* 1998; 79(3): 317–322.

10. Pernot M, Luporsi E, Hoffstetter S, Peiffert D, Aletti P, Marchal C, Kozminski P, Noel A, Bey P. Complications following definitive irradiation for cancers of the oral cavity and the oropharynx (in a series of 1134 patients). *Int J Radiat Oncol Biol Phys* 1997; 37(3): 577–585.

11. Scottish Intercollegiate Guidelines Network. Control of pain in patients with cancer. A national clinical guideline. *Scottish Intercollegiate Guideline Network* 2000; 61 (SIGN publication no. 44).

12. Casey D. Carotid 'blow out'. *Nurs Stand* 1988; 2(47): 30.

LONG-TERM TRACHEOSTOMY AND CONTINUING CARE

Claire Scase

INTRODUCTION

As a result of developments in medical care and technology, individuals with long-term or lifelong respiratory health care needs, such as a tracheostomy,[1] are becoming increasingly common. If clinical indications suggest that the patient will continue to require their tracheostomy tube after their discharge, plans to accommodate this should be instigated.

The aim of this chapter is to consider the unique needs of the individual, both the adult and child who is discharged from hospital with their tracheostomy. To identify the preparation required to enable a smooth transition from hospital to the appropriate discharge destination and avoid re-admission to hospital will also be discussed.

Although most tracheostomies are temporary, there are circumstances where a long-term or even permanent tracheostomy will be necessary due to impaired airway function or unresolved conditions. This reason for and function of having the tracheostomy tube will be central to the specialised and individual needs of the patient and subsequent discharge plan.

When is a long-term tracheostomy tube required?

- To provide ongoing mechanical ventilatory support
- To bypass a long-term or permanent upper airway obstruction to facilitate airflow (e.g. congenital abnormalities)
- To provide access to chest secretions in the event of respiratory insufficiency (i.e. impaired cough reflex/weakened respiratory muscles)
- To protect from aspiration in the event of impaired swallow reflex (e.g. neuromuscular disorders)

What will the aims of the discharge process be?

The advances made in long-term tracheostomy care highlight the health care professionals' role in determining the success and management of this group of individuals. The need for ensuring continuity of care has been defined as 'a philosophy and standard of care that involves patient, family and health care providers working together to provide a co-ordinated, comprehensive continuum of care'.[2,3] This approach can be an effective framework for discharging an individual with a tracheostomy.

Due to the complexities of the tracheostomy patient, an interdisciplinary team approach will benefit the discharge process.[4] This collaborative team approach in discharge preparation can ensure an efficient discharge of the tracheostomy patient is facilitated with appropriate training and support, while avoiding delays in discharge.

The discharge process for an individual with a tracheostomy is just as important as the acute phase of their management and can determine the quality of their life. With the philosophy of 'thriving, not merely surviving',[5] the discharge planning can optimise the patients chances of adapting their lifestyle effectively and efficiently, without the tracheostomy influencing or restricting them unnecessarily. Effective discharge planning has the potential to ensure this quality and continuity of care from hospital to home and avoid re-admission to hospital.[6]

Self-care and independence should be encouraged wherever possible to enable the individual to return to their previous lifestyle as much as possible without depending on others. However, the prospect of learning the skills required to be independent in tracheostomy management can be daunting and even overwhelming.

The following can be used as a framework to guide the process of discharging the individual with a long-term tracheostomy:

- How to determine the appropriate discharge destination
- Preparation of the community team
- Information and education provision
- Emergency situation management
- Discharge of the child with a tracheostomy
- Follow-up care provision

HOW TO DETERMINE THE APPROPRIATE DISCHARGE DESTINATION

Before the discharge process can begin, the destination needs to be established. A home discharge is usually the patients preferred discharge location.

However, there may be factors which delay or prevent this. The discharge setting must be considered to be safe and appropriate to accommodate care and future management of the tracheostomy. Examples of discharge settings include:

- Home
- Continuing care
- Residential home
- Nursing home
- Spinal unit
- Hospice

With a discharge co-ordinator and the patient and/or carer(s), a realistic evaluation will be made of the individual's situation to choose the most appropriate setting. The factors, which will influence the appropriate care setting for the long-term tracheostomy patient, include:

1. Medical condition, prognosis and clinical needs
2. Ability to self care
3. Carer preparation

Medical condition, prognosis and clinical needs

The clinical stability of the tracheostomy will be the primary consideration in determining a discharge destination and plan.[1] This can also determine the level of health care support, the type of environment that can deliver these requirements and the extent of equipment/supplies required to manage the clinical needs.

The discharge planning will need to establish the following tracheostomy related needs:

- Respiratory function/stability and ventilatory support required
- Suctioning requirements
- Wound care and tape changes
- Frequency and associated risks of tube changes
- Risk of life-threatening haemorrhage
- Agitation/risk to self

Ability to self care

The patient's capability to maintain and manage their continuing tracheostomy care should be determined. Their ability to carry out day-to-day assessment, routine care and problem-solving must be consistent and reliable. The following questions should be considered.

Physical ability

- Is there impairment of manual dexterity which may hinder the patient's ability to perform the intricacies of tracheostomy care?
- Is a decline expected in the individuals' physical ability?

Mental ability

Is there cognitive impairment and/or predicted deterioration which may influence the patient's ability in decision-making, planning and problem-solving their care?

Social/behavioural predisposition

Does the individual show the ability to accept and adapt to their tracheostomy?

Patient motivation

Does the individual have the incentive and determination required to learn new skills and manage their care consistently and reliably?

Body image

Body image is concerned as much with control and function as well as physical appearance.[7] A tracheostomy results in both physical and functional changes in the individuals self-image. A combination of a hole in the neck with a tube through which sputum is expectorated may increase anxiety and reduce self-esteem.[8] The individual may experience difficulty relating to the change in their voice production. The health care team should be aware of potential:

- Feelings of loss of former self/altered appearance
- Grief responses
- Lack of acceptance of tracheostomy
- Depression, which may result in the individual having difficulties performing the needs of the tracheostomy at home[9]
- Difficulty learning skills required to be independent with their tracheostomy
- Family member(s) experiencing difficulty with the altered body image of the individual

The following may be helpful in managing these issues:

- Address the grieving process before considering home-care education
- Introduce the individual to ways of disguising the stoma with the use of purpose made scarves or high necklines. This may reduce their self-consciousness, improve their self-image and help to make the stoma aesthetically more acceptable.
- Encourage the individual to maintain frequent stoma care to avoid exudate becoming visible through tracheostomy dressing or odour developing
- Support the individual and their family in making the adjustment

- Introduce individual to other long-term tracheostomy users, to share their personal experiences and to provide a support network

In determining the possibility of a discharge with such circumstances, the patient's support network and social situation must be considered.

Carer preparation

Primarily, the level of support required and available will need to be established. This will be the fundamental factor in determining whether the individual can be discharged home. If discharge home is to be pursued as an option for a patient incapable of independent self-care, an individual should be acknowledged and agreed as the key care provider.[1]

Identifying a carer

Determining this caregiver within the patient's existing support structure should not be identified by assumption alone. Studies of the multi-disciplinary team's role in discharge planning from an acute hospital setting found that families felt pressurised by staff to take responsibility for patients discharge home.[10,11] After discharge from an acute setting, continuing care needs can often be viewed as a family responsibility.[5] They may view this extension of their role as being automatically expected of them. To change from spouse or parent to health care provider could be a choice the individual may be unwilling to make, particularly when considering the advanced technical skills they will be required to perform for an undetermined period of time.

Carer support and training

It is unusual for family members to perform skilled clinical care while the individual is still in hospital.[12] Initially the family member may feel very anxious about taking on a role requiring such a large volume of skills and knowledge. It is therefore vitally important to allow sufficient time and provide emotional support in order to achieve these requirements.

The family carer should therefore be willing as well as capable to take on all the aspects of tracheostomy care. Most importantly, the patient himself should be accepting and confident of this family member's role change.

Furthermore, the demands of such a situation can be stressful and exhausting. The caregiver may experience depression or burnout.[13] A second carer who will be reliable should be identified, accessible and approved by the patient and carer. The option of respite facilities should also be suggested.

Financial impact

Depending on the input required by the patient, the family carer may have financial implications to consider. If the patient is to require constant supervision (e.g. if they are unable to carry out emergency care such as self-suction due to physical limitations), the individual concerned may have to give up work. Available resources and support in terms of financial assistance and care giving options should be investigated to aid the family member in committing to this role change.

To summarise, the family carer will need to be:

- Willing
- Capable
- Confident
- Agreeable to individual
- Available
- Financially supported
- Aware of social isolation and restrictions

PREPARATION OF THE COMMUNITY TEAM

Developments in health care will ultimately result in the demand for more complex and home care support and facilities.[13] Community based individuals who are reliant on their tracheostomy to breathe will be classified as a high-risk health care need. It will therefore be important that the community health care team is fully prepared to meet their needs.

It is acknowledged that as a rule nurse training does not necessarily provide the opportunity to learn how to care for and manage a tracheostomy.[14] Although tracheostomy is becoming increasingly common in community settings,[1] they are still a minority and consequently health care teams are likely to require support and education in providing the needs of these patients. Early contact and interaction with the community team will promote continuity of care and help anticipate any potential difficulties. The community team will be a direct link for the individual in monitoring and evaluating their tracheostomy progress and management. It will be important that the team receive adequate support, information and training prior to and following discharge, in order to facilitate an effective and successful care package for their patient, particularly if they have limited experience of tracheostomy management.

Information the community team may require

- Indication for tracheostomy
- Prognosis and management plan
- Ongoing care requirements
- Equipment/supplies
- Identification and first line management of potential complications

- Management of emergency situations
- Basic life support with a tracheostomy

Table 1 is an example of a discharge summary presenting the individual's requirements. This document is a useful tool to assist the communication of vital information to the receiving health care team.

Table 1: Discharge summary
Tracheostomy team transfer form
Name
Hospital no.
D.O.B.
Transfer from
Transfer to
Date of tracheostomy
Type of tracheostomy
Indication for tracheostomy
Type and size of tube
Tube manufacturer
Date of last tube change
Date of next tube change
Comments on tube changes
Suctioning needs/care of inner cannula
Wound care and dressings
Cuff deflation
Communication management
Swallowing management
Contact details

Name	Position	Contact no.

Team involvement

Preparation for a safe discharge should start as soon as the decision to perform a tracheostomy is made. Depending on the clinical needs and the patient's age, the following health care professionals may be involved in the discharge planning:

- Tracheostomy specialist nurse
- District nurse
- Discharge co-ordinator
- Community physiotherapist
- Community occupational therapist
- Community speech and language therapist
- Community dietician
- Paediatric community team
- Health visitor

The discharge process aims to prepare the patient, carer(s) and community team to provide continued clinical care needs in a safe and adequately equipped environment to promote independence and a return to 'normal' family life and activities.

The benefit of a well-prepared discharge is to enable a smooth transition from the hospital setting to the home environment. Provision of knowledge and skills promotes independence and also helps reduce anxieties once away from the safety of the hospital setting.

INFORMATION AND EDUCATION PROVISION

Education needs

In order for the individual and/or family to be able to accomplish all the aspects of care and management required, information giving and education should begin even before the tracheostomy is performed.[8] Appendix 1 details tracheostomy teaching aids which may be useful, even at this early stage. The indication for the long-term or permanent tracheostomy will have a direct influence on the content and emphasis of care and education required following the discharge.[4] If the aim is for the individual and/or their family to be primary caregivers in the home environment, they must be able to assess and evaluate the tracheostomy and use a problem-solving approach to management. This will involve not only learning how to do something, but the indications for doing so.[13] The individual/family carer who is familiar with the 'normal' clinical condition will be able to detect and/or manage complications more rapidly, for example:

- Difficulty in breathing
- Difficulty in passing suction catheter
- Cuff leak
- Changes in secretions
- Inadequate humidification
- Accidental decannulation
- Displaced tube
- Emergency situations (e.g. drowning, significant bleeding, cardiac and/or respiratory arrest)
- Long-term complications: tracheoesophageal fistula, tracheo-inominate artery fistula, tracheal stenosis

In summary, the education will need to provide the individual and/or carer with the following skills:

- Knowledge base

  - Initial and ongoing reason for tracheostomy
  - Clinical and psychological impact of tracheostomy
  - Ongoing management of the tracheostomy
  - Troubleshooting and dealing with emergency scenarios

- Technical skills

  - Proficiency in use of equipment and supplies

- Decision-making

  - Assessment and evaluation skills
  - Awareness of own limitations

- Problem-solving

  - Response to clinical changes
  - Complications and their management
  - Appropriate access to hospital-based medical team
  - When and how to seek further assistance

Initially, the complexity and quantity of knowledge and skills required by the individual/family to learn can be overwhelming. The importance of early identification of individuals who may need additional support and education will be essential.[9] An educational planner and checklist can be useful in documenting and ensuring all relevant aspects of tracheostomy care are provided (Table 2). This system can be used to document the individuals' progress that they are making, and clearly communicates to the health care team aspects that require extra input and support.

Table 2: Education planner

Patient: _____

Relative/Carer: _____

Date of Discharge: _/_/_

Destination: _____

Aspect of care	Demonstrated to patient	Demonstrated to carer	Patient performed with supervision	Carer performed with supervision	Patient competent	Carer competent
Remove/clean/replace inner cannula						
Stoma care						
Stoma dressing						
Tape changes						
When/how to humidify						
When/how to suction						
Disposal of suction and clinical waste						
When to change tube						
How to change tube						

Complication	Could identify?	Aware of further action/management?
Wound infection		
Chest infection		
Blocked tube		
Accidental decannulation		
Haemorrhage/trauma		
Aspiration		

District nurse:

Telephone number: _____

Training required?   Yes/no

Equipment list sent to district nurses?   Yes/no

Quantity of supplies to be provided on discharge:

Follow-up appointment: Date arranged: _/_/_

Hospital helpline contact telephone number:

Suction equipment servicing: Date: _/_/_

Next tube change due-date: _/_/_

Inform: Electricity board   Yes/no   Ambulance control   Yes/no   By: _____   Identified escort for transfer   Yes/no

295

The following skills will be required:

- Suctioning
- Humidification
- Tube changes
- Tape changes
- Wound care
- Identification and management of problems, e.g. chest infection, aspiration, tube problems and cuff patency

Equipment needs

The use of technological equipment to facilitate the discharge of individuals to their own home is increasing.[15] A supply of both non-disposable and disposable equipment will be required for the individual's discharge home or alternative care setting (Table 3). The level of resources required and available will need to be established in considering a home discharge. Community teams should be given details to pre-order stores prior to discharge. Countryside Supplies Ltd (Appendix 2) are a company who supply and deliver tracheostomy products available on prescription. The service delivers

Table 3: Tracheostomy equipment list

Non-disposable items	Tick if required	Disposable items	Tick if required
Suction pump (mains)		Suction catheters	
Portable suction unit (internal battery)		Suction tubing	
Nebuliser (portable)		Nebuliser tubing and reservoir	
Tracheal dilators		Tracheostomy mask	
Cuff pressure manometer		Spare tracheostomy tubes (including smaller tube as an alternative)	
		Velcro holders/ribbon ties	
		Inner tube cleaning brushes	
		Heat moisture exchanger (HME)	
		Stoma dressings	
		Stoma protectors	
		Speaking valves	

Table 4: Essential equipment list

- Two spare tracheostomy tubes (one size smaller than usual tube as the tract can narrow over time)
- Tracheal dilators
- Fully charged portable suction machine with tubing
- Suction catheters
- Portable nebuliser and saline nebulisers
- Spare humidifiers (Swedish nose, Buchanan bibs)
- Spare dressing and collar/tapes
- Emergency contact telephone numbers
- Emergency information card specifying 'neck breather' and their requirements to be carried with the patient at all times

items to the home for an easy and convenient provision of supplies. It is recommended that at least a seven-day supply of equipment be provided on discharge to smooth the transition between hospital environment and home.

Once discharged, the following recommendations should be practised:

- Keep spare tracheostomy tubes in a designated space both upstairs and downstairs
- Ensure suction units are always fully charged and readily accessible
- Provision of a portable suction unit for use outside the home and in the event of main suction unit failing or electricity power cut
- Ensure patient and/or carers know where items and equipment are stored in the house
- Compile a checklist of essential items to take out and about on every trip (Table 4)

Activities of daily living

The individual will need to plan and organise their day-to-day lifestyle to incorporate their clinical needs. It will also be important to make the individual aware of any activities in their lifestyle, which must be avoided, as airway protection from everyday hazards will be compromised. Some safety tips and advice for tracheostomy care include:

- Commercial coverings/scarves/neckties[16] are available to provide some protection from foreign substances or objects (e.g. sand, dust, during a haircut) from entering the tube or stoma
- The use of water shield for protection in shower/bath[16] can protect against water or toiletries entering the tube or stoma

- Avoid swimming[16] as there will be a very high risk of water entering tracheostomy tube
- Avoid contact sports as they could result in the displacement or dislodgement of the tracheostomy tube
- Avoid toxic substances such as powders or aerosols which, if inhaled, can cause airway/chest damage or infection, e.g. talcum powder, hairspray
- Avoid smoky/polluted environments; smoky particles cannot be filtered by the tracheostomy and can cause increased secretion production
- Avoid contact with animals with fine hair as their hair can easily be inhaled via the stoma
- Choose clothing with loose-fitting necks and front openings to allow easy access to the tracheostomy for care or suctioning
- Sudden changes in temperature (e.g. cold dry atmosphere or central heating) can irritate the airway causing coughing or dry secretions. A dampened bib positioned over the stoma can help moisten dry air.[16]
- Regularly check supplies to avoid running out

EMERGENCY SITUATION MANAGEMENT

The individual and carer(s) will require preparation and guidance to ensure they are able to appropriately manage a range of emergency scenarios.

Resuscitation

The family carer/community team needs to be instructed in mouth to stoma or bag to stoma resuscitation in the event of respiratory arrest.[16] Examples include:

- Occluded tube
- Accidental decannulation
- Problems passing the tracheostomy tube
- Drowning/immersion in water
- Haemorrhage from tracheostomy
- Aspiration

An 'Action Card' can be a useful reminder for carers to use in the event of a respiratory arrest.

Emergency action card in event of respiratory arrest

1. Ring 999 and inform operator that patient is a neck breather
2. Loosen any tight neck wear or clothing

3. If stoma is permanent or upper airway is obstructed, commence mouth to neck resuscitation
4. If upper airway is patent or if tube has fallen out and unable to replace commence mouth to mouth resuscitation (sealing stoma with your finger)

Other considerations

1. Inform Ambulance Control before discharge that the individual has a tracheostomy in the event of requiring their services in the future
2. Inform Electricity Board of clinical situation who will be able to:

    – inform individual in advance of planned power cuts
    – place home on 'at risk' list, to ensure priority electricity supply/reconnection

3. Access to battery-powered equipment (e.g. suction unit, torch) in the event of a power cut
4. Installation of a generator for essential equipment, e.g. ventilator
5. Emergency equipment to be kept fully stocked and in a designated position in the house
6. The use of an identification bracelet specifying that the patient is a 'reckbreather' to alert an emergency team.[16]

DISCHARGE OF THE CHILD WITH A TRACHEOSTOMY

Many aspects included within this chapter can be applied to discharge of a child with a tracheostomy. However, it is important to bear in mind that the child with a long-term tracheostomy presents specific considerations for discharge. The age of the child will determine their level of understanding and ability to participate in their own tracheostomy care. Furthermore, they will require a high level of continuous care and supervision from their parent(s)/guardian(s) to ensure a safe and effective discharge. The ultimate aim for the health care team will be to allow the child and family as normal a life as possible within their existing family structure.

Children may require a tracheostomy for the following indications/conditions:

Diagnosis	Effect
Laryngomalacia ('Floppy larynx')	Softening of supporting cartilage rings, causing collapse of the airway wall on inspiration.
	Characterised by a noisy breath (stridor) which is exacerbated by crying.

Tracheomalacia	As laryngomalacia, but occurring within the trachea.
Haemangioma	Cluster of blood vessels within the airway which cause swelling and airway obstruction.
Papilloma	A wart growing within the airway causing an obstruction to the airflow.

Many of these conditions are detected at a very early age and will resolve as the child grows (i.e. the airway will increase in size, the cartilage will strengthen).

The following points need to be considered in discharge planning:

1. Clinical needs
2. Training needs for others
3. Communication development
4. Promoting normal family life
5. Reaction of the child to the tracheostomy
6. Impact on the parent
7. Attending school
8. Play activities
9. Safety requirements

Clinical needs

- The narrow dimensions, and therefore the absence of an inner cannula, of a paediatric tracheostomy tube is more likely to block with secretions. This necessitates weekly tube changes, and more frequently if the child has a cold or chest infection. Ideally, paediatric tube changes should be performed with two people, particularly with a baby or younger child who may not remain still for the procedure. The use of a blanket to wrap a child may make this situation easier and quicker. Alternatively, consider planning tube changes while the child is asleep (see Chapter 13, Tracheostomy Tube Changes).
- Regular reassessments of the tracheostomy tube will be required to establish whether the tube type and size is still suitable. If the child is to require a tracheostomy tube over a number of months or years, the tube will be upsized at intervals in relation to the increasing size of the airway. Plans to wean and decannulate the child's tracheostomy will require a re-admission to hospital.
- Velcro collars may be an inappropriate method of securing the tracheostomy tube if the child or another child can loosen or remove it. Consider the use of ribbon tapes as a safer alternative.

Training needs for others

All individuals who have been identified as carers will require information and education in the needs of the child. All significant carers will require the skills necessary to ensure the child is safe in their environment. This will include baby-sitters, teachers and other family members.

Communication development

The tracheostomy tube is likely to affect the child's ability to produce their normal quality and volume of voice. They may have difficulty expressing themselves using their pre-existing communication methods. This will include their ability to cry or laugh. Speech therapy can introduce the child and their family to alternative methods of communication to supplement a loss of voice production. This can include speaking valves, communication aids and gesturing/sign language.

Promoting a normal family life

Having a child with a tracheostomy does not need to stop normal family life, but there will have to be changes. Frequent medical needs can make the child 'over adult-orientated'.[17] The family may have to adjust having carers in the home and living surrounded by medical supplies. The danger of focusing on and overprotecting the child with a tracheostomy can evoke sibling reactions of jealousy and resentment. Treating the child normally and equally to their siblings can avoid this. With planning, preparation and support normal activities can resume, including holidays and returning to school.

Reaction of the child to the tracheostomy

The child who has a tracheostomy from a very young age will not recall life without the tube. The tracheostomy will become a normal aspect of their life. Older children may benefit from associating 'child-friendly' terminology for the tracheostomy, which can be developed by the family. For example, suctioning has been referred to as 'hoovering' and a Swedish nose resembles a 'bonio'.

Involving the child in the care of their tracheostomy as soon as possible makes it part of their daily routine. The use of a teaching aid or favourite toy/doll with a tracheostomy can provide an effective pre-operative introduction to tracheostomy and a learning aid for the child and their siblings (Appendix 1). Encourage normal social interactions to avoid isolation and incorporate the tracheostomy and its care within the child's activities.

Impact on the parents

The initial reaction of a parent whose child needs a long-term tracheostomy will undoubtedly be profound. They may experience an emotional response to the loss of their 'normal' child, which manifests with a grief like reaction.

An initial anxiety experienced by most parents and designated carers will be the prospect of tube changes. As these are required frequently it would be impractical and potentially unsafe for parents to be reliant on others to perform this. Frequent tube changes with support from the hospital team can help the parents to overcome fears and concerns.

Long-term effects, particularly after discharge, can include stress, social isolation and exhaustion. While the parent may feel confident to perform tracheostomy care in the home environment, they may feel self-conscious about doing so outside the home.

It will be important to consider the need for respite care either in the form of other family members/friends who can be trained in tracheostomy care, or from within the community or hospital nursing service. This will enable the parent to take breaks and feel less indispensable to the child's needs. However, while it will be preferable to have this respite care provision at home rather than in hospital, the parents may view this as a loss of privacy and intrusion into their home life.

Practical issues will include the financial burden, especially if a parent has to give up work or job flexibility to accommodate care needs/hospital visits. Alterations may need to be made to the home environment if there are accessibility difficulties or limited space for equipment and supplies.

Support networks and organisations, which provide contact with families in similar circumstances, can be beneficial for all involved. Support groups (e.g. *'Aid For Children With Tracheostomies'*, Appendix 1) can provide an exchange of new ideas and experiences to supplement existing knowledge.

Attending school

Safety and supervision requirements need to be established prior to attending/ returning to school or nursery. This will include identifying environmental hazards and training requirements for teachers and supervisors. A supervisor may need to be specifically identified for safety and management of the tracheostomy. Other children may require preparation in the appearance and needs of the child. Storage and access to tracheostomy equipment and supplies will need to be planned. Transport arrangements must include the need for appropriate supervision and the potential for skilled intervention during the journey.

Play activities

Due to the potential hazards during play, supervision will be important. Provide safe play activities with no small objects/toys, which could enter the tracheostomy tube. Contact sports could be dangerous with a risk of the tube becoming displaced or dislodged. Play involving sand or water will be extremely hazardous.

Safety requirements
- Provision of continuous, skilled supervision for routine care needs, monitoring and emergency situations
- Use of a baby intercom system can detect the need for suctioning without the carer being in the same room
- Apnoea alarm systems can alert parents to a blocked or displaced tube
- Pulse oximeter monitoring with alarm system can be useful when the child is asleep
- During bath/feeding times ensure a portable suction unit is readily accessible
- A plastic feeding bib can be useful as a shield during bathing or feeding
- Use of a tracheostomy guard to avoid accidental occlusion by small objects

FOLLOW-UP CARE PROVISION

Once successfully discharged, the patient will require medical consultation, regular follow-up and review by the community and hospital teams to determine their ongoing and changing medical needs. Potentially, this can identify and manage problems, anticipate difficulties and reduce the risk of re-admission to hospital. This contact will also provide a contact and resource for information regarding long-term proposals, expectations and prognosis regarding the need for the tracheostomy tube. Arrangements will be required for ongoing tracheostomy tube changes. It may also be necessary to change the type and/or size of the tracheostomy tube or refashion the stoma.

The individual will need an 'action-plan' to cover every eventuality and access to contact services, both in office hours and out of hours. Examples include clinical complications/deterioration and/or equipment failure. The local hospital service (if different from the treating hospital) will require knowledge of the patient and their needs and be prepared for the possibility of admission. A discharge summary (Table 1) will provide the information relevant in such circumstances. It will be useful for the individual to have a list of the following telephone contacts:

- General practitioner
- District nurse/community nurse team
- Carers
- Local hospital
- Treatment hospital
- ENT consultant
- Tracheostomy/ENT specialist nurse (if available)

Checklist summary of key points

- Involve patient and carer in discharge decisions
- Implement early patient/carer education programmes
- Consider home circumstances when planning a home discharge
- Provision of training and education for community team
- Ensure community team is informed of current and ongoing health care needs
- Co-ordinate provision of equipment/supplies for discharge
- Identify access to specialist advice
- Devise action plan to manage potential problems

REFERENCES

1. Diehl B, Dorsey L, Koller C. Transitioning the client with a tracheostomy from acute care to alternative settings. In: Tippett D (ed.). *Tracheostomy and Ventilator Dependency*. New York: Thieme Medical Publishers Inc., 2000; 237–265.
2. Beddar S, Aikin J. Continuity of care: A challenge for ambulatory oncology nursing. *Seminar Oncol Nurs* 1994; 10(4): 254–263.
3. Gilbert M, Counsell C, Ross L. *Evolution of a Role to Enhance Care Co-ordination*. Lippincott-Raven Publishers, 1997; 2(1): 19–22.
4. Wilson EB, Malley N. Discharge planning for the patient with a new tracheostomy. *Crit Care Nurs* 1990; 10(7): 73–74, 76–79.
5. Russell S. Continuity of care after discharge from ICU. *Prof Nurs* 2000; 15(8): 497–500.
6. Driscoll A. Managing post-discharge care at home. *J Adv Nurs* 2000; 31(5): 1165–1173.
7. Price B. Living with altered body image. *Br J Nurs* 1992; 1(3): 641–645.
8. Serra A. Tracheostomy care. *Nurs Stand* 2000; 14(42): 45–52.
9. Mason J, Murty G, Foster H, et al. Tracheostomy self-care: The Nottingham system. *J Laryngol Otol* 1992; 106: 723–724.
10. Tierny A, Macmillan A, Worth A. Discharge of patients from hospital. *Health Bulletin* 1994; 52(6): 479–491.
11. Adam J. Discharge planning of terminally ill patients home from an acute hospital. *Int J Palliat Nurs* 2000; 6(7): 338–345.
12. Haddad A. Ethics in action. *Regist Nurs* 2001; 64(7): 21–22.
13. Nace A, Fox A. Longterm care of tracheostomy patients. In: Myers E, Johnson J, Murry T (eds). *Tracheostomy Airway Management, Communication and Swallowing*. London: Singular Publishing Ltd, 1998; Chapter 7: 67–73.
14. Schreiber D. Tracheostomy care at home. *Regist Nurs* 2001; 64(7): 43–44.
15. Woollons S. Ambulatory suction equipment for home use. *Prof Nurs* 1996; 11(6): 373–376.
16. Sigler B. Nursing management of the patient with a tracheostomy. In: Myers E, Johnson J, Murry T (eds). *Tracheostomy Airway Management,*

Communication and Swallowing. London: Singular Publishing Ltd, 1998; Chapter 6: 57–65.

17. Cooper H. Tracheostomy care in an edcuational setting. *Health Visitor* 1989; 62(11): 348–349.

APPENDIX 1

Educational aids available	
Aid available	**Supplier**
Tracheostomy patient support guide (for patients and carers) *Sims Portex Ltd*	Sims Portex Ltd
Educational support guide (for health professionals) *Sims Portex Ltd*	Sims Portex Ltd
Guidelines for the care of patients with tracheostomy tubes *St Georges Healthcare NHS Trust*	Sims Portex Ltd
Adult home care guide *Shiley Tracheostomy Products*	Mallinckrodt UK Ltd
A parents guide to paediatric tracheostomy home care *Shiley Tracheostomy Products*	Mallinckrodt UK Ltd
Emergency Resuscitation for laryngectomy and tracheostomy patients leaflet	National Association of Laryngectomee Clubs
'Going down the tubes' training video *St Georges Medical Television*	St Georges Healthcare Trust
Tracheostomy head (for demonstration of percutaneous tracheostomy procedure and tube changes) *Sims Portex Ltd*	Sims Portex Ltd
Tracheostomy teaching aid model (cross-sectional head and neck) *Passy Muir Kapitex Healthcare Ltd*	Kapitex Healthcare Ltd
Patient education tracheostomy care set manikin	Adam Rouilly
Paediatric communication therapy toys: (tracheostomy toy, tracheostomy colouring book, exhalation kit)	Passy Muir Inc Kapitex Healthcare Ltd
Aid for children with tracheostomies (ACT) Charity organisation for parents, carers and health professionals.	Tel: 02920 755932

APPENDIX 2

Manufacturer address	
Adam Rouilly	Castle Road Eurolink Business Park Sittingbourne, Kent ME10 3AG Tel: 01795 471378
Countryside Supplies Ltd	26 Meadow Road Netherfield Nottingham NG4 2FR Tel: 0800 737 1659
EMS Medical Group Ltd	Unit 3 Stroud Industrial Estate Stonehouse Gloucester GL10 2DG Tel: 01453 791791
Hudson Intersurgical Ltd	Crane House Molly Millars Lane Wokingham Berkshire Tel: 0118 965356
Kapitex Healthcare Ltd	1 Sandbeck Way Wetherby LS22 7GH Tel: 01937 580211
Judd Medical	Highfield House 53 Worcester Road Bromsgrove Worcs B61 7DN Tel: 01527 559010
Laerdal Medical Ltd	Laerdal House Goodmead Road Orpington, Kent BR6 OHX Tel: 01689 876634
Mallinckrodt UK Ltd	10 Talisman Business Centre London Road Bicester Oxfordshire OX26 6HR Tel: 01869 322700

National Association of Laryngectomee Clubs	Ground Floor 6 Rickett Street Fulham London SW6 IRU Tel: 020 7381 9993
Rusch UK Ltd	PO Box 138 Cressex Business Park High Wycombe Buckinghamshire HP21 3NB Tel: 01494 532761
Seton Healthcare Group	Tubiton House Oldham OL1 3HS Tel: 0161 652 2222
Sims Portex Ltd	Portex House Military Road Hythe, Kent CT21 6JL Tel: 01303 260551
St Georges Healthcare Trust	St Georges Medical Television Tel: 020 8725 2701
Tyco Healthcare	154 Fareham Road Gosport Hampshire PO13 OAS Tel: 01329 224114

PAEDIATRIC TRACHEOSTOMY

Francis Vaz

INTRODUCTION

Paediatric tracheostomy insertion is a challenging but rewarding procedure. However, while it provides a safe protected upper airway, it is associated with a significant morbidity and mortality.[1,2] The anatomy of the paediatric upper airway is altered in comparison to the adult. The size and age of the child is critical when deciding on insertion and the care of the tracheostomy. The range of age is significant, from the pre-term baby to a child in their late teenage years. Also the psychosocial implications of a child with a paediatric tracheostomy must not be underestimated and it is for all these reasons that when managing a paediatric tracheostomy or undertaking one, the medical staff concerned are well aware of these factors in order to decrease the complications and difficulties associated with them.

INDICATIONS FOR TRACHEOSTOMY

Upper airway obstruction

A tracheostomy is needed in cases of upper airway obstruction when laryngeal intubation is not possible and the airway needs to be secured (see Table 1).

Ventilatory support

A tracheostomy may be indicated for the provision of positive pressure ventilation in patients with long-term requirements specifically the pre-term neonate but also other conditions such as brain damage, CNS diseases and severe burns. It may also be used to support respiratory failure secondary to prematurity, CNS disease and/or poor pulmonary reserve. Intubation may be employed for the short-term but for prolonged treatment the tracheostomy becomes easier to manage.

Table 1: Indications for tracheostomy: upper airway obstruction

Congenital	Bilateral vocal cord paresis	An immobility of the vocal cords leaving them fixed in the paramedian position limiting the airway.
	Congenital subglottic stenosis	Narrowing in the subglottic region.
	Laryngeal webs/atresia	A web is classically anteriorly sited in the larynx and may be of variable severity and thickness.
	Subglottic haemangiomas	A similar entity to a cutaneous strawberry naevus that grows in the early months of life but usually recedes with time.
Acquired	Acquired subglottic stenosis	Typically associated with long-term intubation causing a narrowing of the subglottis.
	Papillomas	A warty like growth secondary to the presence of human papilloma virus that can obstruct the upper airway.
	Subglottic cysts	A cyst that sometimes is associated with previous intubations.
	Tracheal stenosis	
	Vocal fold paresis	
	Burns/trauma to the head and neck region	

Pulmonary toilet/decreasing dead space

In conditions such as aspiration associated with neurological diseases or tracheal/laryngeal clefts and respiratory problems such as broncho-pulmonary dysplasia and chronic lung disease. A tracheostomy can be of use by easing pulmonary toilet and decreasing the dead space.

ANATOMY

Paediatric tracheostomy provides the surgeon with an intricate problem, not only because of the relative difference in size but the variation that exists in the anatomy. In the paediatric population the hyoid bone, thyroid cartilage and the cricoid cartilage lie higher in the neck. In addition these structures in the neck may be difficult to palpate or distinguish, in particular, the cricoid cartilage from the first tracheal ring or the thyroid cartilage. It is also common to find a pre-tracheal pad of fat that prevents the surgeon palpating normal structures with clarity and it is important to be aware of when surgically approaching the neck for a tracheostomy.

Other structures lower in the neck or superior mediastinum that are not often viewed in the adult tracheostomy procedure may be more easily encountered in children such as the innominate artery, left brachiocephalic vein and the apices of the lungs. The presence of such structures in the neck can be accentuated with hyperextension of the neck and consequently a low tracheostomy is rarely formed in a child. Interestingly the recurrent laryngeal nerves are positioned just lateral to the trachea in the child and are more easily encountered during the procedure particularly if the dissection accidentally deviates from the midline.

It is also important to remember that the trachea is a developing structure and as such should be surgically treated with a view to minimising long-term damage. A vertical tracheotomy with no loss of cartilage is chosen so as to prevent tracheal stenosis. The tracheotomy should not extend to or higher than the first tracheal ring so as to decrease the chance of subglottic stenosis.

TECHNIQUE OF TRACHEOSTOMY

The child is placed supine with extension of the neck provided by a sandbag under the shoulders and a headring to ensure head immobility. The child is usually ventilated with an endotracheal tube. Lidocaine/adrenaline is infiltrated where the incision is to be placed, one fingers breadth above the suprasternal notch. A horizontal incision is made that will allow safe and easy access to form the stoma. The superficial fat is often removed to expose the strap muscles. These midline muscles are picked up and the midline is dissected in layers. If the underlying thyroid gland cannot be retracted superiorly it may be divided with electrocautery or suture-ligated. The trachea is then visualised and two monofilament stay sutures are placed either side of the intended vertical tracheotomy. The tracheotomy is a vertical incision performed in the midline between the second and fourth tracheal rings encompassing at least two tracheal rings. The endotracheal tube is then withdrawn so as to allow the insertion of the pre-chosen, checked and prepared tracheostomy tube. The new tracheostomy is connected to the anaesthetic machine and the tube secured with tapes. The stay sutures are fixed to the chest and marked 'do not remove' and 'right' or 'left' as appropriate.

If in the first week there is an accidental decannulation the stay sutures provide safe control of the tracheotomy and easier reinsertion of a new tube.

COMPLICATIONS OF PAEDIATRIC TRACHEOSTOMY

Early (immediate to 1 week)

Obstruction – Obstruction of the tracheostomy tube is a potentially fatal complication. The most common cause of obstruction is accumulation of mucus and crusts in the tube lumen.[2,3] This can be prevented by adequate humidification and suctioning together with adequate systemic hydration.

Accidental decannulation – This is a serious complication in the first two to three days because the fistula track has not yet formed, and the vertical tracheotomy in children makes early tube replacement difficult. The stay sutures either side of the tracheotomy are of great use in this situation.

Air leak – Surgical emphysema is seen but usually it resolves without any treatment. It is most often caused by leakage of air through the tracheotomy into the underlying soft tissues of the neck. The position of the tube and tightness around the stoma should be checked. Pneumomediastinum is to be managed in a similar manner as surgical emphysema. A low tracheostomy does predispose to pneumothorax and should be treated appropriately.

Apnoea – Children with chronic airway obstruction are more likely to suffer with this with the sudden decrease in dead space. Sedation should be avoided in such children.

Creation of a false passage – The changing of the tube or its reinsertion may lead to creation of a false passage, more so if the procedure is done before the tract is well formed. The creation of a false passage may lead to obstruction or pneumothorax.

Haemorrhage – Early haemorrhage may occur from the wound edge or a small previously unnoticed blood vessel not recognised and cauterised at the time of tracheostomy.

Late complications (usually after 1 week)

Obstruction – This may be caused by a granuloma or by a mucous plug. Granulations can appear at the site of the stoma and within the tracheal lumen above the stoma.[3] These granulations lead to the obstruction of the tracheal lumen or the tube. These granulations can also cause bleeding during a tracheostomy tube change. This may require surgical intervention.[4] The obstruction of the tube or the lumen by a mucous plug can be avoided by adequate humidification and suctioning.

Haemorrhage – Haemorrhage due to erosion of the anterior tracheal wall and into the innominate artery may occur as a result of a poorly positioned tube. This is a rare but catastrophic complication.

Chest infections – Infections are more common in children with tracheostomies and should be treated symptomatically.

TYPES OF TUBE

A wide variety of tracheostomy tubes for children exist and each paediatric unit favours specific types. Both plastic (Fig. 1) and silver tubes exist but most small paediatric tubes are single lumen because of the small diameter of the trachea they are in, and also if an inner tube were present then the size of functioning airway decreases. Tubes are selected according to the age of the child (Table 2). Although cuffed tubes are available the majority of paediatric tracheostomy tubes used are uncuffed and function well for the patient with spontaneous ventilation or assisted ventilation. Speaking valves do exist for paediatric tubes but should be used in appropriate cases under the surgeon's, speech and language therapists (SLT) or the specialist nurses advice.

TUBE CHANGES/HOME CARE

Care of the tracheostomy is an essential skill that must be learnt by the primary carer(s) of the child. Appropriate understanding and proficiency in suctioning, humidification techniques and cardiopulmonary resuscitation skills are essential requirements for the carer before discharge of the child.[4] It is

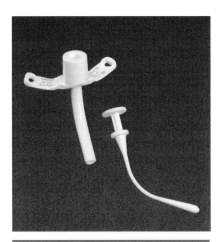

Fig. 1: Shiley paediatric tracheostomy tube.

Table 2: Comparison of endotracheal tube size with tracheostomy tube size relative to age

		<1/12	1/12–6/12	6/12–18/12	18/12–3 year	3–6 year	6–9 year	9–12 year	>12 year
Tracheal diameter (mm)		5.0 6.0	5.0–7.0	6.0–8.0	7.0–9.0	8.0–10.0	9.0–13	10–	13+
Shiley	Size/I.D.	3.0	3.5	4.0	4.5	5.0	5.5	6.0	6.5
	O.D.	4.5	5.2	5.9	6.5	7.1	7.7	8.3	9.0
Alder hay	12–14	16	18	20	22	24			
Broncho-scope	Size	2.5	3.0	3.5	4.0	4.5	5.0	6.0	6.0
ETT (Portex)	Size	3.0	3.5	4.0	4.5	5.0	6.0	7.0	8.0

because of these skills being learnt while in hospital together with appropriate contact details in case of emergency that the longer-term outcome in the home environment for a child with a tracheostomy has improved.

The frequency of tube changes is variable. However, maybe from once a week to once a fortnight. How often a tube change should be undertaken can be judged by the degree of resistance on suctioning which is caused by a build up of secretions within the tube. A rapid tube change should be contemplated in the event of the inability to pass a suction catheter through the tracheostomy tube, if the tube has been displaced, if there is severe respiratory distress that is not able to be resolved with suctioning or if there is no airflow through the tube and the child is becoming cyanotic.

Helpful hints for tube changes

- It is helpful to keep the neck extended when changing a tracheostomy tube therefore a small towel rolled and placed under the shoulders is effective.
- For the writhing child or very young children it is better to swaddle them prior to a tracheostomy tube change.
- Tube changes are best performed 2–3 h post feeding to reduce the likelihood of regurgitation.
- It is often better to have tracheostomy tapes already attached to the flange of the tube and if appropriate to have a dressing mounted on the tube so as not to cause too much tracheal stimulation once the tube is inserted.
- It is essential to have a good light source not only to see where to insert the tracheostomy but to inspect the stoma on changing the tube.

- Occasionally it is easier to commence the tube change while the child is asleep. However, the child is likely to wake on tracheal stimulation and the carer must be prepared for this.
- A play therapist may be helpful in relaxing the child having tracheostomy tube changes and also may help the child come to terms with the need for tube changes.

IMPLICATIONS ON LIFE AND DEVELOPMENT

The child with a tracheostomy will obviously require more supervision and care in comparison to a child without. However, development and growing up need not be overly affected. Communication is an important issue for parents although initially a child cannot speak following tracheostomy. Children rapidly learn to occlude the tube with their fingers or chin to vocalise words. It is important to continue as normal with speech and language development in a child with a tracheostomy and they hopefully should develop without problems. Should language delay become an issue then the SLT should be involved to assist with the further management.

Feeding and eating is not usually restricted, however, care should be taken with the younger child. It is useful in the young child to cover the tracheostomy with a bib to prevent aspiration of foodstuffs that drop down or that a child might insert.

Bathing and playing in water are very important and it is essential to supervise children in these situations as water can easily enter a tracheostomy and the risk of drowning is a real one.

Small toys, beads, sand and anything that is small enough to enter the opening of the tracheostomy tube should not be easily accessed by children as inhalation can cause significant respiratory distress. Children's playtime should not be limited and they should enjoy themselves without being constrained by a tracheostomy.

Decannulation

Before tracheostomy decannulation can be considered, the primary pathology necessitating the tracheostomy should have resolved or been treated. Ventilated children should be breathing room air and those who require regular respiratory toileting should be able to cope with their secretions without suctioning. There is less room for error with paediatric decannulation than in an adult due to the relative size difference. It is for this reason that most children have a diagnostic endoscopy in advance of decannulation and then a ward decannulation is organised.[4] For adolescents the procedure is often similar to adults. For younger children there are a variety of protocols most often involving down sizing of the tube followed by monitored capping, of the tracheostomy tube.[5] If capping off is tolerated decannulation can occur followed by a period of observation as an inpatient on the ward.

The stoma site will be dressed until no air leakage is observed, with an airtight dressing which can be easily removed.

An ENT follow-up will usually be carried out approximately 1 month following decannulation to assess the child's ability to cope without the tracheostomy. Ongoing review will depend on the indication for the tracheostomy and any co-existing conditions.

Conclusion

Paediatric tracheostomies are unusual events in a peripheral hospital and more often seen in hospitals with dedicated paediatric ENT departments or large paediatric intensive care units. They present different problems not only because of the smaller sizes of the tubes but also the varied anatomy and developmental issues associated with the children who undergo this procedure. The use of a multidisciplinary approach in the management of a child with a tracheostomy will include the surgeon, specialist nurse, SLT, play therapist and community team. This team approach is essential to improve the overall quality of care for the child and family. Tracheostomies are extremely rewarding, as they can be life saving for the patient. However, good experience and understanding of them is essential to decrease the morbidity and mortality associated with them.

REFERENCES

1. Midwinter K, Carrie S, Bull P. Paediatric tracheostomy: Sheffield experience 1979–1999. *J Laryngol Otol* 2002; 116: 532–535.
2. Gianoli G, Miller R, Guarisco J. Tracheotomy in the first year of life. *Ann Otol Rhinol* 1990; 99: 896–901.
3. Carter P, Benjamin B. Ten year review of pediatric tracheotomy. *Ann Otol Rhinol* 1983; 92: 398–400.
4. McMurray J, Prescott C. Tracheotomy in the paediatric patient. In: Cotton R, Myer C (eds). *Practical Pediatric Otolaryngology*. Philadelphia: Lippincott-Raven, 1999; 575–593.
5. Wadell A, Appleford R, Dunning C, Papsin BC, Bailey CM. The Great Ormond Street protocol for ward decannulation of children with tracheostomy: Increasing safety and decreasing cost. *Int J Pediatr Otorhinolaryngol* 1997; 39: 111–118.

18

NURSING CARE OF THE CHILD WITH A TRACHEOSTOMY

Teresa Johnson and Lucy Andrews

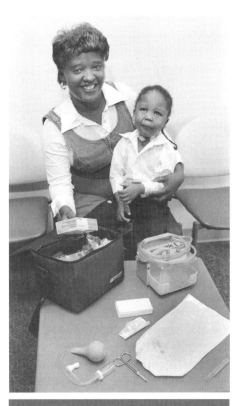

Courtesy of Shiley, Mallickrodt.

INTRODUCTION

Although paediatric tracheostomy is mentioned in other chapters, this book would not be complete without dedicated chapters for children. Children are unique in not only the medical reasons for a tracheostomy but also their care and needs following the procedure. Due to medical advances, more children with chronic medical conditions are surviving, often with a technological dependency, including tracheostomy. The benefits of paediatric tracheostomy, which were not realised until the beginning of the 19th century,[1] have now evolved into a common and successful means of treatment and support. The vast majority of children are able to live and develop within their own homes. The equipment and resources available are continuing to expand providing health care professionals, children and their families with a greater choice for care.

INDICATIONS FOR PAEDIATRIC TRACHEOSTOMY

There are numerous reasons why infants and children require a tracheostomy, many are unique to the paediatric population. Categorisation by medical condition is difficult, as they often fit into more than one. However, four distinct categories do emerge; central nervous system impairment, respiratory dysfunction, congenital and genetic abnormalities and acquired airway obstruction. A summary of each category and the associated medical conditions can be viewed in Table 1.

In addition to the categories listed, a tracheostomy can be used to assist weaning from mechanical ventilation, by reducing the amount of airway resistance or 'dead space'. Furthermore, a tracheostomy can be used for many of the aforementioned conditions to facilitate suctioning or, to provide long-term mechanical respiratory support. It is beyond the scope of this chapter to discuss this latter aspect of care. Some disease processes such as croup require a child to have a tracheostomy for only a short duration others, for an indefinite period of time.

PRE-PROCEDURE PLANNING

Fortunately, a paediatric tracheostomy is rarely performed in an emergency. Usually, it is a planned procedure whereby both the child and parents are adequately prepared. Play is how children learn and understand about their world and therefore, developmentally appropriate play therapy is essential to the pre-procedure care. Play specialists have many innovative means of enabling, even very young children, to gain an understanding of what is going to happen to them.

Being informed that their child requires a tracheostomy can be devastating for parents.[2] In fact, it is common for parents to progress through a grieving

Table 1: Summary of paediatric conditions associated with tracheostomy

Reasons for tracheostomy	Associated conditions
Congenital/genetic abnormalities	Laryngomalacia/tracheomalacia/ bronchomalacia Tracheoesophageal anomalies Haemangioma Cystic hygroma Subglottic stenosis Pulmonary atresia Congenital heart disease Bilateral vocal cord paralysis Laryngeal web Craniofacial – Pierre Robin syndrome Treacher Collins syndrome Metabolic disorders – Leigh's disease
Acquired airway obstruction	Direct airway trauma Burns Smoke inhalation Corrosive chemicals Epiglottitis Obstructive sleep apnoea Foreign body Croup Tumour Subglottic stenosis
Central nervous system impairment	Brain stem or posterior fossa tumour Congenital central alveolar hypoventilation (Ondoine's curse) Spina bifida with Arnold-Chiari malformation Spinal cord trauma (particularly above C4) Spinal muscular atrophy Viral encephalitis Head injury Cerebral palsy
Respiratory dysfunction	Congenital myopathies Congenital thoracic rib cage abnormalities Chest wall injury Diaphragm dysfunction Duchenne's muscular dystrophy Bronchopulmonary dysplasia

process, grieving for the loss of the child they have known.[3] Additionally, parents will have many questions such as will they lead a normal life and will they talk.[4] It is vital that health care professionals have an understanding and knowledge of the child's medical condition and paediatric tracheostomy in order to provide support and facilitate understanding.

INITIAL MANAGEMENT FOR CHILDREN WITH A TRACHEOSTOMY

For the initial few days children should be continuously monitored and observed. It is recommended that they will be routinely managed in a paediatric intensive care or high dependency unit depending on their individual needs. Children should only be cared for in a paediatric ward area if all the necessary emergency equipment and personnel are consistently available. Personnel should consist of an ENT surgeon, paediatrician, paediatric ward nurses with tracheostomy experience and the ability to provide high intensity nursing care. The hospital paediatric cardiac arrest team should be trained to paediatric advanced life support standard. Additionally, there should be the provision for the child to be transferred or retrieved to a paediatric high dependency or intensive care unit if necessary.

Nursing emphasis should be upon: maintaining a patent airway, cardio-pulmonary assessment, providing airway humidity, maintaining hydration and fluid balance, preventing infection, tracheostomy care, promoting child's comfort, effective pain management, emotional and educational support for the child and family.[3]

Early post-procedure complications include; haemorrhage, subcutaneous emphysema, obstruction, accidental removal and infection. All complications are potentially life threatening. There is an increased susceptibility to infection as many of the body's natural defences are bypassed. Infants are particularly prone to infection due to an immature immune system. Additionally, they are particularly prone to obstruction due to the small tracheal tube diameter. Suctioning may need to be frequent in the initial few days to remove mucous and blood. Some bleeding from the site is expected. Suctioning technique will be discussed later in this chapter.

Children are naturally inquisitive and depending upon their developmental stage it is often difficult for them to understand the significance of the tracheostomy. Consequently, there is an increased risk of accidental removal. Pre-procedure play preparation can assist with preventing this serious complication. A pair of 'stay' sutures are placed on either side of the vertical incision in the trachea. These can assist with an early tube change by applying lateral tension which will hold open the tracheal opening allowing the insertion of the tube.

Between five and seven days post-procedure an appropriately trained and skilled professional will perform the first tracheostomy change. This tends to be an ENT surgeon or a tracheostomy clinical nurse specialist. 'Stay' and skin sutures will be removed at this stage. Following a successful tube change children can be cared for in the most appropriate hospital setting for their needs. In many situations care will be continued within an intensive care or high dependency area however, a transfer to a paediatric ward as soon as is clinically possible is usually advocated for the child's and families benefit.

DAILY MANAGEMENT AND CARE FOR THE CHILD WITH A TRACHEOSTOMY

Introduction

Following the first successful tracheostomy tube change the emphasis often moves away from providing acute medical and nursing interventions to that of safe day-to-day management of the tracheostomy and support for the child and family. It is beyond the scope of this chapter to include every component of individualised care however, the essential aspects of paediatric tracheostomy management will be discussed.

Infection control

Any child with a tracheostomy has a high susceptibility to both stoma and respiratory infection. Effective hand washing is the single most important barrier to preventing infection and should be completed prior to any aspect of care. Parents and carers must be made aware of the importance of hand washing and taught the correct procedure. Gloves should be worn as a protective barrier but cannot substitute effective hand washing. During hospitalisation an aseptic or non-touch aseptic technique is recommended for tracheostomy care, once a child is within their home environment a clean technique is satisfactory.[3]

Suctioning

Children are at a greater risk from the complications of suctioning than adults. There is an increased risk of obstruction with secretions during suctioning due to the smaller airway sizes. Additionally, children have a higher oxygen demand per kilogram of body weight due to a high basal metabolic rate. Oxygen consumption in infants is 6–8 ml/kg per min compared with 3–4 ml/kg per min in adults. Consequently, they are at a greater risk of hypoxia and associated bradycardia during suctioning.[5]

Table 2: Calculating size of suction catheter		
3.0 I.D.	–	6 Fg
3.5 I.D.	–	7 Fg
4.0 I.D.	–	8 Fg
4.5 I.D.	–	8 Fg
5.0 I.D.	–	10 Fg
6.0 I.D.	–	12 Fg

There is an increasing array of suction catheter sizes available for children. The diameter of the catheter should be half the internal diameter (I.D.) of the tracheostomy tube. A simple calculation to determine the French gauge (Fg) size is to double the I.D. of the tracheostomy tube and use the closest catheter size available (Table 2).

Depending on their medical condition children may be able to cough and clear secretions adequately and this should always be encouraged. Secretions can be cleaned with a tissue, or from the proximal end of the tracheostomy tube using a large bore suction or Yankeur catheter.

Routine suctioning on a stable non-ventilated child with a tracheostomy is no longer advocated. However, it is advisable to suction a child first thing in the morning and before going to bed. Additionally, children require suctioning when secretions are visible in the tube, for noisy breathing, continuous coughing, increased work of breathing and at the child's request. If secretions are not cleared adequately, the tube may obstruct and there is an increased risk of infection.[6] To maintain the patency of an infant's small airway more frequent suctioning, often 6 hourly, may be required. There is little evidence to support the effectiveness of saline during routine suctioning.[6] However, 0.9% saline may be effective for dealing with secretions that are particularly tenacious especially in infant airways. The amount needed depends on the child's size but as a guide use 0.2 ml with neonates, 0.5 ml with infants and up to 2 ml with children.[7]

If a child requires invasive suctioning insert the catheter without applying suction to a depth of no further than 1.0 cm beyond the length of the tube.[8] A measuring tape can be placed at the cot or bedside to assist with accuracy. Withdraw the catheter while applying suction. The amount of suction should be a negative pressure of 50–100 mmHg[8,9] using the lowest possible to facilitate clearance. The entire process should take between 5 and 10 seconds.[7] Unless during an emergency allow at least 30 seconds for recovery between each attempt. Deep suctioning until you feel resistance of the carina is not recommended as it leads to mucosal damage and can be uncomfortable.[7]

Humidification

In normal respiration inspired air is warmed, filtered and moistened.[8] A tracheostomy bypasses this natural system and artificial humidification is often required. Failure to provide adequate humidification may lead to secretions becoming thick and sticky resulting in tube occlusion and respiratory infection.

The types of humidification available include a heat moisture exchange (HME) device attached onto the connector of the tracheostomy. These also have the advantage of allowing the child to remain mobile and active and are recommended for the majority of children during the day. Young children have very short necks and a HME device can cause irritation beneath the chin, however, there are now several different types available for this age group. Some HME filters are also designed to administer low flow oxygen and have inbuilt speaking valves.

Additional methods of humidification are heated water systems delivered via a tracheostomy mask. This is ideal for when a child is unwell, has particularly thick secretions or overnight. Room humidification systems may also be useful.

Chest physiotherapy

The aim of chest physiotherapy is to loosen secretions and prevent infection. Encouraging children to remain as ambulant as possible will, in most instances, provide adequate physiotherapy. Children who require regular chest physiotherapy are those who are less mobile and/or with weak respiratory muscles. All children are likely to require additional physiotherapy when they are unwell.

Stoma care

Care of the stoma includes daily observation of the site and accurate documentation of the findings. Observations should note any redness or swelling, evidence of granulation tissue, exudate or increased discomfort during care. Daily cleaning of the stoma is recommended. Cleaning should be with 0.9% sterile saline solution and the skin allowed to dry.[8] Gauze can be used but mouth care sponges wet with saline can be very effective. A swab of the stoma for infection only needs to be done if the child is pyrexial, displays signs of being unwell or has increased/offensive wound exudate.

Changing tapes and dressings

You only have to observe a toddler or young child eating to realise that daily tape and dressing changes will become an essential part of routine tracheostomy care. Two people are often required, especially if a child is less compliant, making the tape change difficult. A play therapist's involvement may allow the procedure to pass uneventfully. Prior to starting, emergency equipment should be checked and readily available.

One person should support and position the child. A soft blanket can be placed beneath the shoulders to facilitate a slight neck extension. The head should not be over extended as, due to the short length of both neonatal and paediatric tubes, this extreme position/movement can cause tube displacement. The second person is responsible for changing the ties. During the process it is important to examine skin integrity. Once secure the carer should be able to place one finger between the neck and the tie.[3]

The range of ties will vary but generally consist of either cotton tapes or Velcro fastening. The latter are quicker and easier to use but are not suitable for all children, particularly toddlers and those with special needs, as they can be easily undone. Parents sometimes find their own suitable substitute including colourful ties or ribbons.[2] It is essential that any tie used is resistant to fraying and has soft padding to protect skin integrity. Children are often more prone to skin breakdown and pressure sores because they cannot always communicate discomfort and are more reliant on others to meet their needs.

A tracheostomy dressing is used to provide absorbency of any exudate keeping the skin clean and dry and to also promote comfort. Stoma dressings are usually changed at the same time as tapes. A pre-cut keyhole foam absorbent dressing is recommended and placed under the flanges of the tracheostomy tube. The dressing should be inserted from below the tube.[8]

Changing a tracheostomy tube

From experience, this is the aspect of care that causes the most anxiety to health care professionals and parents alike. The child's tracheostomy is essentially life sustaining and removing and replacing the tube is naturally a daunting prospect. The frequency of a tube change will depend on the type used and the thickness of secretions. The maximum time a tube should remain in place is four weeks. All equipment should be prepared including a replacement tube of the same size and one of a smaller size. Tracheostomy tube changes should not be performed following meals as this can precipitate vomiting and aspiration.[6,8]

Two people are recommended when performing a routine tube change,[6,8–10] this is particularly important with children who may be less compliant requiring diversion therapy and additional reassurance. With the child supported by one person and the neck slightly extended, the second carer cuts the ties and gently removes the tube following the natural curve.[6,9] Please note that while children tend not to have cuffed tracheostomy tubes, due to their funnel shaped airways creating a natural seal, adolescents might and therefore these should be changed using the adult method. Following removal, careful suction of the stoma may be required. A new tube is then replaced using the same natural curve, introducer removed if used, position confirmed and held firmly until securely tied.

If insertion is very difficult use the next smallest tube size and inform your paediatric community nurse or doctor (see Chapter 13, Tracheostomy Tube Changes).

Emergency tracheostomy care

Signs of respiratory distress include an inability to pass a suction catheter, stridor (noisy inspirations), decreasing saturations and increasing respiration rate.

This situation requires an immediate tube change following the guidelines for a routine tracheostomy change.

If a tracheostomy cannot be reinserted during a routine or urgent tube change then, contact a paediatric anaesthetist if in hospital. At home the carer needs to call the emergency services for immediate transfer to hospital. Transfer of a child in this circumstance should always be via ambulance, never by car. The child's condition should be carefully monitored and basic life support (BLS) commenced if necessary.

DISCHARGE PLANNING

There is now accepted awareness that technology dependent children should be able to live within their home environment.[11] This is fundamental to a child's development and family integrity[3] and yet it is only relatively recently that children with tracheostomies have been living outside of hospital.[9] It can also prove cost effective for the health service to support children at home, although the financial impact upon the family should not be dismissed. A number of essential criteria should be met before discharge; the child must be medically stable, family/carers involvement is needed, support accessible, equipment and resources available and financial considerations.[9]

The transition from hospital to home can be a daunting experience for any child and parent, perhaps even more so when the child has a tracheostomy, which in essence, is life sustaining. Discharge planning should begin as early as possible, in many instances prior to the procedure. The discharge process is complex and generally involves a myriad of professionals and agencies working in partnership with the child and family. It has been highlighted in several retrospective studies that parents of technology dependent children, expressed an unfulfilled need for a named person, to take responsibility for the orchestration of their child's care from discharge home and beyond.[12–16] It is therefore advisable that a professional is nominated and responsible for the overall co-ordination of the discharge plan, in order to make the transition as trouble free as possible. This professional can also act as an advocate for the child and family. The Community Children's Nurse (CCN) may be in the best position to take on this responsibility as their experience lies in the intricacies of life at home and the services which may be of use to the family. It has been found the involvement of CCN services facilitated a more rapid transition home, which was welcomed by children and families.[17]

Every child will require an individualised plan of care. It is recommended that a multi-professional/agency meeting be called, prior to discharge, in order to clarify who is responsible for what. It is fundamental that the family is central to the planning process and cognisance is taken of their needs and concerns.

It is imperative that parents who are caring for their child are confident in all aspects of their child's care prior to going home, from tracheostomy tube replacement to Basic Life Support (BLS), as invariably parents provide the majority of their child's care from day-to-day. It is advisable that one or two people are responsible for this training in an effort to offer a consistent approach, and prevent duplication or omission in the training process. An outline of the training requirements of parents and carers are represented in Table 3.

Training for parents may involve videos, bedside teaching and practice with manikins. It is suggested that a minimum of two people learn all aspects of tracheostomy care and management. Written information has been found to be beneficial to parents[17] as it constitutes a reference point and gives parents an opportunity to revisit what they have learned. The goal for parents is to provide safe care while promoting the growth and development of their child.

It may be of considerable benefit to arrange a trial visit home prior to discharge. Often the realities of taking a child home become evident at this time and any problems encountered can be resolved prior to the actual discharge date.

The ultimate aim of discharge planning is to facilitate a gradual shift in the balance of care to the parents and child thus creating a partnership in care.

Training children

With focus upon the training needs for parents, developing children's competence can be overlooked. It is suggested that children with a cognitive

Table 3: Training requirements

Knowledge based:
- Understanding of child's underlying medical condition
- Anatomy of airway and tracheostomy placement
- Respiratory physiology and assessment

Practice/knowledge based:
- Routine tracheostomy care – hand washing, cleaning, changing tapes and dressings, skin care
- Chest physiotherapy and aerosol treatments/humidification
- Suctioning
- Tracheostomy tube change
- Emergency tracheostomy procedures
- Oxygen delivery
- BLS

Equipment training:
- Equipment care and use
- Monitoring equipment
- Other issues including gastrostomy feeding

Other needs:
- Developmental needs
- Medications
- Promoting actives of daily living – communication, play, dressing
- Psychosocial needs

developmental age of more than four years without any additional disabilities and who are emotionally ready can become proficient in many aspects of tracheostomy care.[2] Obstacles to learning can include fear, anxiety and parental unwillingness. Often time and patience is all that is needed to overcome these barriers.

Training for children can be commenced in hospital but many children will learn more effectively in familiar surroundings. Children need clear steps to assist them with learning and a timeframe for completion.[2] Play specialists are invaluable in helping children learn through play and practice. Positive reinforcement and motivation tools, such as star charts, work well to support children through the learning process.

Conclusion

Children with tracheostomies have a complex array of needs. The care available for these children is continually evolving and health care professionals need to keep pace with these changes, working in partnership with children and families, to facilitate expert care. The equipment and resources, once adapted from adult provisions, are now specifically tailored to meet children's needs. Children with tracheostomies are no longer restricted to the hospital environment but can be cared for and supported within their own home. The ultimate goal of caring for a child with a tracheostomy is to provide safe, specialist care while enabling a child to grow and develop and ultimately achieve their full potential.

REFERENCES

1. Irving RM, Jones NS, Bailey CM, Melville J. A guide to the selection of paediatric tracheostomy tubes. *J Laryngol Otol* 1991; 105: 1046–1051.
2. Bissell CM. *Pediatric Tracheostomy Home Care Guide*. MA: Twin Enterprises Inc., 2000.
3. Fitton CM, Myer CM. Practical aspects of pediatric tracheotomy care. *J Otolaryngol* 1992; 21(6): 409–413.
4. Bleile KM. *The Care of Children with Long-Term Tracheostomies*. CA: Singular Publishing Group Inc., 1993.
5. Chameides L, Hasinski MF (eds). *Pediatric Advanced Life Support*. TX: American Heart Association, 1997.
6. Great Ormond Street Hospital for Children NHS Trust. *Your Child's Tracheostomy*. Great Ormond Street Hospital for Children NHS Trust, 1996.
7. Runton N. Suctioning artificial airways in children: Appropriate technique. *Pediat Nurs* 1992; 18(2): 115–118.
8. St. George's Healthcare NHS Trust. *Guidelines for the Care of Patients with Tracheostomy Tubes*. St. George's NHS Trust, 2000.
9. Adamo-Tumminelli P. *A Guide to Pediatric Tracheotomy Care*, 2nd edn. IL: Charles C. Thomas Publisher, 1993.
10. Jennings P. Caring for a child with a tracheostomy. *Nurs Stand* 1990; 4(30): 24–26.
11. Whaley LF, Wong DL. *Nursing Care of Infants and Children*, 4th edn. MO: Mosby Year Book, 1991.
12. Goldberg AI, Faure EAM, Vaughn CJ, Snarski RRT, Seleny F. 'Home care for life supported persons: An approach to program development'. *J Paediat* 1984 (May); 104(5): 785–795.
13. Kirk S. Caring for a technology-dependant child at home. *Br J Nurs* 1999; 4(8): 390–393.
14. Kirk S, Glendenning C. *Supporting Parents Caring for a Technology-Dependent Child*. National Primary Care Research and Development Centre, University of Manchester, 2000.
15. Noyse J. Barriers that delay children and young people who are dependent on mechanical ventilators from being discharged from hospital. *J Clin Nurs* 2000; 11(1): 2–11.
16. O'Brien ME. Living in a house of cards: Family experience with long-term childhood technology dependence. *J Pediat Nurs* 2001; 16(1): 13–22.

17. Rehm R. Creating a context of safety and achievement at school for children who are medically fragile/technology dependent. *Adv Nurs Sci* 2002 (Mar); 24(3): 71–84.

BIBLIOGRAPHY

Engleman SG, Turnage-Carrier C. Tolerance of the Passy Muir speaking valve in infants and children less than 2 years of age. *Pediat Nurs* 1997; 23(6): 571–573.

Friedberg J, Giberson W. Failed tracheotomy decannulation in children. *J Otolaryngol* 1992; 21(6): 404–408.

Jennings P. Caring for a child with a tracheostomy. *Nurs Stand* 1990; 4(32): 38–40.

Kirk S. Negotiating lay and professional roles in the care of children with complex health care needs. *J Adv Nurs* 2001; 34(5): 593–602.

Marcellus L. The infant with Pierre Robin sequence: Review and implications for nursing practice. *J Pediat Nurs* 2001; 16(1): 23–33.

Murphy G. The technology-dependent child at home. *Paediat Nurs* 2001; 13(7): 14–18.

Wyatt ME, Bailey CM, Whiteside JC. Update on paediatric tracheostomy tubes. *J Laryngol Otol* 1999; 113: 35–40.

USEFUL ADDRESSES

Contact a family	209–211 City Road London EC1V 1JN Tel: 020 7608 8700 Help-line: 0808 808 3555
Action for sick children	Argyle House 29–31 Euston Road London NW1 2SD Tel: 0717 833 2041
Aid for children with tracheostomies (ACT)	Lammas Cottage Stathes Bridgewater Somerset TA7 0SL Tel: 01823 698398
Pierre Robin syndrome support group	83 Swallow Field Road Charlton London SE7 7NT
Treacher Collins family support group	114 Vincent Road Thorpe Hamlet Norwich Norfolk NR1 4HH

Cystic hygroma and haemangioma support group	Villa Fontane Church Road Worth Crawley West Sussex RH10 4RA
Climb	Climb Building 176 Nantwich Road Crewe CW2 6BG

USEFUL WEB SITES

www.tracheostomy.com
One of the leading tracheostomy web sites
Aaron's tracheostomy page

www.tracheostomy.com/trachkids
Aaron's page for children

www.bissells.com
Aaron's family

www.actfortrachykids.com
Aid for children with tracheostomies (ACT)

www.cafamily.org.uk
Contact a family
For families with disabled children

www.specialneedsbooks.com
Books for families of children with special needs

www.climb.org.uk
National information and advice regarding children with metabolic diseases

CHILDREN'S TRACHEOSTOMY CARE WITHIN THE COMMUNITY

Lucy Andrews

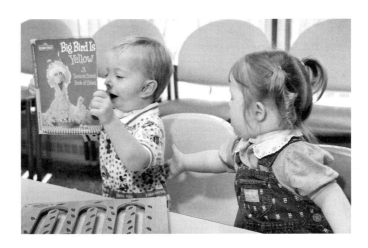

CHILDREN'S COMMUNITY NURSING

Children's community nursing (CCN) services have historically been sparse.[1] The consequent impact of this has been that help available for families caring for a child with a tracheostomy has been limited. However, rapid development and expansion of CCN services nationwide has enabled many families to receive varying amounts of support depending on local provision, which has been reported as beneficial.[2] The input from CCN team services described in this chapter is very much a gold standard of care, which could be aspired to where such resources are available. The discharge process can be fairly protracted as equipment and supplies need to be procured, therefore it is recommended that discharge planning begin as soon as possible.

Table 1: Discharge planning for a child with a tracheostomy/Monthly equipment and supplies

Equipment	Supplier	Amount	Date ordered	Cost	Signed
Tracheostomy tubes					
Tracheostomy tapes					
Tracheal dilators					
Suction units × 2 (one portable)					
Suction tubing and sterile water					
Swedish noses (thermovents)					
Suction catheters					
Small Yankeur suction catheter					
Emergency bag and equipment					
Disposa gloves					
Lyofoam or similar dressings					
Cavilon					
Saline and gauze for trache care					
Lubricating jelly					

EQUIPMENT AND SUPPLIES

The equipment list is lengthy and it is useful to draw up an itinerary, stating where items are purchased from, how many are needed, when it needs servicing as a reference point. This practice ensures that no omissions are made and fresh supplies are ordered when needed. A copy of this can be kept in the notes and if appropriate, given to parents (Table 1).

It is generally recommended that families have two suction machines, one of which is portable, a supply of suction catheters and sundries, tracheostomy tubes, tapes, humidifiers and other tracheostomy care paraphernalia. Provision must also be made for emergency equipment (Table 2). Parents must also be confident in the procedure of emergency tracheostomy replacement. Provision also needs to be made for the regular servicing of equipment and users need to be aware of daily cleaning and maintenance. It is vital that parents have access to a workable telephone at all times.

IMPACT ON DAILY LIFE AND THE NEED FOR RESPITE CARE

The day-to-day care for a child with a tracheostomy however cannot be underestimated. It should not be forgotten that a technical failure or a lapse in human attentiveness or judgement can result in disastrous consequences

Table 2: Emergency equipment	
Item	**Size**
Tracheostomy tube	
Tracheostomy tube (smaller size)	
Tracheal dilators	
Lubricating jelly	
One large suction catheter	
Suction catheters	
Ambu-bag with attachments and mask	
Suction unit (ensure charged)	
Suction tubing	
Gloves	
Tracheostomy tapes/collar	
Stethoscope	
Gauze and saline	
Scissors	
Telephone nearby or charged mobile phone (with credit)	

for the child and that can be a heavy burden for parents. Family and friends can feel ill equipped to offer any child-minding support and so any sort of time out for parents can be elusive. Literature and common sense tell us that what parents want is for carers, competent in their child's care to be available to offer flexible respite care, which is sensitive to their needs (Association for the care of children with life threatening or terminal conditions and their families).[3–5] Carers need to be trained and confident in all aspects of tracheostomy care before they are able to offer such support. A robust package of care, which takes into account the unique needs of each family, needs to be organised, usually by the CCN team as early on as possible so that families are not left to cope alone without a much needed break. Effective respite care should, in essence, enable families to continue to care.[2,6]

COST TO THE FAMILY

The awesome responsibility that parents experience when looking after a child who has a tracheostomy is evident. The impact on all family members can be far reaching. While making valiant efforts to live an ordinary life, day-to-day, the difficulties faced by families can be multi-faceted, incurring a cost to the family personally, socially, financially and physically. Parents face enormous strain attempting to find the time (and energy) to meet the needs of other family members, primarily the brothers and sisters of the affected child and marital discord is not uncommon.[7] Adequate respite care and educational provision may go some way to alleviate this by offering parents time which is not solely dedicated to the care of the child with a tracheostomy. Parents have also reported a feeling of social isolation,[2] resulting from a lack of friends and family who are able to offer baby-sitting favours, commonly enjoyed by families of unaffected children. Again, respite care is a solution but cannot seek to recoup the spontaneity of life enjoyed by other families. It is also pertinent to consider financial costs. Generally speaking, it is usual for one parent to be at home to look after their child, this situation may have arisen after a parent was forced to give up paid employment, substantially decreasing the family income. If the child is cared for in a single parent household, the financial implication may be even more evident. It is vital that professionals are equipped to advise families on financial help that is available. Virtually all children with a tracheostomy should be able to receive higher rate disability living allowance (DLA). The application process can be complicated and confusing, therefore it is suggested that a person with experience of this process be that a CCN, social worker or other professional is available to offer guidance and support with a DLA application. There are also alternative routes of financial support, which may be explored, such as the Family Fund Trust, which provides grants to families of disabled children, to help with additional costs that may be incurred.

SLEEP DEPRIVATION

The physical demands of caring for a technology-dependent child must also be acknowledged. Parents commonly report the phenomena of sleep deprivation. Kirk and Glendinning (2000), Watson et al. (2002) Studies[8,9] have found that parents felt that they could not relax, as any omission on their part could be of grave significance to their child. Repeated nights of broken sleep, understandably, have a negative impact on parent's ability to cope. Respite care resources come in several guises, there is home based care, hospice care and link family schemes, to name but a few and it is recommended that parents are offered choices that take their individual needs into consideration, where such resources are available.

PLAY AND WELL-BEING

The all-encompassing well-being of the child is paramount, and it is generally accepted that children thrive in a warm, loving, nurturing environment where they can develop and grow. Play, as we are aware, is the centre of a child's world and children with tracheostomies are encouraged to play as usual, with a few adaptations and limitations here and there. Considerations arise to ensure that nothing unwanted enters the tracheostomy tube. Children are advised to avoid swimming, playing with dry sand (wet sand may be permissible under very close supervision), fluffy toys, small beads, in fact, any toy that is small enough to pass into the tube. Tracheostomy bibs may go some way to preventing unwanted tracheostomy emergencies, relating to inhaled foreign objects. Play can also be extremely useful in alleviating some of the stress that arises during tube changes and other unpleasant procedures. Trained play professionals are adept in devising strategies to enable the child to lay still during such procedures, which can have a positive impact on the people, especially parents, who are changing the tube. Parents cite that it goes against their nurturing instincts to perform unpleasant and uncomfortable procedures on their child and therefore any attempt to alleviate the parental disquiet is welcomed.

EDUCATION

All children are entitled to an education,[10] and robust preparations should be made as early as possible. The child will need a full time carer at school, who is fully competent to meet all of the child's care needs. To access such support, the child will require a statement of educational needs (SEN), and the statementing process is lengthy. It is therefore advisable that preparations are made as soon as logistically possible. The benefits of education are wide spread. The child is able to enjoy skill and academic attainment, a feeling of normality and belonging, socialisation with his or her peers and the family can benefit from a well-earned break. Delays in the schooling process, which may result from mismanagement, are detrimental and need to be avoided by thorough planning at the earliest opportunity.

THERAPY SERVICES

The child's speech and language development may not necessarily be affected. Some children learn to speak spontaneously, others may require some professional help from speech and language therapy services. Children should be assessed on their individual need. It is a similar picture from a dietetic perspective, some children may manage perfectly well and some may require support with swallowing difficulties. From a practical point of view, bibs are recommended to prevent inhalation of food or drink and plenty of fluids are encouraged to keep secretions thin.

Conclusion

The complexities of caring for a child with a tracheostomy and their families cannot be given justice within a chapter but these are guidelines to be used in conjunction with prior knowledge and experience, while cognisance is given of each child and families unique needs. The families whom I have encountered, have all expressed a wish for a life, which is as normal as possible for their children and themselves. The commitment and dedication of these families should be recognised and admired and we should never forget that the parents are the true experts in the care of their child. It is up to us as health care professionals to ease their load, by providing appropriate care and support, which is tailor-made to suit their needs.

REFERENCES

1. Muir J, Sidey A (eds). *Textbook of Community Children's Nursing*. London: Bailliere Tindall, 2000.
2. Murphy G. The technology dependent child at home. Part 1: In whose best interest? *Paediatr Nurs* 2001 (Sep); 13(8): 14–18.
3. ACT. *The Act Charter for Children with Life Threatening and Terminal Conditions and their Families*. Bristol: ACT, 1993.
4. Hall S. An exploration of parental perception of the nature and level of support needed to care for their child with special needs. *J Adv Nurs* 1996; 24: 512–521.
5. Department of Health. *Evaluation of a Pilot Project Programme for Children with Life Threatening Illnesses*. London: NHS Executive, 1998.
6. Kirk S. Caring for a technology-dependent child at home. *Br J Commun Nurs* 1999; 4(8): 390–393.
7. O'Brien M. Living in a house of cards: Family experiences with long term childhood technology dependence. *J Pediatr Nurs* 2001 (Feb); 16(1): 13–22.
8. Kirk S, Glendinning C. *Supporting Parents Caring for a Technology-dependent Child*. National Primary Care Research and Development Centre, University of Manchester, 2000.
9. Watson D, Townsley R, Abbott D. Exploring multi-agency working in services to disabled children with complex healthcare needs and their families. *J Clin Nurs* 2002 (May); 11(3): 367–375.
10. Rehm R. Creating a context of safety and achievement at school for children who are medically fragile/technology dependent. *Adv in Nurs Sci* 2002 (Mar); 24(3): 71–84.

BIBLIOGRAPHY

Goldberg AI, Faure EAM, Vaughn CJ, Snarski RRT, Seleny F. Home care for life supported persons: An approach to program development. *J Pediatr* 1984 (May); 104(5): 785–795.

Noyse J. Ventilator dependent children who spend prolonged periods of time in intensive care units when they no longer have a medical need or want to be there. *J Clin Nurs* 2000a (Sep); 9(5): 774–783.

Noyse J. Barriers that delay children and young people who are dependent on mechanical ventilators from being discharged from hospital. *J Clin Nurs* 2000b (Jan); 11(1): 2–11.

EVIE'S STORY

Carol Phillips and Kate Bamkin

I have an 18-month-old daughter called Evie, who at 13 months was admitted to hospital with severe respiratory distress. After being admitted to the ward she was transferred to the Paediatric Intensive Care Unit (PICU) as she was deteriorating rapidly. The doctors were fairly sure she had picked up a virus and she ended up spending 2–3 weeks on CPAP – I think this stands for continuous positive airway pressure. She was breathing for herself but just getting a bit of extra help, as she had become very tired. Evie's upper airway is very tiny and she also has laryngomalacia (floppy larynx). This really hindered her and her recovery seemed to get 'stuck'.

When the word tracheostomy was mentioned I have to say I was truly devastated. All I could think about was a memory from when I was a little girl, of a lady who lived in my village whom I knew was different and that she wore a funny thing around her neck and she spoke with a very robotic voice. I thought how weird she was, but only in a child-like not understanding kind of way as she was always very nice. So many thoughts and fears went through my mind – the operation, a hole in her throat, not being able to talk etc.

I did make it very clear to the doctors that this was the last thing I wanted for Evie and they said it would be a last resort. By the time it was agreed that the operation should be done I was almost desperate and would have agreed to almost anything just to have Evie back. It's funny how your goalposts move and with time you just accept the situation you are in.

Everyone was very helpful and I already knew of two other children on PICU who had trachys. One little boy didn't speak as he wore a Swedish Nose which he preferred, but there was a little girl who had just had the surgery and was talking by using a speaking valve. I think my biggest dread was that Evie would not be able to gurgle at me and quite how I would cope with a silent cry. I would have liked to have a chance to talk about it with another mum but it all happened fairly quickly and that opportunity never really arose. We had a meeting with the tracheostomy nurse who explained various things to us and was very helpful and gradually it didn't seem to be such a horrific thing at all.

Having said that, nothing could have prepared me for seeing Evie when she came back from theatre. Apart from the fact that she was ventilated, hooked up to the monitor for heart rate etc., she was also sedated and paralysed. Worst of all, her little neck and chin was all blood splattered as cleaning up is not one of the priorities. That really upset me, but I guess that's just a mum thing.

The first few days after the surgery were quite stressful. This was because there were other issues with Evie, which were quite unusual and finding the best tube that suited the width and length of her trachea was quite difficult. The doctors fitted a different tube for the change at one week and she didn't react at all well to this but thankfully things settled down after a few days.

TUBE CHANGES

I certainly didn't hang around for the first tube change and thought I would never be able to even look at the stoma let alone clean it daily and change the tube weekly. Suctioning secretions I was never so fearful of because it's just a piece of plastic with a black hole – just like another nose really – that's how I think of it. Now, cleaning the stoma and changing the tube is almost second nature, although I still get jittery when it's time to do the change. Evie has a habit of sucking in her stoma when you remove the old tube so it's a question of biding your time and although it seems like an eternity when you're waiting for her to breathe out and for the little hole to appear I know it's only a matter of seconds. The only thing on my mind is that I've just got to hold my nerve and get that piece of plastic in my little girl's throat so she can breathe. I think determination is the key and I manage not to shake like a leaf until it's all over.

The tube change is weekly but the foam which protects her neck we change daily just to make sure it's clean and as dry as possible. This does take the two of us, neither of us have attempted this on our own, so get some friends and relatives trained so you've always got someone on hand to assist. We always used to do this at bath time as it can obviously get wet, especially with hair washing but this started to spoil what was a lovely time for us before as she was anticipating the change and getting really distressed. So now we've found that it's much better to wait for Evie to be asleep instead of setting aside a regimented time to change it. This is far less distressing for all of us and much easier to do, as we do not have to cope with flailing arms and legs as well.

It doesn't always work as it can wake her but it's a really good feeling if we manage the change and she didn't know a thing about it.

GETTING HOME

When we were given a date to go home with Evie, our emotions were all over the place – excitement and terror. Changing the trachy in the security of the hospital is one thing but doing it at home alone is a completely different ball game. The first couple of times we did the change a community nurse came around to the house just to be there while we did it. It was OK and now we do it on our own but of course the conditions are completely different. You don't have your sterile chrome trolley to have everything set out nicely on. I have to say that now we just open the tube packet, apply the gel and pop it in. But, every single time it comes to the change – even five months on we still get quite nervous. Evie hates it and cries so we try to wait until she is asleep and we find this works for us best.

We are very lucky when it comes to suctioning in public. We rarely have to do this and I think this is because she wears the speaking valve, which suppresses her secretions a little. In fact I have to take off the speaking valve and put on a Swedish Nose just to encourage her to cough as her Consultant said that we should really suction her every 3–4 hours.

Our house has become a bit like a hospital ward with the consumables we need to have in stock such as suction catheters, foam dressings, cleaning packs, new trachys and replacement tubing for suction equipment. We particularly need more equipment because of Evie's reluctance to produce secretions, so every night she is hooked up to a humidifier that keeps everything moist and stops her from plugging off which due to her dryness she would probably do. The Consultant explained that the nose is a very sophisticated thing in the way it filters and humidifies the air we breathe which of course having the trachy bypasses and we have found having this machine works well for her. This has made us a little afraid to travel far just because of the equipment we'd need to take with us, but as we grow more confident this is becoming less and less daunting.

OUT AND ABOUT

Everywhere we go we have to take portable suction and everything you would need in an emergency including a couple of new trachy tubes in case the old one becomes blocked or comes out. Coming out is very unlikely, I think, as the Velcro on the tapes that secure the tube is quite hard to loosen. However, I won't speak too soon as Evie's little fingers could become curious as she gets older. Sometimes going out into the cold air can make Evie cough so we have to give her a quick 'hoover'. Doing this in public is quite daunting but you do get used to it. I think of it as wiping her nose!

SPEECH

Evie wears a speaking valve and manages very well with this – I would say her voice sounds normal and it's pink to match her outfits – technology has come a long way since the 60's!

CLOTHING

Clothing can be a problem as V-necked T-shirts for little girls don't seem to be the height of fashion at the moment so finding tops with suitable necklines is difficult. We can get away with her wearing round necked tops (even tight ones) but we have to leave the buttons open at the back. This is rather irritating and I've even been tempted to go into 'trachy friendly' baby clothes design.

I can honestly say the tracheostomy has helped Evie tremendously. She is well, she now gains weight easily (as she is not using all her calories on trying to breathe) and she doesn't wheeze when she is sleeping. Even though she recovered well from her infection that originally landed us in hospital, they say that she'll benefit from having the trachy until she is around 3-years-old as it will help her until she has outgrown her upper airway problems. Of course now if she does get a virus it's easy to manage which is reassuring.

Obviously we are used to things the way they are now, but what will stay with me is how a friend who used to baby-sit Evie came to visit for the first time and she just burst into tears when she saw her. I must admit I had some photographs developed from earlier on in the summer and there is Evie looking up smiling with her pretty little neck intact – that hurt. But it's no good looking back with sadness because at the end of the day Evie is safe and well and life is easier for her and that's all that matters.

INFECTION CONTROL ISSUES IN THE CARE OF PATIENTS WITH A TRACHEOSTOMY

Cheryl Trundle and Rachel Brooks

INTRODUCTION

Historically, respiratory infections such as *Mycobacterium tuberculosis* and pandemic influenza have caused significant morbidity and mortality, emphasising the need for robust infection control measures (IC) in caring for patients.

Maintaining a high standard of IC is the responsibility of *all* health care personnel. All employers and their employees should ensure a safe environment for patients, staff and visitors. With the emphasis moving from primary to secondary care provision, it is becoming increasingly recognised that the consequences of infection affect not only the hospital, but the community as a whole. The role of infection control in facilitating the delivery of high quality care and in preventing and controlling the transmission of infection cannot be over-emphasised.[1–3]

HEALTH CARE ACQUIRED INFECTION (HCAI)

The second National Prevalence Survey undertaken in 1993 revealed that 9% of patients admitted to hospital in the UK acquired an infection.[4] The risk of hospital acquired infection (HAI) has increased in line with the greater complexity of medical procedures, and survival of patients with multiple risk factors for infection (see Table 1). Patients with tracheostomies will often have many of these risk factors. The emergence of antibiotic-resistant organisms further complicates the issue, making effective treatment more difficult.[5]

Table 1: General factors associated with increased risk of infection

Extremes of age
Reduced immune status
Hospitalisation/institutional care
Presence of invasive devices
Clinical investigations
Concurrent underlying conditions
Multi-organ impairment (associated with critical care situations)

Studies into the socio-economic burden of infections estimate the cost to the National Health Service (NHS) to be around £986 million per annum; with £930 million spent on in-patient treatment and care and a further £55 million in the community. The study also highlighted that 19% of infections were identified post-discharge.[6] These infections increase morbidity and mortality amongst patients and it is estimated that 10% of patients with HAI die.[6,7] Patients who suffer a HAI cost 2.5 times more than non-infected patients and have a three-fold increase in their length of stay. Therefore a 10% reduction in HAI would save a hospital trust nearly £362,000, make available an extra 1,413 bed days, thus enabling the completion of the equivalent of 191 consultant episodes. Costs of providing a more robust IC service, with management support and adequate resources, would be outweighed by the savings made by preventing HAI.[6,8]

Infections of the respiratory tract, pneumonia in particular, are serious and life-threatening. Intubation, mechanical ventilation and other invasive procedures including insertion of a tracheostomy will render the patient more susceptible to such infection by inhalation or aspiration of micro-organisms from the oropharynx or gut, either due to the underlying condition for which the procedure was performed or due to the patient's current health status. In addition, in hospitalised patients the microbes may multiply and are drug-resistant. Pulmonary infection accounts for nearly 23% of all hospital acquired infection[4] and is a significant cause of morbidity and mortality in both adults and children. Costs per infection have been estimated at £2,080 for each patient, with national figures of £103.77 million per annum. In intensive care units (ICU), up to 50% of patients who acquire pneumonia die, and nearly one-third of deaths are directly attributable to pneumonia (see Table 2).[9] Patients with a tracheostomy are at similar risk of airborne infection as those orally or nasally endotracheally intubated. Infection spread via the airborne route should not be any more of a risk to patients with a tracheostomy than those who are intubated orally or nasally, as long as closed systems are maintained with ventilated patients and appropriate filters (e.g. 'Swedish noses') are in place for self ventilating patients.

Table 2: Costs of hospital-acquired infection

Site of infection	Additional costs (£ per patient)	Ratio of costs (compared to non-infected)	Additional days in hospital	Incidence of HAI (%)
Lower respiratory tract infection	2,080	2.3	8	1.2
Multiple infections	8,631	6.3	29	1.4
Any infection	3,154	2.8	11	7.8

Source: Data from Plowman, 1999.

Table 3: Risk factors for hospital acquired pneumonia in intubated patients

Endotracheal tube impedes the cough reflex and clearance mechanisms
Endotracheal tube damages the mucosal lining of the respiratory tract
Biofilms form on the surfaces and lumens allowing for growth of micro-organisms
Respiratory equipment provides an ideal environment for the growth of Gram-negative organisms
High risk of aspiration
Patients are exposed to and dependent on many HCWs
Patients are exposed to many antibiotics
Risk of ventilator associated pneumonia increases by 1% for each day of ventilation

Source: Data from Wilson, 2001.

NORMAL FLORA

The normal upper respiratory tract is colonised with *Streptococcus viridans, Neisseria catarrhalis* and diphtheroids. Also known as *Streptococcus oralis, Strep. viridans* can be involved in dental caries and in serious infections such as infective endocarditis and deep seated abscesses in the brain and liver which have seeded from the dental caries via the blood supply.[10] It is not usually implicated in pulmonary infections despite the fact that it is normal oral flora. *Neisseria catarrhalis* and diphtheroids are non-pathogenic (i.e. they do not cause disease).

In fit individuals the oropharynx is often colonised by *Streptococcus pneumoniae* and *Haemophilus influenzae* and these organisms are the most common cause of community acquired pneumonia. In healthy people the lower respiratory tract by contrast to the upper is normally sterile in health, no commensals/normal flora colonising this anatomical area (Table 3).

In hospitalised patients the body's normal flora can become altered. Patients who are seriously ill are exposed to antibiotics and endotracheal and tracheostomy tubes can irritate the respiratory mucosa and allow Gram-negative bacteria to colonise the oropharynx. These Gram-negatives such as *Pseudomonas, Proteus* and *Klebsiella* spp. normally colonise the gut and do not attack healthy tissue. Once they are established in the oropharynx they become 'opportunistic bacteria' and will colonise or infect the area and can cause infections, particularly if the tissue has been traumatised by suctioning or insertion of foreign bodies such as endotracheal tubes or a tracheostomy. These organisms also cause pulmonary infections when they are aspirated into the lungs.

COMMON PATHOGENS CAUSING PULMONARY INFECTIONS

Respiratory secretions pool around the cuff of the tracheostomy tube and will gradually leak past the cuff down into the lungs (Fig. 1). Gastric contents, heavily colonised with Gram-negative organisms may also be aspirated into the lungs. Although many cases of pneumonia are viral, antibiotics are given to treat cases due to the severity of the patient's condition. The diagnosis of pneumonia is often made on the clinical features in the patient of fever, purulent respiratory secretions, failure to maintain adequate blood gases and changes to the lung fields on chest X-ray.

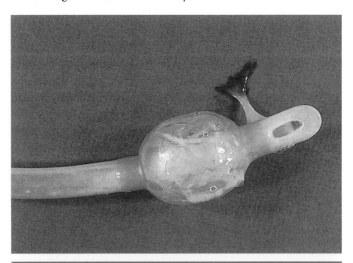

Fig. 1: Evidence of bacteria in secretions around the cuff of an extubated endotracheal tube.
Reproduced with permission from the Current Science Group. From Atlas of Infectious Diseases, Part II: Pleuropulmonary and Bronchial Infections, Simberkoff, 1996, *Current Medicine*.

BACTERIAL INFECTIONS

Gram-negative organisms are responsible for 50% of deep infections in patients with tracheostomies. *Streptococcus pneumoniae, Haemophilus influenzae*, Staphylococci (20%),[9] and *β Haemolytic Streptococcus Group A* are also common causes of bacterial infection in the patient.

Streptococcus pneumoniae

Strep. pneumoniae, also commonly known as pneumococcus, is part of the normal flora but is also an important pathogen. It is more abundant in normal flora during the winter. It is the most common cause of pneumonia normally due to aspiration of the pneumococci from the upper to the lower respiratory tract. Pneumococci migrate through the bronchial mucosa and cause inflammation and the production of purulent secretions. This results in stiff, congested and consolidated lungs.[11] Hospitals are finding increasing numbers of patients with resistant strains of streptococci. Staff therefore need to be aware that this may have implications for their infection control management. For example most ICT's will request that units isolate patients with highly resistant strains of *Strep. pneumoniae*. Patients with a tracheostomy would be a particular infection control risk because of the large numbers of aerosols generated during their care (Fig. 2).

Haemophilus influenzae

H. influenzae is the common causal organism of epiglottitis, otitis media and was previously a major cause of meningitis before the introduction of the

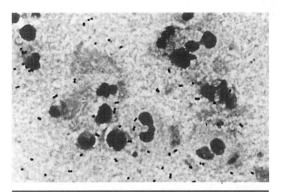

Fig. 2: Sputum from a case of suspected pneumonia.
Reproduced from Infection Control in Clinical Practice, J. Wilson with permission from Elsevier.

HIB vaccine. *H. influenzae* is exclusively a human pathogen living in the upper respiratory tract. The respiratory epithelium in the upper respiratory tract becomes traumatised by an invading pathogen, often a virus, preventing normal clearance of secretions and micro-organisms. This predisposes to a secondary infection with the normally resident *H. influenzae.*[12]

Pseudomonas aeruginosa

This is a common pathogen in hospitalised patients causing infections in a wide range of sites which include the urinary tract, chronic wounds and the respiratory tract. It is an organism that survives well in moist and wet environments and is therefore abundant in the ICU environment (Fig. 3). Children with cystic fibrosis are particularly vulnerable to infection and because they are often asymptomatic carriers, they are prone to repeated chest infections. The mortality rate in this group of patients is high. Respiratory equipment which is generally wet and warm is an ideal environment for pseudomonas to proliferate. Patients with pseudomonas pneumonia expectorate green, purulent sputum and generally respond well to appropriate antibiotic treatment, although some resistant strains are emerging.

Klebsiella

Together with other Gram-negative organisms bacteria such as *Proteus*, *Klebsiella* is becoming a more important pathogen for respiratory patients over recent years. It can cause severe bronchopneumonia and as with other bacteria, resistant strains are emerging. Outbreaks of *Klebsiella* have been reported in ICU and contaminated equipment such as water traps[13] and poor hand hygiene have been implicated.[14,15]

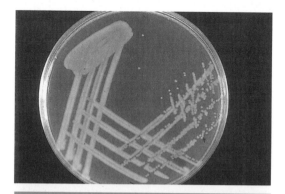

Fig. 3: Picture of Pseudomonas.
Reproduced from Infection Control in Clinical Practice, J. Wilson, with permission from Elsevier.

Streptococcus pyogenes (β Haemolytic Streptococcus Lancefield Group A)

Patients with streptococcal throat infection usually present with sudden onset of a sore throat, pyrexia, tonsillitis or pharyngitits and enlarged/tender cervical lymph nodes. This primary infection responds well to appropriate antibiotic treatment. However, if untreated in tracheostomy patients it can cause severe infection. If the pathogen gains access to the stoma site and penetrates the tissue the patient would be at risk of a localised superficial infection or more seriously a deep necrotising fasciitis. This is extremely difficult to treat due to its rapid and aggressive progression to underlying tissues which require extensive debridement and excision. Obviously this cannot be done due to the close proximity of vital structures. Fortunately it is very rare (Fig. 4).

Staphylococcus aureus (Staph. aureus)

Staph. aureus is commonly found on patient's skin. Therefore infection of tracheostomy sites with this organism may be a problem. Staphylococcal pneumonia has a significant mortality rate and staff must be equally vigilant not to transmit both sensitive and resistant strains of *Staph. aureus* between patients.

Methicillin-resistant *Staph. aureus* (MRSA) is no more pathogenic than methicillin-sensitive *Staph. aureus* (MSSA) although management is more complex. A broad range of antibiotics are available for MSSA whereas patients who are clinically infected with MRSA can only be treated with a limited range of glycopeptide antibiotics such as vancomycin or teicoplanin. It is helpful to carry out topical MRSA treatment concurrently with systemic

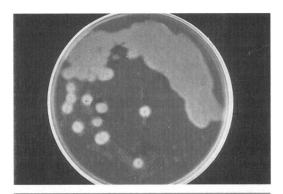

Fig. 4: Picture of blood agar plate with *Streptococcus Group A*.
Reproduced from Infection Control in Clinical Practice, J. Wilson, with permission from Elsevier.

349

treatment. Staff are recommended to refer to their local policy for the topical treatments available. The Working Party report on MRSA in 1998[16] recommended that patients found to be colonised with MRSA should be treated to try to prevent progression to clinical infection. This would be very relevant for tracheostomy patients especially when they are in a critical care area or receiving many invasive procedures.

If patients are known to be MRSA positive at their tracheostomy site it may be beneficial to apply mupirocin ointment to the site itself if it is well healed and there are no signs of tissue breakdown. Mupirocin ointment can only be used on superficial wounds (not more than 5 cm in diameter) and it needs to be applied two or three times daily. Staff should seek advice from their local ICN on the use of mupirocin on such sites. Prolonged or repeated use of mupirocin also leads to the development of resistance so repeatedly treating a colonised area such as a tracheostomy stoma is not desirable. Alternatives to mupirocin are available if resistance develops and the patient requires topical treatment. In the community setting patients who are colonised with MSRA should not need any additional or special care apart from good hand hygiene and the use of appropriate protective equipment for management of the tracheostomy.

Mycobacterium tuberculosis (MTB)

Pulmonary TB is contracted by inhaling droplets expelled by an infected patiént during coughing, sneezing or talking. It is not highly communicable but is likely to spread amongst those with prolonged close contact such as those in the same household. Tracheostomy patients should therefore not be at significant risk unless they are in close contact with an infected person.

Legionella pneumophilia

Legionnaires disease can be severe with a case fatality of 39% in hospitalised cases[17] but it is not communicable. *L. pneumophilia* has to be inhaled in aerosol form directly from the infected source. Patients present with general malaise, a non-productive cough and then develop rapid fever associated with patchy pulmonary consolidation. A particular source is contaminated water such as poorly maintained cooling towers, ventilation systems and jacuzzis. Tracheostomy patients are no more at risk than others but it would be prudent to advise patients to run showers for a few minutes before use when staying in hotels.

VIRAL INFECTIONS

Viruses are responsible for the majority of community acquired respiratory infections. Viruses are responsible for up to 20% of lower respiratory tract infections in hospitalised patients.[18] However they are rarely isolated from clinical specimens and do not generally cause severe debilitating illness in patients with tracheostomies. Respiratory viruses are spread by droplets from the respiratory tract which can be picked up on the hands, from the environment or equipment. The respiratory syncytial and parainfluenza viruses are of real concern in children.

Respiratory syncytial virus (RSV)

RSV affects 69% of children by the age of one year and 83% by the age of two. Although it is the most common cause of bronchiolitis and pneumonia in children, it is associated with low mortality ($<1\%$). RSV can however cause severe infections in neonates and babies but is not usually problematic in older children with long or short term tracheostomies. Children infected with this virus need regular suctioning and oxygen therapy. IC precautions are extremely important, and isolation or cohort nursing is required in hospitals to prevent outbreaks. RSV can survive for up to 7 h outside the body so thorough environmental cleaning is required to reduce transmission by direct and indirect contact.[18]

Parainfluenza

A seasonal viral illness transmitted directly by oral contact or droplets, and also indirectly via hands and contaminated equipment. Illness is more severe in infants, children, the elderly and patients with compromised respiratory or immune systems. Again tracheostomy patients with parainfluenza are at more risk of transmission to others via droplets so isolation is desirable in hospital. Specific antibodies to the infection have a short life so reinfection is common although it is often milder on subsequent exposures.[18]

GENERAL INFECTION CONTROL MEASURES

IC prevents the transmission of micro-organisms between patients and from and to staff. Special precautions may be necessary for those patients known or suspected to be suffering from particular infectious conditions. Key procedures which contribute to this end are discussed below.

Hand hygiene

Semmelweis in the 1850s was one of the first people to postulate that hands may be vectors of infection.[19] The rate of maternal mortality amongst mothers examined by medical students was much higher than in women in the maternity ward cared for by midwives. By the introduction of hand washing using Chlorine of Lime after the medical students had examined the cadavers in the mortuary and before going onto the wards, the maternal mortality rate was reduced from 22 to 3%.

Microbes are acquired on the surface of the skin by every day contact with people, objects and the environment and it is now universally accepted that direct contact is the mode of spread for the majority of health care-associated infections. Pathogens are most likely to be transferred to the hands when handling moist, heavily contaminated substances and areas of the body, such as a tracheostomy site. However the majority of these organisms may be removed by adequate and timely hand hygiene.[14,15,20]

There is evidence which links unwashed hands and cross-infection in health care settings.[21] Many pathogenic organisms (e.g. *Clostridium difficile*, MRSA, Vancomycin-resistant enterococci, RSV) survive well in dust and on surfaces and equipment. The gap between how many times health care workers (HCW) think they perform hand hygiene and how many times it is actually performed show a large degree of self delusion. Tibballs in 1996[22] asked doctors how many times they thought they decontaminated their hands and the perceived rate was 73% whereas the actual rate was only 9%. Bartzokas[23] observed that senior doctors only washed their hands twice during 21 h of patient ward rounds!

Contaminated hands or equipment pose a direct threat when introduced into susceptible sites such as tracheostomy wounds, during tube manipulation or suctioning. These pathogens may establish themselves as temporary or permanent colonisers[a] of the patient and can go on to cause local or systemic infection.[b]

However in spite of the overwhelming body of evidence, compliance with hand hygiene remains poor. Various educational initiatives have produced temporary improvements but these have not been sustained long-term. Introduction of alcohol handrubs which are easy to use, kind to the skin and less time consuming to use, have resulted in some improvement when used in conjunction with a multi-modal approach to the problem.[24] Rao[25] demonstrated that following the introduction of an alcohol hand gel cases of hospital-acquired MRSA were reduced from 50 to 39%. Hand hygiene remains an integral part of patient care to minimise transmission of infection and consideration should be given to what you are about to do and what you have just done which may put the patient at increased risk of infection (Fig. 5).

---

[a] *Colonisation* – The presence of a potentially pathogenic organism with little or no adverse effect on the host.

[b] *Infection* – Acquisition of a pathogenic organism which establishes itself, multiplies and causes an adverse effect on the host. The effects may be local or systemic.

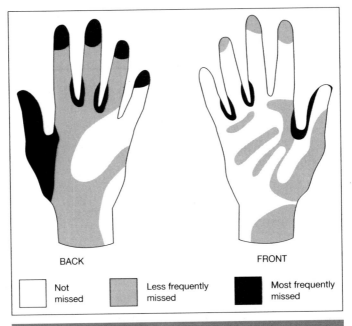

BACK   FRONT

☐ Not missed   ▨ Less frequently missed   ■ Most frequently missed

Fig. 5: Pictures of how to do hand hygiene. Reproduced from Infection Control in Clinical Practice, J. Wilson, with permission from Elsevier.

Use of personal protective equipment (PPE)

Body secretions and excretions are the major source of pathogenic micro-organisms and use of PPE is essential to protect the patient from acquisition of infection from another patient and to protect the HCW themselves. Type of equipment used should be ascertained by risk assessment of the type of patient, the procedure to be performed and the anticipated degree of contact with blood or body fluids. PPE should include aprons or water-repellant gowns, gloves (well-fitting non-powdered latex or equivalent, e.g. nitrile), goggles, masks, or masks with integral visors. The mucous membranes of the eye absorb aerosols very readily and consideration to eye protection and availability of goggles should be paramount. Activities such as suctioning therefore will require gloves, possibly a protective apron and staff may consider a mask and eye protection necessary if the patient is suffering from an infectious condition, e.g. TB or there are copious secretions which may result in splashing or aerosol spray.

Waste, linen and sharps management

Correct disposal of clinical waste, management of soiled or infected linen and safe sharps handling are all key to protecting the patient and the HCW from infection. By adhering to the principles of Universal Precautions and following locally agreed IC policies and procedures the chances of infection in patients with a tracheostomy and the transmission of infection to others is minimised. If the patient is known to have an infection, for example an MRSA positive sputum culture, or an infected tracheostomy wound additional measures may be required to prevent cross-infection. Safe systems of work and sharps disposal, as well as a clear policy on management of sharps injuries should also follow local guidelines. Staff training, for all types of HCW should address this topic, and inclusion in induction and statutory refresher sessions should be a minimum requirement. It is essential that all staff are aware of how to correctly manage a sharps incident.

Decontamination of equipment

There are numerous examples of infections transmitted from patient to patient via contaminated equipment.[26,27] With the emergence of new diseases variant Creutzfeldt–Jakob Disease (vCJD), changing epidemiological patterns and the increases in multi-drug-resistant organisms (multi-drug-resistant *Mycobacterium tuberculosis*, MDR-TB) there has been an increasing awareness of the importance of decontamination and sterilisation. In order to protect the patient from cross-contamination 'single use' or 'single patient use' items should be used wherever possible.

Staff should be aware of how to care for and adequately clean 'single patient use' items. Local policy (which is based on manufacturer's guidelines, research recommendations and best practice) should give clear guidance as to how often cleaning is required; what solutions should be employed; the methods necessary to ensure adequate levels of decontamination are reached; and how long each item may be used for. This would include some equipment used for patients with tracheostomies such as inner tubes, speaking tubes, humidification or oxygen circuits, suction equipment etc. Nebuliser circuits (which are generally 'single patient use') should be cleaned with hot water and neutral detergent between uses and thoroughly dried. Damp or narrow lumened equipment with globules of water inside provide an ideal medium for the proliferation of Gram-negative organisms which can cause serious respiratory tract infections in vulnerable patients. If adequate drying is not possible it may be necessary to use a new circuit for each episode of nebulisation.

Where re-usable items are used, they should be adequately decontaminated between uses, by autoclaving centrally in the Sterile Supplies Department (SSD). In a hospital environment this may include such equipment as silver tracheostomy tubes. In a community setting different guidelines may be followed and these instances will be discussed later. Current legislation[27] recommends that benchtop sterilisers are removed from all other areas as it has been shown that some staff are unaware of correct procedures for their use, maintenance is not always carried out in accordance with regulations, instruments cannot be adequately tracked and it is impossible to verify that instruments are being adequately sterilised.

Education and training

This is a vital component in assuring that both patients and staff are protected. HCW should be aware of how infections are transmitted; which patients are particularly vulnerable to acquiring infections; those most likely to spread infection to others and the measures necessary to ensure that a safe environment is provided for everyone involved in patient care. Local policies and procedures should be written in clear and concise terms; be practical and achievable; readily accessible to the work force; revised and up-dated regularly and practice evaluated to ensure adherence. IC education is essential to ensure that all HCW's practice is delivered in a timely and effective manner.

SPECIFIC IC MEASURES FOR TRACHEOSTOMY PATIENTS

Stoma site infection

In the immediate post-operative period the tracheostomy wound is closely observed for bleeding and then the site should be inspected daily for signs of infection. These include increasing erythema or cellulitis around the tracheostomy itself, purulent discharge from the site and any breakdown of tissue surrounding the stoma site. The patient may also complain of undue or increased pain at the site. Systemic signs of sepsis such as pyrexia with possible signs of systemic sepsis such as raised C-reactive protein, white cell count and erythrocyte sedimentation rate may develop if an infection establishes itself.

Types of wound dressing have already been addressed (see Chapter 10, Wound Care). From an IC point of view it is important to keep the wound and surrounding skin as dry and free of secretions as possible as the presence of moisture predisposes to infection and tissue breakdown.

Suctioning

Bacteria can readily contaminate the hands of HCW and respiratory equipment therefore to prevent transmission of organisms a sterile suction technique must be used.[28] A closed suction unit is preferable for ventilated patients. These systems are changed every 24 h and are beneficial as they prevent unnecessary exposure of the trachea and pulmonary system to foreign objects, including bacteria, by inhalation and limit HCW's exposure to sputa. Hand hygiene should be performed before and after suctioning and non-powdered latex gloves must be worn if the closed system is broken for example when the system is changed or the patient is to be hand ventilated.

Open suctioning generates aerosols of body fluids which can contaminate both the HCW performing the task and the environment.[29] If open suctioning is carried out HCWs should wear gloves and apron as minimum protective clothing, facial protection is also recommended. Local policy may require a sterile glove to be used on the suctioning hand to maintain a good sterile procedure although experienced staff could argue that a sterile procedure can be maintained with a non-sterile glove.

A good suctioning technique must be maintained to prevent damage to the mucous membranes which creates an opportunity for bacteria to gain access to tissues. Poor technique has been shown to result in patients acquiring serious eye infections from spraying of sputum.[30]

Tracheostomy tube care and maintenance

Short-term tracheostomy tubes with removable inner tubes allow for easy cleaning. The inner tubes are recommended to be removed and cleaned every 4–6 h using running warm water. This helps prevent sputum adhering to and occluding the inner lumen. Brushes are available to clean inner tubes but should be used with caution, not routinely, as they could abrade the luminal surface, making it easier for sputum and micro-organisms to adhere. After use these brushes may harbour micro-organisms and should be disposed of at least daily, see manufacturer's instructions for specific product guidelines.

Historically, nursing procedures advocated the use of hydrogen peroxide for cleaning and disinfecting inner tubes. However, the use of a general purpose detergent and tap water to clean tubes is now deemed acceptable. For patients in hospital using re-usable tube system, they should be sterilised in the sterile services department prior to re-use. Patients in the community are advised to wash spare tube sets as normal and then boil them in water for 10 min to decontaminate them ready for the next tube change.

Humidification and nebuliser equipment

Humidifiers and nebulisers are particularly prone to colonisation by Gram-negative bacteria which may go on to cause respiratory tract infection or local wound contamination. To prevent this risk nebulisers that are not single use should be rinsed out and dried thoroughly after each use. Saline may be nebulised to loosen secretions and medication may need to be administered by this method. Gram-negative bacteria readily contaminate fluids exposed to handling and the environment and therefore could pose a risk to patients receiving nebulised fluids. It has been shown that HCW are unaware of the necessity of adequate cleaning and correct storage of nebulisers to prevent contamination and cross-infection when these machines are used by several patients in a ward.

Whether in the hospital or the community, IC procedures are vital to protect the patient with a tracheostomy from acquisition of pathogenic organisms, and to minimise the possibility of spread to other vulnerable individuals. These also serve to protect staff caring for the patients. The rate of health care acquired infection may be seen as an indicator of the quality of care provided[31] and each Trust has a fundamental role in the prevention and control of infection for its patients and staff. IC is an integral part of *all* care delivered to patients by HCWs. Prominent on the political and public agenda, it forms part of the clinical governance framework, ensuring that appropriate evidence-based IC measures are in place, and that these are regularly audited and evaluated.

REFERENCES

1. National Audit Office. *The Management & Control of Hospital Acquired Infection in Acute Trusts in England*. Report by the Comptroller and Auditor General. London: Stationery Office, 2000.
2. NHS Executive. *The Management and Control of Hospital Infection: Action for the NHS for the Management and Control of Infection in Hospitals in England*. HSC 2000/02.
3. NHS Executive. *Controls Assurance Standard: Infection Control*. London: HMSO, 2000.
4. Emmerson AM, Enstone JE, Griffin M, Kelsey MC, Smyth ETM. The second national prevalence survey of infection in hospitals – An overview of results. *J Hosp Infect* 1996; 32: 175–190.
5. House of Lords Select Committee on Science & Technology. *Resistance to Antibiotics and other Anti-Microbial Agents* (HL Paper 81–I, 7th Report Session 1997–1998). London: Stationery Office, 1998.
6. Plowman R, Graves N, Griffin M, Roberts JA, Swan AV, Cookson B, Taylor L. *The Socio-Economic Burden of Hospital-Acquired Infection*. London: Public Health Laboratory Service & London School of Tropical Medicine, 1999.
7. Hayley RW. *Managing Hospital Infection Control for Cost Effectiveness. A strategy for Reducing Infectious Complications*. Chicago: American Hospital Publishing, 1986.

8. Wilson J. *Infection Control in Clinical Practice*, 2nd edn. London: Balliere Tindall, 2001.
9. Fagon Y, Chastre J, Hance AJ, Montravres P, Novara A, Gilbert C. Nosocomial pneumonia in ventilated patients: A cohort study evaluating attributable mortality and hospital stay. *Am J Med* 1993; 94(3): 281–288.
10. Ross PW. Streptococcus and enterococcus. In: Greenwood D, Slack R, Peutherer J (eds). *Medical Microbiology*, 15th edn. London: Churchill Livingstone, 1997.
11. Finch RG. Pneumococcus. In: Greenwood D, Slack R, Peutherer J (eds). *Medical Microbiology*, 15th edn. London: Churchill Livingstone, 1997.
12. Slack RCB. Infective syndromes. In: Greenwood D, Slack R, Peutherer J (eds). *Medical Microbiology*, 15th edn. London: Churchill Livingstone, 1997.
13. Gorman LJ, Sanai L, Notman AW, Grant IS, Masterton RG. Cross infection in an intensive care unit by *Klebsiella pneumoniae* from ventilator condensate. *J Hosp Infect* 1993; 23: 27–34.
14. Larson E. A causal link between handwashing and risk of infection? Examination of the evidence. *Infect Cont Hosp Epid* 1988; 2: 28–36.
15. Reybrouk G. Role of hands in spread of nosocomial infection. *J Hosp Infect* 1983; 4: 103–110.
16. Working Party Report. Revised guidelines for the control of methicillin-resistant *Staphylococcus aureus* infection in hospitals. *J Hosp Infect* 1998; 39: 253–290.
17. Valenti WM, Hall CB, Douglas RG. Nosocomial Viral Infections I: Epidemiology and significance 1981. In: Wilson J (ed.). *Infection Control in Clinical Practice*, 2nd edn. London: Balliere Tindall, 2001.
18. Chin J (ed.). *Control of Communicable Diseases Manual*, 17th edn. Washington: APHA, 2000.
19. Newsom SWB. Ignaz Philip Semmelweis. *J Hosp Infect* 1993; 23: 175–188.
20. Gould D. Nurses' hands as vectors of hospital-acquired infection: A review. *J Adv Nurs* 1991; 16: 1216–1225.
21. Casewell M, Phillips I. Hands as route of transmission of *Klebsiella* species. *Br Med J* 1977; 2: 1315–1317.
22. Tibballs J. Teaching hospital medical staff to handwash. *Med J Australia* 1996; 164: 395–398.
23. Bartzokas J. Motivation to comply with infection control procedures. *J Hosp Infect* 1991; 18(Suppl A): 508–514.
24. Pittett D, Hugonnet S, Harbath S, et al. Effectiveness of a hospital-wide programme to improve compliance with hand hygiene. *Lancet* 2000; 356: 1307–1312.
25. Gopal Rao G, Jeanes A, Osman M, Aylott C, Green J. Marketing hand hygiene in hospitals – A case study. *J Hosp Infect* 2002; 50: 42–47.
26. Advisory Committee on Dangerous Pathogens (ACDP) and the Spongiform Encephalopathy Advisory Committee (SEAC) Joint Working Group. Transmissable Spongiform Encephalopathy Agents: Safe Working and the Prevention of Infection. London: HMSO, 1998.
27. Health and Safety Executive. *Control of Substances Hazardous to Health Regulations 1994 (COSHH) SI: 3246*. London: HMSO, 1994.
28. Ayliffe GAJ, Fraise AP, Geddes AM, Mitchell K. *Control of Hospital Infection*, 4th edn. London: Arnold, 2000.

29. Cobley M, Atkins M, Jones PL. Environmental contamination during tracheal suction. *Anaesthesia* 1991; 46: 957–961.
30. Hilton E, Adams AA, Uliss A, Lesser ML, Samuals S, Lowry FD. Nosocomial bacterial eye infections in intensive care units. *Lancet* 1983; 1: 1318–1320.
31. Glynn A, Ward V, Wilson J, Taylor L, Cookson B. *Hospital Acquired Infection: Surveillance, Policies and Practice.* London: PHLS, 1997.

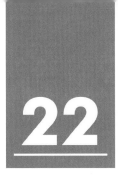

NUTRITIONAL ASSESSMENT AND MANAGEMENT OF PATIENTS WITH TRACHEOSTOMIES

Vicky Gravenstede

Good nutrition is vital to maintain health and well-being, appropriate nutritional intake is therefore an important aspect of patient care.

The patient who requires a tracheostomy will often be acutely unwell and/or have a chronic difficulty with swallowing, therefore making it impossible to meet their nutritional requirements. See Chapter 11, Swallowing.

The management of these patients will not differ from the patient without a tracheostomy, however the patient with a tracheostomy will most certainly need nutritional support to some degree while they have an unsafe or absent swallow.

This chapter aims to discuss the prevalence of malnutrition, assessment tools used, types of nutritional support and the complications and benefits of different types of feeding.

MALNUTRITION

The problem

Studies have shown that 40% of patients are malnourished on admission to hospital.[1-4] Malnutrition may be secondary to increased nutritional requirements, decreased dietary intake, increased nutrient losses and drug nutrient interactions.[5-8] All of these can be experienced by the patient with a tracheostomy. Diminished nutritional status may contribute to increased risk of morbidity and mortality.[8-11] Malnutrition should be identified and treated as efficiently as possible to promote rapid recovery and minimise unnecessary hospital costs.

Identifying malnutrition

The Kings Fund Report identified the importance of the early recognition of malnutrition in hospital patients and recommended that 'only when the assessment of every patients' nutritional status has become routine will the full benefits of nutritional treatment be recognised'.[12] The Malnutrition Advisory Group highlighted the use of screening tools to assess individual nutritional status on admission to hospital in response to this report. The aim of these tools is to identify those high-risk patients. Parameters used to score risk include Body Mass Index (BMI), weight loss, ability to eat, appetite, and stress factors. The ability to eat is often restricted in patients with tracheostomies and the presence of multiple stresses place this group at high risk of malnutrition.

Factors affecting patients' requirements[13,14]

- Diet induced thermogenesis (DIT) activity:
  - Bedbound immobile – 10%
  - Bedbound mobile/sitting – 15–20%
  - Mobile on ward – 25%
- Stress:
  - Surgery/trauma – 10%
  - Long bone fracture – 10%
  - Persistent pyrexia – 10%
  - Acute pancreatitis – 20%
  - Inflammatory bowel disease – 10%
  - Burns – 10–70%
  - Head injury – 20–30%
  - Sepsis – 20–50%

Biochemical markers, commonly albumin, have been used as an indication of malnutrition. However, due to its long half-life (~20 days) and the influence of other stress factors on serum levels it cannot be used accurately as an independent marker. Other proteins, such as retinol binding protein or transferrin, have a shorter half-life and are therefore more accurate. They are, however, still influenced by existing stress factors and should be used with discretion and in combination with other indicators.

Assessing nutritional status

The tracheostomy patient who has been identified as 'high risk' of poor nutritional status will require ongoing accurate assessments and monitoring.

Weight history is the most important method of assessing long-term nutritional status. If weight loss has been gradual it is more likely that fat tissue has been

Table 1: Calculating and grading BMI[8,13]

$BMI = \dfrac{Weight\,(kg)}{Height^2\,(m)}$	
BMI	**Grading**
>40 kg/m²	Morbid obesity
35–39 kg/m²	Severe obesity
30–34 kg/m²	Moderate obesity
25–29 kg/m²	Overweight
18–25 kg/m²	Desirable
<18 kg/m²	Underweight

lost. If weight loss is rapid it is muscle tissue that is predominantly lost. The significance of weight loss is assessed using the following scale:[15]

- <5%: Not significant unless likely to continue
- 5–9%: Not serious unless rapid or patient already malnourished
- 10–20%: Clinically significant – Nutritional support required
- >20%: Severe – Long-term aggressive nutritional support required

BMI is valuable in assessing nutritional status. It demonstrates body composition on a weight for height basis[8] (Table 1), an accurate weight and height are therefore necessary to calculate BMI.

Weight can be measured simply and accurately on the ward. All wards should have access to stand-on, sit-on and hoist scales to ensure that all stable patients can be weighed on admission and then on a weekly basis. If the patient is clinically unstable an estimate of weight must suffice until it is possible to weigh them.

Height is equally simple to measure using a wall-mounted scale for mobile patients. In immobile patients a tape measure can be used to determine height or, alternatively, the demi-span. This involves measuring the distance from the right sternal notch to the base of the 3rd finger on the left hand. The following equation can then be used to calculate height.[13,15]

$$Height = 0.73\,(2 \times demi\text{-}span) + 0.43$$

Anthropometric measurements may also be used to assess nutritional status. This may include measuring skinfold thickness using callipers, and mid-arm muscle circumference to assess fat and muscle stores. Body composition may be estimated using Bioelectrical Impedance Analysis.

This involves passing an electrical current through the body to measure percentage body fat by calculating resistance against the current. Anthropometrics are not commonly used in practice due to time limitations and the physical constraints of completing them on the ward.

Assessing nutritional requirements

Individual nutritional requirements differ depending on multiple factors including activity and the stresses of acute and chronic illness. Direct calorimetry is an accurate method of assessing energy expenditure. This system measures heat emitted from the body to calculate energy needs.

Indirect calorimetry may be used to assess calorie requirements. A 'hood' is fixed over the patients' head and the volume of carbon dioxide gas expelled is analysed to determine energy expenditure. Indirect calorimetry is expensive and, like direct calorimetry, not commonly used in hospitals. Consequently, other methods of estimating energy requirements have been developed.

Over 200 equations are available to calculate energy requirements. Schofield[14] and Elia[15] are the equations most commonly used to calculate energy and protein requirements in the acutely and chronically ill. Age, weight and gender are used to calculate a patients' Basal Metabolic Rate (BMR) onto which activity and stress factors are added (Table 2).

Table 2: Estimating nutritional requirements – Equations for BMR[14]

Females	kcal/day	Males	kcal/day
15–18 years	$13.3W + 690$	15–18 years	$17.6W + 656$
18–30 years	$14.8W + 485$	18–30 years	$15.0W + 690$
30–60 years	$8.1W + 842$	30–60 years	$11.4W + 870$
Over 60 years	$9.0W + 656$	Over 60 years	$11.7W + 585$

W = Weight in kg.

Estimation of nitrogen requirements[15]		Nitrogen g/kg/day
Normal		0.17 (0.14–0.20)
Hypermetabolic	5–25%	0.20 (0.17–0.25)
	25–50%	0.25 (0.20–0.35)
	>50%	0.30 (0.25–0.35)
Depleted		0.30 (0.20–0.40)

NUTRITIONAL SUPPORT

Diet

A patient who has a tracheostomy is at higher risk of swallowing difficulties and aspiration. The patient will have an assessment, often carried out by a speech and language therapist, to ensure that they can swallow safely prior to commencing oral diet. A modified consistency diet may allow the patient to take oral diet and reduce the risk of aspiration. The speech therapist can advise on the consistency required. The dietitian in turn supports nutritional intake by maximising the nutritional value of the diet. By fortifying the diet (Table 3) and encouraging nutrient dense food and fluids the patient may be able to meet their nutritional needs orally.

Artificial nutritional support

Patients who are unable to tolerate tracheostomy cuff deflation are at a high risk of aspiration with oral diet. Artificial nutritional support (ANS) is required to meet the nutritional needs of these patients.

If the gastrointestinal tract is functioning it should be used. Nasoenteric feeding will provide short-term nutrition to the patients who are temporarily unable to meet their requirements orally. In those who are unable to return to full oral intake, longer term feeding routes such as gastrostomy or jejunostomy feeding tubes should be considered.

There are many routes available for artificial feeding (Fig. 1). Once the most appropriate route has been selected by the multidisciplinary team the dietitian recommends a suitable regime to meet the patient's needs.

Table 3: Methods of fortifying diet	
Nutritional support	**Examples**
Food fortification	• Whole foods, e.g. butter, cheese, cream, sugar etc. • Modular fortifiers, e.g. Maxijul, Polycal, Calogen, Protifar etc.
Supplement drinks	• *Non-prescribable*, e.g. Build-up Milkshakes or Soups, Complan, Nourishment. • *Prescribable*, e.g. Ensure, Enlive, Resource, Fortisip, Fortijuce, Scandishake.
Supplemental puddings	• *Non-prescribable*, e.g. Yoghurt, Custard, Milky puddings. • *Prescribable*, e.g. Forticreme, Clinutren Dessert, Resource Pudding etc.

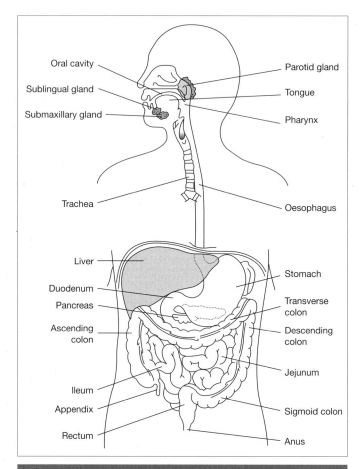

Fig. 1: Sites of feeding tubes in the gastrointestinal tract.[8,13]

Enteral or Parenteral

There is much debate surrounding the risks and benefits of enteral nutrition (EN) and parenteral nutrition (PN). Practice should no longer focus on PN versus EN but on the most appropriate method of meeting individual nutritional needs. Enteral nutrition is the optimal method of meeting nutritional requirements as it is the most physiological way of delivering nutrients. It is the safer and cheaper form of ANS and should, therefore, be used where possible. However, PN is a valuable route of feeding when the gastrointestinal tract is unavailable for use.

The choice between enteral and parenteral nutrition is not always black or white. Each route has its risks and benefits (Table 4). By assessing these risks

Table 4: Risks and benefits of artificial nutritional support[7,8,16–19]

	Indications	Benefits	Complications
Enteral	• Functioning and accessible gut	• Prevents gut atrophy • Decreases gut permeability* • Increased mucosal immunity • More physiological • Cheap • May reduce the risk of bacterial translocation** • Associated with less life threatening complications	• Poor gastric emptying • Diarrhoea • Constipation • Nausea/vomiting (though rarely due to the feed, if occurs contact your ward Dietitian) • Pulmonary aspiration • Tube displacement or blockage • Mucosal erosion • Feed-Drug interactions
Parenteral	GIT not available, e.g. • Short bowel syndrome • Obstruction • Diffuse peritonitis • Multiple bowel perforations • High output fistula • Fistulae situated in or distal to jejunum • Confirmed, prolonged paralytic ileus (CT Abdo, Abdominal XR) • Malabsorption syndromes	• Allows gut rest • More likely to achieve complete delivery of prescribed nutrients	• Vessel perforation • Pneumothorax • Embolism • Catheter occlusion • Line sepsis/ infection • Hyperglycaemia • Altered liver function • Gut atrophy

*A measure of the ability of molecules to pass across a membrane, e.g. high permeability – molecules can pass freely across the membrane, low permeability – movement of molecules across the membrane is restricted.
**The movement of bacteria from one source to another, e.g. from the gut into the blood stream.

and benefits, nutritional status, GI function and disease state, the multidisciplinary team will advise on the most appropriate route for the patient.

Complications of artificial feeding

Enteral feeding

Pre-existing malnutrition, elective or emergency surgery, medications and the underlying disease may all contribute to a reduced tolerance of enteral feeding. A patient who requires a tracheostomy may have a combination of these factors. Close monitoring of enterally fed patients allow complications to be recognised quickly (Table 5). The feed itself is often not the cause of the complication therefore other aspects of the patients condition and treatment should be examined. By monitoring and adjusting these were possible and manipulating the feed, many of these problems can be resolved.

Table 5: Complications of enteral feeding[7,8,16]

Complication	Possible causes	Solution
Aspiration of gastric contents	Risk increases with gastric residuals >200 ml Can occur as a result of: • Injury/trauma sustained • Disease process • Medications • Incorrect tube positioning • Gastro-oesophageal reflux • Raised intracranial pressure • Faecal impaction • Prone position	• Check gastric residuals regularly • Ensure patients head elevated 40°C (unless contra-indicated) • Check tube position before each feed • Review medications • If patient repeatedly pulling out tube, consider short-term bolus feeding or gastrostomy if requiring long-term feeding • Consider prokinetics, e.g. Metoclopramide, Erythromycin • Consider post pyloric feeding • Ensure cause being treated
Diarrhoea	The most commonly reported complication: • Infection, e.g. *Clostridium difficile* • Antibiotic treatment • Enteral administration of electrolytes, e.g. Magnesium • Hypertonic feed • High feed rate	*Do Not Stop Feed* Determine cause: • Send stool samples for culture • Review medications, e.g. broad-spectrum antibiotics • Ensure adequate fluids to replace those lost • Ensure feed at room temperature • Consider a fibre feed

Table 5 (continued)

Complication	Possible causes	Solution
Tube blockage	• Drugs, e.g. syrups, crushed tablets via the tube • Inadequate flushes • Stagnation of feed in the tube	*Do Not Reinsert Guidewire* • Regular water flushes • Flush tube with extra water or bicarbonate of soda. Use a 3 way tap to create a dead space • Alternate short bursts of pressure (push/pull action with a small syringe) • Massage visible particles in the tube to break up obstruction
Constipation	• Reduced gut motility secondary to medications • Inadequate fluids • Inactivity	• Compare to normal bowel habit • Ensure adequate fluids • Consider fibre feed • Review medications that may cause/relieve constipation • Discuss with motility nurse
Nausea and vomiting	• Delayed gastric emptying • Raised ICP • Incorrect tube position • Medications, e.g. morphine based drugs • Excessive feed rate	• Check tube position • Check gastric aspirates • Consider anti-emetics • Consider transpyloric feeding

Parenteral feeding

Parenteral nutritional support is associated with mechanical, infectious and metabolic complications (Table 6). These complications may be minimised by ensuring the involvement of trained personnel, by following hospital protocols and by regular patient review by the multidisciplinary team. Feed manipulation is valuable in controlling the metabolic complications associated with parenteral feeding. By altering the rate of feed, the concentration and the content of the feed these complications can be minimised.

Monitoring artificial feeding

Regular monitoring is essential in both enteral and parenteral feeding (Table 7). In enteral feeding the body controls the absorption of nutrients according to its requirements. Regular review focuses on patients' tolerance to feed and ensures

Table 6: Complications of parenteral feeding[8,13,20]

Complication	Cause	Solution
Hydro/pneumo/ haemo-thorax, embolism, central vein thrombosis	• Malposition of line • Damage to blood vessel	• Dedicated personnel to insert lines • Follow evidence based protocols for line insertion and care • Careful monitoring post insertion
Peripheral vein thrombosis (PVT) in PPN	• Irritation of the vein by infusion of a hyperosmolar solution	• Use dedicated fine bore midline catheter • Use all in one solution to reduce osmolality • Inspect site 6 hourly: redness or discomfort – remove catheter
Incompatibility/ precipitation	• Additives to PN made on ward • No pharmacy involvement	• Single use of feeding line • Pharmacy based provision of PN
Infection	• Interruption during feeding • Multiple source of bacterial entry	• Use strict non-touch aseptic technique • Ensure line kept clean • Do not interrupt feed • Dedicated, single use feeding line
Hyperglycaemia	• Concentrated dextrose infusion • Inadequate endogenous insulin	• Reduce dextrose concentration of PN • Maintain PN infusion over 24 hours • Adapt insulin infusion
Electrolyte imbalance	• High GI output • Inadequate/excess provision of electrolytes • Excess/inadequate fluid provision • Renal dysfunction	• Monitor electrolytes daily and decrease or supplement accordingly • Monitor additional sources of electrolytes, e.g. medications
Fluid overload	• Excess fluids given for clinical condition or body weight • Renal dysfunction	• Adapt fluid provision accordingly • Monitor fluid balance strictly

Table 6 (continued)

Complication	Cause	Solution
Vitamin/trace element deficiency	• Inadequate provision of micronutrients	• Monitor levels • Ensure PN solution adequately supplemented
Hypo-phosphataemia	• Altered metabolism • Inadequate provision • Re-distribution of PO_4 to cells	• Monitor plasma levels • Ensure pharmacists involved in PN provision
Biliary stasis	• Secondary to lack of stimulation of bile production	• Encourage small enteral intake in long-term PN patients where possible
Fatty liver	• High circulating levels of insulin prevents the use of fat for energy which results in deposition in the liver	• Monitor liver function • Minimise intake of excess carbohydrate in long-term PN patients

Table 7: Monitoring artificial nutrition[13]

Monitor	Comments
Tolerance of feed	To ensure no vomiting, diarrhoea, abdominal discomfort, bloating since starting enteral feeding.
Bowel pattern	Monitor daily. Normal bowel habit should be taken into consideration when monitoring bowel pattern.
Gastric aspirates	Initially 4–5 hourly until established or consistently if on critical care unit. Upper limits on gastric aspirates vary between hospitals, e.g. >200 ml.
Biochemistry • Electrolytes • BFT's • LFT's • Urea and creatinine • Albumin • Glucose	 • Daily, 2× weekly when stable • 2× weekly • 2× weekly • Daily, 2× weekly when stable • 2× weekly • Regular BM's or daily glucose, daily in parenteral feeding

Table 7 (continued)	
Monitor	**Comments**
Body temperature	Daily. A consistently raised temperature may affect your patients nutrient requirements, or indicate infection in parenterally fed patients.
Weight	Minimum weekly. Weight is important as it is the best indicator of whether your patient is being over or under fed, and if their requirements are being met. Fluid balance should be taken into account. Daily weights are required in PN.
24 h fluid balance	Daily, including stoma/drain output, nasogastric aspirate/drainage, oral intake. To ensure that patient is receiving appropriate fluid volumes.
Medications	Medications are reviewed regularly as some drugs may: • Interact with the nutrients in the feed and alter absorption of either the nutrient or the drug, e.g. Calcium in feed decreases absorption of Phenytoin. Sucralfate interacts with feed to form a solid bezoar that can block the nasogastric tube or oesophagus. • Cause side effects that can potentially be attributed to the feed, e.g. broad spectrum antibiotics – diarrhoea. • Contribute to energy intake, e.g. Propofol contains 1.1 kcal/ml if a patients is being sedated with 18 ml/hr of propofol this will provide 475 kcal/d which has a significant contribution to daily energy input. In lipid containing PN the lipid:carbohydrate ratio may become unbalanced.

full estimated requirements are being delivered. In PN the body does not have the opportunity to control the absorption of nutrients as they are delivered directly into the circulation. Daily review is necessary to monitor blood biochemistry and fluid balance to ensure serum levels are within normal ranges.

Artificial feeds available

The enteral feeds that you see in each hospital vary depending on which company your hospital is contracted with. However, except in name, the general feeds differ very little from company to company (Table 8). Your dietitian will advise on the most appropriate feed depending on the patients needs.

Table 8: Enteral feeds currently available on the market

Feed	Description	Example
Standard	1 kcal/ml basic feed. Used as first choice in most cases.	• Nutrison Standard • Osmolite • Isosource Standard
Fibre	1 kcal/ml with fibre. Often used in gastro or long-term patients. May help to control blood sugars in diabetic patients.	• Nutrison Multifibre • Jevity • Isosource Fibre
High energy	1.2–1.5 kcal/ml. Used in patients with particularly high requirements or who are unable to tolerate higher volumes.	• Nutrison Energy • Nutrison Energy Multifibre • Ensure Plus • Osmolite Plus • Jevity Plus • Isosource High Energy
Low sodium	1 kcal/ml reduced sodium. For patients with raised sodium levels.	• Nutrison Low Sodium • Isosource Low Sodium
Low carbohydrate/ respiratory	1.5 kcal/ml with reduced carbohydrate content. Fat content is increased to compensate for calories. Often used in ventilated patients.	• Pulmocare
Semi-elemental elemental	1 kcal/ml. For those who are unable to tolerate standard feeds or breakdown nutrients properly, e.g. pancreatic patients, irritable bowel disease (IBD).	• Peptisorb • Peritive • EO28
Low volume	2 kcal/ml. For those patients on fluid restrictions.	• Nepro • Concentrated • Concentrated 40
Immune enhancing	1–1.2 kcal/ml with combination of nucleotides, glutamine, arginine or omega 3 fatty acids. May diminish the body's inflammatory response to trauma and enhance immune function.	• Impact • Oxepa • Stresson

Provision of parenteral feeds also varies between hospitals. Options are dependant on facilities available (Table 9). The multidisciplinary team will review the patient and advise on appropriate PN depending on your hospital system.

In summary, the optimal management of a patient with a tracheostomy will consider the impact that the tracheostomy has on the patients ability to manage an adequate oral diet. While a patient has a tracheostomy, the patient will have an increased risk of aspiration and/or swallowing problems. Therefore the effective assessment and management of the patient's dietary intake will require a multi-professional approach to ensure truly holistic care and management. The role of the dietician within this team is to optimise the dietary intake according to their needs and ability.

Table 9: Parenteral feeds available

System	Uses	Advantages	Disadvantages
Multibottle	Bottles of dextrose, amino acids and lipid are hung separately. Vitamins, minerals and trace elements added on the ward	• Flexible components • Longer shelf life • Cheaper than 3 chamber bags	• High risk of infection due to multiple manipulations • Micronutrients need to be added on ward • Risk of errors • Time consuming
3 Chamber	Single bag with 3 separate chambers for dextrose, amino acid and lipid that are mixed before use	• Long shelf life • Cheaper than in-house compounding • Reduced risk of infection single infusion over 24 h • No refrigeration needed	• Reduced flexibility of nutrient choice • Micronutrients need to be added separately due to the stability and extended shelf life of the bag • More expensive than multibottle
All-in-one	Single standard bag containing dextrose, amino acid and lipid	• Reduced risk of infection as single infusion over 24 h • Close monitoring of stability possible • Choice of formulations	• Reduced flexibility nutrient choice • Limited shelf life • Needs refrigeration on ward for storage

System	Uses	Advantages	Disadvantages
Table 9 (continued)			
Compounded, in-house, all-in-one bag	Single bag containing all macro and micronutrients compounded by pharmacy in sterile conditions	• Reduced risk of infection as single infusion over 24 h • Flexible according to individual needs • Close monitoring of stability possible	• Limited shelf life once compounded • Needs refrigeration for storage on the ward • Most expensive option
Vitrimix	Mixture of 20% Intralipid, Vamin 9 and Glucose. Contains: Energy – 1000 kcal/L Protein – 45 g/L Na^{2+}, K^{2+}, Ca^{2+}, Mg^{2+}, Cl^{2+}	• If PN is not available in the short-term can be used in the interim period. • Long shelf life • Cheaper than all-in-one bag	• It is not nutritionally complete and therefore should not be used for more than 5 days as a means of providing nutritional support.

REFERENCES

1. McWhirter JP, Pennington C. Incidence and recognition of malnutrition in hospital. *B Med J* 1994; 308: 945–948.
2. Naber TH, Schermer T, de Bree A, et al. Prevalence of malnutrition in non-surgical hospitalised patients and its association with disease complications. *Am J Clin Nutr* 1997; 66: 1232–1239.
3. Zador DA, Truswell AS. Nutritional status on admission to a general surgical ward in a Sydney hospital. *Aust NZ J Med* 1987; 13: 234–245.
4. Hendrickes W, Reilly J, Weaver L. Malnutrition in a childrens hospital. *Clinical Nutrition* 1997; 16: 13–18.
5. Pinchcofsky GD, Kaminski MV. Increasing malnutrition during hospitalisation: Documentation by a nutrition screening program. *J Am Coll Nutr* 1985; 4: 471–479.
6. Elia M. Undernutrition in the UK. *Clinical Nutrition Update* 2000; 2(5): 14–15.
7. Edwards S, Mangat P. TPN versus EN: Divided loyalties without a clear solution. *Complete Nutrition* 2001; 1(5): 9–13.
8. Thomas B (ed.). *Manual of Dietetic Practice*, 3rd edn. Oxford: Blackwell Science, 2001.
9. McCalve SA, Snider HL, Spain DA. Preoperative issues in clinical nutrition. *Chest* 1999; 11: 645–705.

10. British Association of Parenteral and Enteral Nutrition. *Hospital Food as Treatment*. Maidenhead: BAPEN, 1999.
11. Griffin RD. Supplemental nutrition; how much is enough? *Intensive Care Med* 2000; 26: 838–840.
12. Lennard-Jones J (ed.). *A Positive Approach to Nutrition as Treatment*. Report of a working party. Kings Fund Centre, 1992.
13. Todorovic VE, Micklewright A (ed.). *A Pocket Guide to Clinical Nutrition*. 2nd edn. London: British Dietetic Association, 1997.
14. Schofield WN. Predicting basal metabolic rate, new standards and review of previous work. *Hum Nutr Clin Nutr* 1985; 44: 1–19.
15. Elia M. Artificial nutritional support. *Medicine International* 1990; 82: 3392–3396.
16. Scott A, Skerrat S, Adam S. *Nutrition for the Critically Ill: A Practical Handbook*. London: Arnold, 1998.
17. Raper M. Feeding the critically ill patient. *British Journal of Nursing* 1992; 1(1): 273–280.
18. Jolliet P, Pichard C, Biolo, et al. Enteral nutrition in intensive care patients. *Clinical Nutrition* 1999; 18(1): 47–56.
19. Tait J. Going nasogastric: Current thinking in nasogastric tube techniques. *Complete Nutrition* 2001; 1(2): 27–29.
20. Torence A. *Metabolic Complications of PN*. PENG update course, 1992.

APPENDIX 1

Examples of these tables in use:

1 Mrs Smith, 56 years old, admitted to the critical care unit following AAA repair. Initially did well following surgery but developed sepsis source from her chest. Has had a tracheostomy placed after 2 failed attempts to wean from the ventilator. Requires artificial feeding via a nasogastric tube.

Ventilation: CPAP/ASB	Sedation: None
Temperature: ~38°C + spiking to 39.5°C	Activity: Bedbound immobile
Weight: 63 kg　　Height: 1.6 m	BMI: 24.6 kg/m^2

Estimated Requirements:
BMR = $8.1 \times 63 + 842 = 1352$ kcal
DIT + Activity: 10%
Stress: 10%　　　　　　　　　　　　Total Calories = 1622 kcal/d
Protein = 0.14–0.2 g Nitrogen/d
　　　　　$0.14 \times 63 = 8.8$ g N_2, $8.8 \times 6.25 = 55$ g protein
　　　　　$0.20 \times 63 = 12.6$ g N_2, $12.6 \times 6.25 = 79$ g protein
　　　　　　　　　　　　　Total Protein = 55 g–79 g/d

INDEX